MEDICAL STATISTICS

MEDICAL STATISTICS
PRINCIPLES & METHODS

Dr K.R. Sundaram, M.Sc., Ph.D., FSMS
Professor & Head, Department of Biostatistics, Amrita Institute of Medical Sciences,
Cochin- 682041 (Kerala) & Ex. Professor & Head, Department of Biostatistics,
All India Institute of Medical Sciences, New Delhi-110029

Dr S. N. Dwivedi, M.Sc., Ph.D., FSMS
Additional Professor, Department of Biostatistics,
All India Institute of Medical Sciences, Ansari Nagar, New Delhi-110029

Dr V. Sreenivas, M.Sc., Ph.D.
Associate Professor, Department of Biostatistics,
All India Institute of Medical Sciences, Ansari Nagar, New Delhi-110029

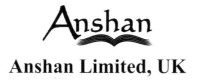

Anshan Limited, UK

Published in the UK by

Anshan Ltd

11a Little Mount Sion
Tunbridge Wells
Kent. TN1 1YS

Tel: +44 (0) 1892 557767
Fax: +44 (0) 1892 530358

e-mail: info@anshan.co.uk
Website: www.anshan.co.uk

ISBN: 978 1848290 310

British Library Cataloguing in Publication Data
A catalogue record for this book is available from the British Library

Not for sale in India, Pakistan, Nepal, Sri Lanka and Bangladesh

This edition is co-published by BI Publications Pvt Ltd and Anshan Limited, and printed at Saurabh Pritners Pvt. Ltd., Noida, India

Preface

The Medical Council of India has acknowledged the need to cultivate logical thinking among the doctors, otherwise busy with their day-to-day clinical and laboratory work. Biostatistics is recognized as a basic tool to achieve this objective. Indeed, during the last three or four decades, remarkable advances have taken place in biological and medical sciences, which have made 'decision making', particularly in the fields of health care and medical treatment, more and more complex. The medical and biological scientists have to base their decisions on carefully planned, executed, analyzed and interpreted investigations, which may include epidemiological studies, clinical trials, biological assays, laboratory experiments, hospital and community based registries and even operational research. Today, a medical student's training would be considered incomplete without a reasonable acquaintance with the principles of scientific research and applications of biostatistical techniques to enable him/her to plan his/her research studies with scientifically and statistically valid designs and to arrive at valid and meaningful conclusions.

The content and character of the discipline of Biostatistics itself have undergone a radical change during the last few decades and it is difficult to find all the information at one place. We were encouraged to write this book by frequent requests for a single source of getting information on the basic principles and methods by many undergraduate, postgraduate, doctoral and post-doctoral medical students during our teaching of medical statistics at some of the premier medical institutions in India. The questions that we faced during our teaching and the numerous interactions that we had with the medical/clinical faculty during the planning, monitoring, analysis, interpretation of the results of research projects, and reviewing of articles submitted for reviews gave us an ample understanding of the difficulties of an average bio-medical student and researcher in understanding the Biostatistical principles and methods. We decided to focus on the explanation of the logic behind the statistical principles and applications of the techniques and the interpretation of the results rather than on theoretical or mathematical details. Almost all the explanations in the present book are supported with relevant examples based on medical and biological data.

There are 15 chapters in this book. They cover mainly basics of measurement scales; study designs; study of population, sample and its size, sampling methods and methods of data collection; methods of exploring and understanding data using descriptive statistics; logic of statistical inferences; parametric and non-parametric methods of statistical inference; multivariable analysis in view of various types of outcomes like quantitative, qualitative and time to event data; design and analysis of randomised controlled trial; diagnostic and screening tests; medical demography; hospital statistics, commonly used statistical software; and misuses of statistics. This book focuses on basic concepts before discussing public health and clinical implications under each topic. At the end of each chapter, a few MCQs have been included to allow the readers to test their understanding of various topics after going through each chapter. Answers, and explanatory hints in some cases, are provided, chapter-wise, in an Appendix at the end. We generated various Statistical Tables, viz., Normal distribution, Student's t-distribution, chi-sqaure distribution and Fisher's F-distribution using version 9.1 of STATA.

Building on our practical experience, the chapters in this book are written in such a way as to provide a clear overview of the topics in an easy to understand language. The arrangement of chapters and topics in the book can be followed while teaching the graduate and postgraduate medical students. This arrangement will ensure greater effectiveness not only in teaching, but also in understanding by the students. The book will also be useful to the research workers in allied areas in designing their research projects and analyzing the data, applying various statistical methods and in interpreting the results with scientific validity.

This book is meant to be primarily used as a text for teaching undergraduate, postgraduate and paramedical course students in Medical, Nursing and Dental colleges; Ayurveda, Unani and Homeopathy colleges; and Universities. This book will also be very useful for the research students and scientists in medical, biological, pharmaceutical, agricultural and industrial research institutions; administrators and policy decision makers in hospitals & hospital administration and Health, Agricultural, Industry & Social Welfare Ministries.

We thank the Institute of Mathematical Statistics for permitting us to reproduce the Statistical Tables on the critical values and probability levels for Wilcoxon rank sum test and Wilcoxon signed rank test. We are also grateful to the publishers of *Lancet* for granting us the permission to reproduce revised checklist of items and also revised flow diagram from the Consolidated Standards of Reporting Trials (CONSORT) statement.

We also thank Mr. Ashish Kumar Upadhyaya who generated and organized various Statistical Tables in the book. We are immensely thankful to Dr. B.C. Sharma and Mr. Y.R. Chadha of BI Publications, Pvt. Ltd., New Delhi for taking up publication of our book and for going through each chapter thoroughly and carefully and suggesting very useful editorial modifications in the text. Without their deep involvement and support, publication of this book would not have been possible.

Last, but not the least, we thank our respective family members for their encouragement and forbearance throughout the period of preparation of this book.

June, 2009

K.R. Sundaram
S.N. Dwivedi
V. Sreenivas

Contents

1 | Introduction to Medical Statistics

- Origin and definition of statistics
- Biostatistics: Medical statistics, health statistics, vital statistics, history of biostatistics, specific uses of statistical methods in medicine, public health and biology
- Branches of statistical methods: Design methods, analysis methods
- Basic statistical concepts: Scales of measurement, observation & data, parameter & statistics, ratio, proportion and rate
- Variation: Biological variation, experimental variation & environmental/behavioural factor/intervention variation
- Accuracy, precision & unbiasedness of the estimate

1.1. Origin and Definition of 'Statistics'

Most undergraduate students of medicine may feel that mathematics in general and statistics in particular are an unnecessary burden on their curriculum. Hopefully, their attempt to evaluate research being reported in various journals—which should start at this stage and is definitely a part of their postgraduate study—should prove it otherwise and unravel the importance and relevance of statistics in their chosen career, whether it is clinical practice, administration or medical research. The pertinence of this field of study in medicine is elaborated further in the section entitled 'Uses and applications of medical statistics' of this Chapter.

The word 'statistics' has originated from the Greek word 'status' meaning 'state' or 'position'. In the olden days 'statistics' was mainly used for administering the affairs of a country in relation to the status of various administrative requirements. For example, estimating budget requirements, amount of tax to be collected, the labour and military force required, and the amount of clothing, food, schools and hospitals required, etc. However, in the modern sense, statistics has a much wider meaning. The Webster's Dictionary[1] defines statistics as 'the branch of mathematics that deals with the collection and analysis of quantitative data'. By this definition, statistics is an applied scientific discipline whose roots lie in mathematics.

The word statistics can be defined both in the plural and singular sense. In the plural sense, it means 'numerically stated facts' or 'facts expressed in figures'. For example, when the following facts are expressed in figures, they become statistics:

1. The population of India, according to the 2001 Census is 1.027 billion.
2. The total outpatient department (OPD)/clinic attendance at the All India Institute of Medical Sciences, New Delhi during 1999-2000 was 19 62 888.
3. The percentage of people who are literate in India according to the 2001 Census is 65.38%.

In the singular sense, it is the 'science' dealing with the methods of data collection, their compilation, tabulation and analysis to provide meaningful and valid interpretations. In other words, it deals with the scientific treatment of data derived from individuals.

From these two definitions, we can understand that statistics implies both 'data' and 'methods'. Keeping these two aspects in mind, statistics has been defined in different ways by different authors. Statistics helps in collecting data scientifically, and in organizing, summarizing and presenting the data collected so that valid and meaningful inferences can be drawn with credibility and reliability.

1.2. Biostatistics

Statistical methods applied in the fields of medicine, biology and public health are termed as 'biostatistics', also called 'biometry', which means the 'measurement of life'. Biostatistics is known by many names—medical statistics, health statistics and vital statistics. Though all these terms may mean the same, one can differentiate between them in the following ways:

Medical statistics: Statistics related to clinical and laboratory parameters, their relationship, prediction after treatment, clinical trials, bioassays, diagnostic analysis, quality control, etc. may be included in 'medical statistics'.

Health statistics: Statistics related to the health of the people in a community; epidemiology of diseases; association of socioeconomic and demographic variables, personality and behavioural variables, environmental factors and nutrition with the occurrence of various diseases; control and prevention of diseases, promotion of health, etc., are included in 'health statistics'.

Vital statistics: Statistics related to the vital events in life—birth, illness, death, marriage, divorce, adoption, etc.—their rates of occurrence, causes of increase or decrease in the vital rates, expectation of life at birth and at a given age, etc., are included in 'vital statistics'.

Population forms the basis of a majority of studies on vital and health statistics. Hence, the study of population, called **'demography'**, also becomes a part and parcel of biostatistics. Accurate information on population with respect to sex, age and other important factors is essential to define the vital statistics rates. Demography pertains to the magnitude, distribution, reasons for increase/decrease in population size, relationship with socioeconomic and environmental factors, etc.

1.2.1. History of Biostatistics

As mentioned earlier, statistics was used in earlier times mainly for affairs related to the administration of various matters in a country. Later, some types of actuarial methods were used by insurance companies to find out the longevity of people in order to fix the insurance premia for various age groups. Thereafter, data on vital statistics, especially on births and deaths, were collected in western countries. John Graunt's Bills of mortality[2] and William Farr's systematic compilation of causes of death in the office of the Registrar General of England[3] are noteworthy in this connection. This was considered a landmark for data collection and the science of vital statistics. Later, this information was related to studies on death rates, causes of death and contamination of water supply. Statistics was also used in forecasting population figures and constructing population growth models. The work of Mendel[4] in genetics related to plants was another path-breaking event in the history of biostatistics. These methods were later extended to studies on human genetics and hereditary factors. Some of the stalwarts in the development of statistical methods for various problems related to plants, agriculture, genetics, biology and epidemiology are Francis Galton, Karl Pearson, E. S. Pearson, R. A. Fisher, Jacques Bernoulli, Abraham de Moivre, P. C. Mahanalobis, P. Armitage, A. R. Feinstein D. J. Finney, G. I. Bliss, C. I. Oscar Kempthorne, D. R. Cox, Brian MacMahon and C. R. Rao. The list is endless and many more statisticians have contributed substantially in developing newer methods for the solution of various problems, and communicating those methods and relevant theories to other statisticians and researchers.

It is not very clear when statistics was introduced in the medical curriculum. The first textbook in biostatistics was authored by Austin Bradford Hill in 1937.[5] In the Johns Hopkins University, a course in biostatistics was taught to the medical students in 1948.[6] Books by Donald Mainland[7] and Huldah Bancroft[8] were followed for teaching biostatistics. At present, numerous textbooks are available on a variety of topics, which can be applied to various problems in different fields. Also available are a number of journals on various topics in biostatistics to keep statisticians and researchers up-to-date in the application of biostatistical methods. Formerly, biostatistics was mainly taught as a part of preventive and social medicine in many universities. However, because of its applications in a variety of fields such as pharmacology, psychology and psychiatry, microbiology, physiology, medicine and biotechnology, biostatistics is no longer restricted only to students of preventive and social medicine. In many medical colleges, especially those with postgraduate courses, there are separate departments of biostatistics with computer facilities and professional staff trained in biostatistics and computer software, directly catering to students and researchers in various specialties. Also, specific courses and workshops in various areas of biostatistics are frequently held by professional bodies for the benefit of statisticians and researchers to update their knowledge and keep pace with the ever-growing techniques in statistical applications and modeling. Many modern techniques such as meta-analysis, bootstrapping and evidence-based medicine are now available for application. It is almost inevitable that a medical student pursuing either a clinical practice, a research career or health management and administration should have a sound knowledge not only in basic statistical methods, but also of specific methods applied to the variety of problems related to medicine, biology and public health. This book attempts to give an insight into these methods, with appropriate illustrations and examples.

1.2.2. Uses of Medical Statistics

Statistical methods are very widely used in both research and administration in almost all fields, such as medicine, biology, public health, agriculture, industry, economics and meteoriology. Although, most of the basic as well as advanced statistical methods are applied in all these fields, there are certain specific methods which are applicable to specific field(s).

One common question medical students or practitioners generally ask is: why should they learn statistics? Generally, a biology or medical student would like to keep mathematics and formulae at a distance. Hence, after choosing medicine as their career, they wonder why they are asked to take the trouble of learning mathematics/statistics. The following sections may provide an answer to this question.

1.2.2.1. Uses of statistical methods in general

Statistical methods, in general, are needed for the following tasks:
- Gathering (collecting) medical and health data scientifically
- Describing (summarizing) the collected data to make it comprehensible
- Generalizing the results obtained from a sample to the entire population with scientific validity
- Drawing conclusions from the summarized data and generalized results
- Understanding and evaluating the published literature

In general, statistical methods are useful in planning and conducting meaningful and valid research studies on medical, health and biological problems in the population for the prevention of diseases, for finding appropriate and effective treatment modalities, and for the promotion of health. Having sound knowledge of basic as well as advanced statistical methods will help the students, practitioners, researchers, administrators and public health managers to understand and evaluate scientific articles and reports as well as to apply various statistical methods in their research projects, to determine priorities for health problems and allocate available resources judiciously and economically.

1.2.2.2. Specific uses of statistical methods in medicine, public health and biology

Statistical methods are needed in medicine, public health and biology:

- To define the normal limits (reference values) of various laboratory and clinical parameters (e.g., blood pressure, pulse rate, cholesterol level, haemoglobin level, blood cell counts, etc.). The normal limits of fasting blood sugar may be 60-110 mg% and that of cholesterol, 150-210 mg%;

- To determine whether various laboratory and clinical parameters are correlated and, if they are, to determine their degree of correlation and statistical significance. For example, correlation of blood pressure with cholesterol (higher the cholesterol, higher the blood pressure); correlation of blood pressure with weight (more the weight, higher the blood pressure) and the correlation of blood sugar level with weight (more the weight, higher the blood sugar level);

- To estimate the magnitude of various diseases and health problems and to **assess** their distribution with respect to age, place, time and other factors and to identify the possible causative factors such as socioeconomic status, lifestyle, behavioural habits and environmental factors. This branch of statistics is called 'epidemiology'. Prevalence (number of persons affected by the disease under consideration expressed as percentage or per thousand of the total number of persons studied) of diabetes in those over 50 years of age in town 'A' in 2002 could be 5%, and some of the possible causal factors for it could be overweight, lack of exercise and excess sugar intake. Hypertension may be positively associated with smoking habits and diabetes may be positively associated with the type of job (sedentary type or field work), while tuberculosis may be negatively associated with socioeconomic class. The chance of developing lung cancer is higher in heavy smokers than in non-smokers or mild smokers and the chance of developing diabetes is higher in those with sedentary type of work compared to those engaged in work requiring movement and labour;

- To develop new, more effective drugs and treatment methods for various diseases and to predict various outcomes (improvement, cure, living or dead) after treatment, based on various factors. This branch of study is called 'clinical trials'. Treatment 'A' may be better than treatment 'B' or no treatment in improving the condition of a disease of the patients, controlling for the effect of various factors, such as age, behavioural habits, diet, etc. Multivariate analysis is applied for this purpose;

- To test the efficacy of new vaccines for the prevention of diseases. This branch of study is called 'prophylactic trials';

- To collect data scientifically on vital events in life (birth, death, fertility, morbidity), to estimate vital statistics rates (birth, death, fertility, morbidity rates) and to evaluate the expectation of life (number of years expected to live) at birth and at various ages by constructing the Life Table based on mortality data. This branch of statistics is called 'vital statistics'. The birth rate, death rate and expectation of life at birth in India in 2001 were 25.8 live-births per 1000 of the population, 8.5 deaths per 1000 of the population and 63.4 years, respectively;

- To estimate the potency and relative potency of drugs, to determine ED_{50} (the effective dose of the drug at which 50% of those responded positively (i.e., showed improvement) and determine the route and frequency of administration of the drug to give the maximum benefit to the patients. This branch of study is called 'biological assays'. If the relative potency of drug A compared to that of drug B is 1.2, then 1 unit of drug A is equivalent to 1.2 units of drug B. Relative potency is computed by applying specific statistical methods;

- To estimate the probability of survival after treatment for a specified period in chronic diseases such as cancer and AIDS. This branch of study is called 'survival analysis'. Based on the treatment and mortality data of cancer patients, the chance of survival of a patient after a certain period of treatment can be computed by applying survival analysis methods and it can be compared with the corresponding chance of survival after treatment with another drug;

- To maintain the quality of drugs and laboratory, surgical and medical instruments, and equipment. This branch is called 'quality control analysis';

- For the validation of new, efficient and economic screening and diagnostic tests in comparison to those already existing. For example, validation of the sputum test with respect to X-ray for detecting tuberculosis and validation of the HbA_1c test with respect to fasting and postprandial blood sugar levels for detecting diabetes. This is called 'validation analysis';
- To study the genetic composition of a population and the changes in the composition with respect to factors such as mutation, migration, etc., and their impact on the health status of the people. This branch is called 'statistical genetics';
- To ensure that the maximum benefit of diagnosis, treatment methods and prognosis reaches the population with minimum cost, based on available resources. This branch is called 'health economics and operational research'.

Although some of the above-mentioned applications may appear redundant to those who aim only at a career in clinical practice, certain aspects are, however, very relevant and important for them also, without which they may not be able to keep pace with medical advances for the betterment of the population in general and the patients in particular. Many of the above-mentioned applications are directly relevant for those who choose a career in medical research, management, public health administration or epidemiology.

1.2.3. Branches of Statistical Methods

Statistical methods can be broadly divided into two branches—design methods and analysis methods (Fig. 1.1).

1.2.3.1. Design methods

Design methods deal with the methods of collecting data scientifically. The role of statistics is not restricted to analyzing data, but also involves planning the study scientifically and executing it properly. There are only

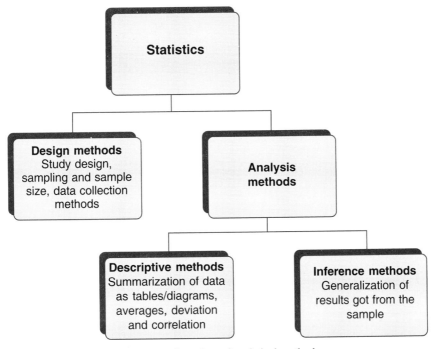

Fig. 1.1: Branches of statistical methods

a handful of ways to carry out a study properly, but innumerable ways to do it incorrectly. Many students are tempted to give more emphasis to the statistical analysis of data applying sophisticated methods, while giving lesser or no importance to the design of studies. If the design of the study is defective, the results of the study will have limited validity or not be valid at all. Hence, designing the study needs care as much as analyzing the data.

In most situations, the data are not collected as complete coverage, but as sample coverage. In case it is possible, complete coverage is ideal. However, in most cases, it is not practically possible or feasible because of lack of time, budgetary restrictions and the large number of personnel required for such studies. For example, for studying the percentage of population of Delhi affected by diabetes within a short period and with a comparatively small budget, it may not be practicable to screen the entire population of Delhi for diabetes. In such situations, data are usually collected from a small representative portion of the total. This helps in getting results in much lesser time, with fewer resources and personnel. The study element in 'totality' (complete coverage) is called 'population' or 'statistical universe' and the small representative portion (sample coverage) is called 'sample'. That is, the population comprises the study elements in totality while the sample is a small portion of the population, representative of various characteristics, which may influence the study variables. One of the important aspects of the design of a study is determining the minimum sample size required to be selected from the population and the appropriate method of selection so as to ensure the 'representativeness' of the sample. Apart from this, choosing the appropriate study method (design)—whether it is an observational or an experimental study and whether it is a one-time (cross-sectional) or follow-up study (longitudinal)—also form part of the design of a study.

1.2.3.2. Analysis methods

Statistical analysis methods are of two kinds—descriptive methods and inference methods.

Descriptive methods: Descriptive methods include the statistical methods used to summarize the data collected in terms of statistical tables, diagrams and graphs and certain summarizing parameters such as averages, variation and correlation. The data collected can be more clearly understood and interpreted in terms of these summarization methods. For example, a table giving data on hypertensive patients with respect to their sex, age group and diet may show that 60% of the sample were males; among the males, more than 70% were 50 years or older while among the females, 80% were in this age group; 70% of males were non-vegetarians and the corresponding figure for females was 60%, the mean diastolic blood pressure of males was 110 mmHg with a range of 90-120 mmHg and that of females was 100 mmHg with a range of 92-115 mmHg.

Inference methods: Inference methods include the statistical methods used to generalize the results obtained from the sample selected from the entire population. 'Science' is an investigation towards truth, supported by experimental evidence. However, experiment and induction do not always lead to the truth. For example, two scientists may arrive at two different conclusions from the same experiment. Statistics provides the means of measuring the amount of subjectivity that goes into the conclusions, in terms of probability. Based on a theoretical model, the probabilities of the various possibilities of the experiment can be estimated and it can be determined whether the effect of the treatment is real or could have occurred by chance alone.

However, statistics cannot prove anything with 100% confidence. It is only a powerful and reliable tool to get as close to the truth as possible. Hence, even if it is concluded that the better outcome of the treatment is real, there will be a chance element (error) in that statement. In statistical inference, the chance element can be estimated and can be made as small as possible by choosing the design of the study appropriately. This is called the 'p' value, or level of significance, or type I error or alpha. While generalizing the results obtained from the sample for the population, this chance element has to be stated.

Studies based on a sample provide results for the sample only; yet, what is required is the results for the population. Inference methods help us to generalize the results obtained from the sample for the entire population with a certain amount of confidence. For example, if the estimate of the percentage of persons affected by diabetes in a Delhi population was 10% based on a sample study, this estimate can be refined by attaching a specific confidence, say 95%, that the true (population) value lies between, say 8%, and 12%. This means that there is a chance of 5% that the true value may lie beyond these two limits. If 40% of 50 tuberculosis patients receiving the standard drugs are cured, while 60% of a comparable group of 50 tuberculosis patients receiving a new drug are cured, and if the statistical test of significance shows that this difference of 20% in the cure rate is statistically significant at a chosen level of significance, say 5%, (95% confidence), then there is a 5% chance that this difference is not due to the better efficacy of the new drug, but, just by chance.

1.3. Some Basic Statistical Concepts

It will be worthwhile to be familiar with a few basic statistical concepts as a starting point.

1.3.1. Scales of Measurements

There are two types of data characteristics one can study—constant and variable (Fig. 1.2).

1.3.1.1. Constant

A constant is a value that does not change with any situation. For example, the value of pie is 22/7, which does not change with time, place or person. Similarly, the value of 'e', the base of the natural logarithm is 2.7183. This is a constant and the value will not change in any situation. These are called mathematical constants.

1.3.1.2. Variable

In contrast, the value of a variable changes. A variable is a characteristic that can take on different values with respect to a person, time or place, or any other factor. For example, blood pressure, height, weight, blood group, cholesterol level, pulse rate, severity of illness and the grade of a student in an examination are variables. Basically, there are two types of variables: **discrete** and **continuous**.

Discrete (categorical) variable: If the characteristic is classified according to a group, class or category, it is called a 'discrete' variable. Examples of discrete variables are blood group (A, B, AB and O), status of a disease (severe, moderate and mild), socioeconomic class (rich, middle class and poor), grades in examination (excellent, good, average and poor), sex (male and female) and diet (vegetarian and non-vegetarian). In this type of variable, the number of persons falling in each group of the variable is counted. Hence, this type of variable is also called 'countable variable'.

There are two types of discrete variables: **ordinal** and **nominal**. If there is an order in the classification of the groups of the variable, it is called an 'ordinal' and if no order is possible in the classification, it is called 'nominal'. Status of disease, grade in examination and socioeconomic class are ordinal variables while sex, diet and blood group are nominal variables.

Another type of discrete variable is the one classified into groups, but having some numerical value. Families classified according to size (one member, two members, three members, etc.) or number of children (no child, one child, two children, three children, etc.) are examples of discrete variables, which can be classified into groups assigned a numerical value If there are only two groups, such as sex, the variable is called 'binary' or 'dichotomous'. If there are more than two groups, it is called 'polychotomous variable'.

Continuous (measurable) variable: If the characteristic is measurable in units of measurement carrying a numerical value, it is called a 'continuous' variable. Examples of continuous variable are weight (kg), height (cm), income (rupees, dollars or pounds), age (years or months), blood pressure (mmHg), time (hours, minutes and seconds) and temperature (Fahrenheit or Centigrade). This type of variable can have decimal point values. The weight of an individual can be 50.8 kg and the height 170.3 cm. Since any interval of this type of variable can still be refined, it is called a continuous variable. Even between 50.5 and 50.6, a value such as 50.57 can be obtained.

There are two types of continuous variables. If the 'zero' point and the unit of measurement are arbitrary (i.e., there is no true zero point), then it is called an **'interval scale'**. In this scale, the starting point (the zero point) is arbitrary. Temperature is an interval type of continuous variable. It is measured in two types of scales—Fahrenheit (F) and Centigrade (C). Though these are two different types of measurements, they contain the same information since they are linearly related by the equation: $F = (9/5) \times C + 32$.

Freezing of water occurs at $0°$ on C scale and its boiling at $100°$. On the F scale, the corresponding values are $32°$ and $212°$, respectively. Readings for some other values are given below:

CG	0	10	30	100
FH	32	50	86	212

The ratio of the differences between the readings on one scale will be the same as that on the other scale. That is, for C, $(30–10)/(10–0) = 2$ and for F, the corresponding ratios are $(86–50)/(50–32) = 2$.

Another example is 'time'. Time can be measured as the Indian standard time (ISI) and Greenwich mean time (GMT), which are linearly related as: $IST = GMT + 5½$ hours.

If the variable has a 'true' zero point independent of the unit of measurement, then it is called a **'ratio scale'**. In this type of continuous variable also, the differences between the readings on one scale are the same as those on another scale. Weight can be measured in kilograms and pounds; they are linearly related and the starting value is always 'zero', irrespective of the scale. The linear equation is 1 kg=2.205 lbs

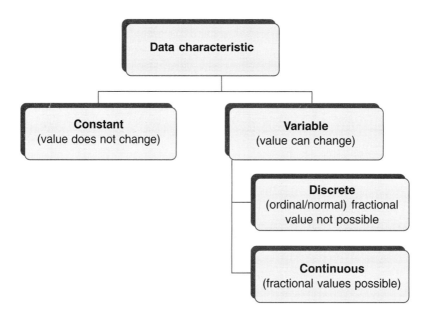

Fig. 1.2: Data characteristics

In the ratio scale, percentages are meaningful (e.g., a decrease of 25% in the weight of an obese person after being on a controlled diet for a month). In the interval scale, percentages are meaningless. For examples, percentage decrease or increase in the clock time or temperature has no meaning.

1.3.2. Observation and Data

Each value of a variable recorded is an 'observation' and a set of observations of one or more variables form the 'data'. If the values of the variable in the population are not affected by any external factor, the data are **homogeneous**; but if they are affected by some external factor, the data are **heterogeneous**. Data on birthweights of babies born to women from a poor socioeconomic class alone are homogeneous. But data on birthweights of babies born to women from high, middle and poor socioeconomic classes are heterogeneous.

Data pertaining to discrete variables are called **'qualitative data'** and those pertaining to continuous variables are called **'quantitative data'**. Most of the data related to biology and medicine could be quantitative data and those for public health and sociology could be qualitative data.

1.3.3. Parameter and Statistic

'Parameter' is the statistical characteristic related to the population and 'statistic' is the statistical characteristic related to the sample. If the percentage of population affected by diabetes is 10%, it is a parametric value. If the corresponding value in the sample selected randomly from the population is 12%, it is a statistic value. The former is usually represented as 'P' and the latter as 'p'. Similarly, if the mean systolic blood pressure (SBP) of the male population is 120 mmHg, it is the parametric value (μ) and if the SBP of a sample of males selected randomly from the population is 122 mmHg, it is the statistic value ($\bar{X}$). *What we are able to get from studies based on samples are the statistic values of the statistical characteristics and those values will be estimates of the corresponding parameters.* When the sample size increases, the statistic value estimated will be as close as possible to the population parameter values and it is then said to be an accurate estimate of the parameter.

1.3.4. Ratio, Proportion and Rate

The parameters ratio, proportion and rate are computed for summarizing data related to discrete variables (qualitative data). Many people consider all these terms to mean the same, but in reality they are different.

1.3.4.1. Ratio

Ratio is obtained simply by dividing one quantity by another, without implying any relationship between the numerator and denominator, i.e., the numerator is not a part of the denominator. Examples are patient/doctor ratio, patient/nurse ratio and student/teacher ratio. If in a hospital there are 100 doctors and 300 nurses, then the doctor/nurse ratio is 100/300 or 1:3. If there are 1000 students in a school and the number of teachers is 50, then the teacher/student ratio is 50/1000 or 1:20.

1.3.4.2. Proportion

Proportion is a type of ratio in which the numerator is included in the denominator. For example, if there are 1000 males and 900 females comprising a total population of 1900, the proportion of females in the population is:

Proportion (P) = 900/(1000+900) = 900/1900 = 9/19

This is usually expressed as a percentage or in multiples of 10s such as 1000, 10 000, 100 000, etc., depending on the number in the numerator relative to the denominator. In this example, the percentage of females in the population is $(9 \times 100)/19 = 47.4\%$. Similarly, the percentage of males in the population is 52.6%. If the number in the numerator is small (number of tuberculosis cases) compared to the denominator (total population), it is expressed per 1000 or 10,000 or even 1,00,000 to avoid expressing it in terms of decimal point. For example, it would be better to express a value as 50 per 10000 instead of 0.5 %.

1.3.4.3. Rate

Rate is a ratio in which a distinct relationship exists between the numerator and denominator and, most essentially, a measure of time is an intrinsic part of the denominator. Rate requires the numerator, e.g., cases of a disease, acquired over a specific time interval and a denominator, e.g., the population which did not have the disease, observed during the same time interval. For example, crude death rate is defined as the number of deaths that occurred during a specific period of time, say one year, divided by the total mid-year (as on 1 July) population of the same area and over the same period of time. It is expressed per thousand of the population. Other common examples of rate are: typing speed (number of words/minute) and speed of a car (kilometers/hour).

1.3.5. Variation

One of the most important and basic concepts in statistics is 'variation'. It can even be said that statistics is nothing but the study of variation. If there is no variation, there is no statistics. Variation is inherent in nature. No two things are alike. There may be at least a slight variation even under the most homogeneous conditions. In studying the blood pressure of persons there could be variation between individuals of the same sex, age and many other factors (individual variation). Variation could also be there in the same person when the reading is taken at two different times/places (within variation). There are basically four types of variation (Fig. 1.3):

1. Biological variation
2. Experimental variation
3. Real (environmental) variation
4. Sampling variation.

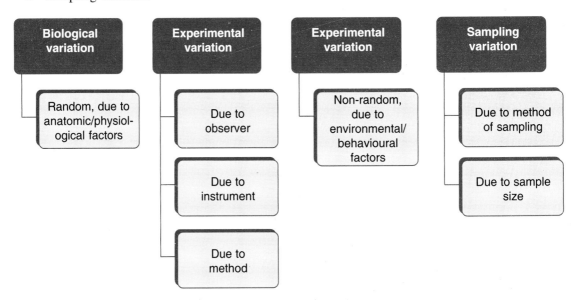

Fig. 1.3: Sources of variation

.3.5.1. Biological variation

Variation that is normal or natural or due to a chance or random occurrence within biological limits is called biological variation. This type of variation can be determined statistically. Variation in blood pressure, height, weight, haemoglobin level, etc., of individuals of the same age, sex, socioeconomic status, environment, etc., would be of biological variation type.

.3.5.2. Experimental variation

Variation due to the observer, instrument or method is called 'experimental variation'.

Observer variability: Variation due to the persons measuring the parameter or recording/collecting the information is called 'observer variability'. Blood pressure or pulse rate or cholesterol values of the same person measured by two observers may not be the same because of differences in their experience, training or concentration. Information obtained by two investigators from the respondent on an item can also vary because of the way the question is asked (age in completed years or actual age; household income per year including only the income of the main earning member in the house or including the income of each earning member in the family and including or excluding income from other sources, etc.). This type of variation can be minimized by giving systematic and uniform training to observers in measuring or reading the variable values, or asking relevant questions.

Instrument variability: Variation occurring due to the type of instrument or equipment used to measure the parameter is called 'instrument variability'. Blood pressure of a person recorded with a sphygmomanometer and aneroid instrument, or two sphygmomanometers may vary, as may the weight of a child using two types of weighing machines (beam balance and spring balance or two beam balance machines) because of the differences (may be minute) in the instruments. This type of variation can be minimized by the standardization of the instruments to be used for measuring the parameter and using accurately tested instruments giving reliable (consistent) readings.

Method variability: Variation may occur with the laboratory procedures used for the estimation/measurement or recording of parameters such as haemoglobin and cholesterol level, and the nutritional status of children due to the different procedures, chemicals, reagents or measurements used. This type of variation can be minimized by the standardization of the techniques, measurements, chemicals or reagents to be used for measurement or recording.

.3.5.3. Environmental/behavioural factor/intervention variation

This is the real variation which is beyond the limits of normal variation. This type of variation is not by chance or random.

Biological variation is mainly anatomical or physiological in nature. However, pathological variation is real variation and is mainly due to environmental factors. Variation in the blood pressure or cholesterol level of individuals according to their smoking habits, type of job (sedentary or active) and diet, variation in the nutritional status of children in accordance with their socioeconomic status, parents' education or diet will not be biological. This type of variation occurs due to the influence of the afore-mentioned environmental and behavioural factors and can be minimized by suitable intervention such as giving treatment by administering a drug or by surgery; quitting smoking; exercising; eating nutritious food; improving the economic standard, etc., as the case may be.

.3.5.4. Sampling variability

Variation occurring due to the method of sampling and/or sample size is called 'sampling variability'. This type of variation cannot be avoided in studies based on samples. This results in error and can be measured statistically. Variation of this type can be minimized by adequately increasing the sample size and/or by adopting an appropriate sampling method.

Statistics is the study of variability and chance. There will be variation in the results obtained from different samples. For example, the prevalence of malnutrition in children from one study of a sample of children may be 10%, while from another study of a sample of children from the same population, it may be 12%, and so on. Similarly, in a clinical trial, the difference in the improvement rate with the standard drug and the new drug may be 5% from one sample study and 6% from another study, and so on. This variation is called random or chance variation. Chance/uncertainty is measured by probability. No conclusion can be drawn with 100% certainty (confidence). A statistical inference method enables us to quantify the extent to which the chance variability can affect the results by computing the probability of the result occurring by chance alone. In clinical trials, if the improvement with a new drug is 80% and that with the standard drug is 60%, to determine whether this difference is real (the additional improvement rate of 20% is due to the better effect of the new drug compared to that of the standard drug) or not, an appropriate statistical test is performed and the probability that the additional improvement rate is due to the effect of the new drug compared to that of the standard drug is computed. This probability value is simply called as the 'p' value and it varies from 0 to 1. As a rule of thumb, if the p value is less than 5%, then it is concluded that the difference is not by chance, but real and that the difference is statistically significant with 95% confidence. The confidence can be increased (the proportion of chance can be reduced) by increasing the sample size of the study.

1.3.6. Accuracy, Precision and Unbiasedness of the Estimate

Ideally, any measurement made is expected to be accurate. An accurate measurement is defined as one that is precise and unbiased. These terms are not the same and each term has a different meaning. **Accuracy** is the closeness of a measured or computed value to its true value and **precision** is the closeness of repeated measurements of the same variable to each other. Precision may also be called as reliability, repeatability, consistency, stability and reproducibility.

If the estimated values of the parameter from different samples are concentrated around a point, then it is precise. If that point is the true value of the variable, on an average, it is also unbiased and may be accurate considering the central point to be an estimate of the true value. That is, on an average, it measures consistently and near to the true value and is, hence, accurate. If the grouping is not around the central value, it causes a systematic error and becomes biased. The reason for this difference may be due to some specific factor. If the measurement is made by two persons, one having a lot of experience and the other not much experience, there may be consistency in the values measured by each person separately, but the measurements made by the experienced person may be unbiased and, hence, accurate. The measurement made by the fresher may also be consistent, but may be biased since his values may be concentrated around a point, which may not be the central point (true value). The difference between the true value and the value obtained by the persons, on an average, is called 'bias'. In the case of an experienced person, the bias may be negligible while in the case of an inexperienced person, the bias may be high.

Multiple Choice Questions

Choose the correct answers in the following multiple choice questions. The correct answers are listed on p. 342.

Q.1. A measurable variable is called:
a. Qualitative variable
b. Nominal variable
c. Continuous variable
d. None of the above

Q.2. Weight measured in kilograms is a:
a. Categorical variable
b. Nominal variable
c. Continuous variable
d. None of the above

Q.3. **A scale used for classification into unordered qualitative categories is:**
a. Ordinal scale
b. Nominal scale
c. Interval scale
d. None of the above

Q.4. **A scale used for classification into ordered qualitative categories is known as:**
a. Ordinal scale
b. Nominal scale
c. Interval scale
d. Ratio Scale

Q.5. **Gender is a:**
a. Nominal variable
b. Ordinal discrete variable
c. Interval type variable
d. Ratio type variable

Q.6. **A physician, after examining a group of patients of a certain disease, classifies the condition of each one as 'normal', 'mild', 'moderate' or 'severe'. What is the scale of measurement that is being adopted for classification of the disease condition?**
a. Nominal
b. Interval
c. Ratio
d. Ordinal

Q.7. **A pathologist examines the tissues received from thyroid specimens and classifies each as 'normal', 'papillary carcinoma, 'follicular carcinoma', 'medullary carcinoma' and 'other'. What scale of measurement is the pathologist using?**
a. Interval
b. Nominal
c. Ordinal
d. Ratio

Q.8. **A continuous variable:**
a. Can have units of measurement
b. Should have units of measurement, but may not take into consideration decimal points
c. Should have units of measurement and takes into consideration decimal points
d. No units of measurement, but takes into consideration decimal points

Q.9. **When a variable is classified according to some ordered attributes, which are not capable of measurement, the scale is known as:**
a. Interval scale
b. Ratio scale
c. Normal scale
d. Ordinal scale

Q.10. **A continuous variable is a:**
a. Qualitative variable
b. Measurable variable
c. Nominal variable
d. Ordinal discrete variable

References

1. Landau SI, ed. *International Webster's Student Dictionary of the English Language.* International Encyclopedic edition. New Delhi: CBS Publishers and Distributors; 2001.
2. Grant J. *Natural and Political Observations Made upon the Bills of Mortality: London, 1662.* Baltimore: Johns Hopkins Press; 1939.
3. Farr W. In: Armitage P, Colton T, eds. *Encyclopedia of Biostatistics. Vol. 2.* New York: John Wiley and Sons; 1998.
4. Mendel GJ. In: Stern E, Sherwood C, eds. *The Origins of Genetics: A Mendel Source Book.* San Francisco: Freeman; 1966.
5. Hill AB. Principles of medical statistics. *Lancet;* 1937.
6. Colton T. Discussion of "teaching biostatistics—past, present and future". In: *Proceedings of the American Statistical Association: Sesquicentennial invited papers session.* American Statistical Association, Alexandria, 1989; 345-49.
7. Mainland D. *Elementary Medical Statistics.* Philadelphia: WB Saunders; 1952.
8. Bancroft H. *Introduction to Biostatistics.* New York: Hoeber–Harper; 1957.

2 | Sampling and Data Collection Methods

- Sampling: Important terms in sampling, important terms in estimation, sampling design/scheme/plan
- Probability sampling methods: Simple random sampling, systematic random sampling, stratified random sampling, cluster sampling, sampling with probability proportional to size (PPS sampling), multistage sampling, multiphase sampling
- Non-probability sampling methods: Volunteer sampling, convenience sampling, quota sampling, judgement sampling/area sampling, snowball sampling
- Other sampling methods: Sequential sampling, double sampling, interpenetrating subsampling (replicated sampling)
- Methods of data collection: Survey instruments, designing of survey instruments, questionnaire, open-ended questions, closed questions, steps in designing a questionnaire
- Systems of data collection, instruments for measuring data, reliability and validity of data measuring instruments, data collection techniques, ethical considerations, reporting population and samples

Medical studies are, in general, based on sampling enquiries, i.e., knowledge about population based on a sample. These enquiries may be broadly categorized into two groups: one that can be answered by carrying out a sampling experiment (randomized controlled clinical trials) designed or controlled by the investigator (described in Chapter 9), and the second based on sample surveys. The latter group comprises enquiries that can only be answered through a sample survey. This chapter is mainly concerned with sample surveys that do not involve any experimental control. The various methods of sampling (including random and non-random) have been described with the help of appropriate examples. Likewise, the various components of data collection methods have also been described. Due emphasis is laid on first understanding the basic terminologies that are commonly used in describing sampling and data collection methods. While describing these aspects, references have been made to the approaches used for community-based public health studies, which are easy to understand. These principles can easily be utilized skillfully while dealing with clinical studies and/ or laboratory-based studies.

2.1. Sampling

The process of drawing a representative sample from the population is known as sampling. There are various methods of sampling. Sample results and the related conclusions rely totally on the selected population. The generalization of these results to a larger or different population is merely a judgement or a guess and may not be valid statistically.

2.1.1. Important Terms in Sampling

2.1.1.1. Population

Population is defined as an aggregate of the sampling units. A finite population has countable number of sampling units. The basic aim of any study is to generally know about the population (i.e., universe). Hence, the meaning of population may vary from study to study. For example, (i) if one wants to know about a specific aspect(s) in the general population of Delhi (e.g., the percentage of people suffering from asthma at a given time), an aggregate of each and every person of Delhi is the population. (ii) If one wants to know about a specific aspect in the geriatric population of Delhi (e.g., say those above 60 years of age) suffering from asthma at a given time, an aggregate of each and every aged person in Delhi is the population. Again, (iii) if one wants to know about a specific aspect in patients coming to a particular hospital in Delhi (e.g., the percentage of patients suffering from asthma during a given time), an aggregate of each and every patient coming to that hospital in Delhi during the considered period is the population. On the other hand, (iv) if one wants to know about a specific aspect of hospitals in Delhi (e.g., the percentage of hospitals with the facility of magnetic resonance investigation (MRI), an aggregate of each and every hospital in Delhi is the population. Better understanding of the study population and its consideration in an appropriate manner may go a long way towards deriving results which can yield better generalizations.

2.1.1.2. Sample

A small portion of the population which truly represents the population with respect to the study characteristics of the population is known as a sample; for example, 100 persons, selected randomly out of a total study population of 1000 persons for estimating the mean blood pressure. Samples may be of two types: probability/random sample or non-probability sample.

Probability/random sample: This is a sample in which the sampling units are selected through a sampling method that ensures knowledge about the probability (described in Chapter 4) of selection (non-zero) of each sampling unit ensures a definite probability of selection of each sampling unit. In this chapter, probability and chance will be used as synonyms. One should always try to use such samples, which allow valid scientific results. Methods with an equal probability of selecting each sampling unit ensure simpler methods of analysis. The various probability-sampling methods will be described later.

Non-probability sample: This sample can be differentiated from the probability/random sample on the basis of a basic assumption about the nature of the population under study. In this approach, there is an assumption of an even distribution of characteristics within the population. In contrast, randomization is a feature of the selection process for probability sample rather than an assumption about the structure of the population. The sampling units for a non-probability sample are chosen arbitrarily and there is no way to estimate the probability of any sampling unit being included in the sample. Also, there is no assurance that each unit has a chance of being included. For example, the consideration of villages, which are easily approachable; individuals who are present during a casual visit; and so on. This makes it impossible to estimate sampling variability or to identify possible bias. Thus, reliability can never be measured in a non-probability sample. Despite these drawbacks, non-probability samples may be useful in many circumstances; for example, when only descriptive observations of a sample are required. When it is not feasible to carry out a probability sampling and the objective is to carry out a preliminary study or questionnaire testing, non-probability sampling may be adopted, for example in market opinion surveys. However, generalization of results obtained from such studies for the population is not possible. Various non-probability sampling methods will be described later.

Representative sample: This is a sample that resembles or represents the population. It does not necessarily have all the possible characteristics of the population and it represents the population with respect to the characteristics under study, thus enabling valid generalizations of the results. For example, in a study on the burden of lung cancer, the considered sample should have an age and sex distribution similar to that of the population.

Sampling unit: An element or a group of elements of the population used for drawing a sample is called a sampling unit. This is generally well defined and identifiable. For example, to select persons, an individual person will serve the purpose of sampling unit; to select families, a family will be the sampling unit; to select villages, a village will be the sampling unit; to select patients, a patient will be the sampling unit; to select wards, a ward will be the sampling unit; and to select hospitals, a hospital will be the sampling unit

Sampling frame: A list of all sampling units with identification addresses in a population is known as a sampling frame. It serves as the base for selecting a sample. A spot-map or other similar physical identification sources may also serve this purpose.

Sample size: This is the size of the subgroup of the population that is finally covered under a study, irrespective of the target size of the sample. For example, if a study was planned to cover a sample of size 500 but the sample size finally covered is either 400 or 600, the sample size of this study will be 400 or 600.

Minimum sample size required: The minimum sample size required is calculated based on the design of the study and its specific objective along with other possible statistical considerations. The methods for estimating the minimum sample size under different designs of studies are given in Chapter 10. Coverage of the minimum sample size is one of the various steps necessary for carrying out a conclusive study. A study covering a sample smaller than the required minimum sample size (e.g., 400 instead of the calculated 500) may not be conclusive. However, coverage of a sample larger than the required minimum sample size (e.g., 600 instead of the calculated 500) is a welcome step that may further enhance the validity of the result. However, covering of sample more than the minimum sample size estimated depends on many factors, such as available resources, time and ethical considerations.

Sampling fraction: The proportion of sample size chosen to the population is known as the sampling fraction. If we have to select a sample of size 100 out of a population of size 500, then the sampling fraction will be 100/500, that is, 1/5 or 20%.

Sampling interval: The inverse of the sampling fraction, taken as the nearest complete number, is known as the sampling interval. If we have to select a sample of size 100 out of a population of size 500, then the sampling interval will be 500/ 100 = 5.

Parameter: This refers to the study characteristics of the population, e.g., mean of a variable and percentage of the population affected by a particular disease, correlation coefficient between two variables, say, height and weight, etc.

2.1.2. Important Terms in Estimation

Estimator: The estimator of a population parameter is a function of the observations in the sample. It may be based on all the observations in the sample (e.g. sample mean and sample variance) or based on only some of the observations in the sample depending on the definition of the parameter (e.g., range).

Unbiased estimator: An estimator of a particular parameter is known as an unbiased estimator of that parameter if its average value is equal to the parameter. For example, if we consider all possible samples of a fixed size out of a population and calculate the average value of the estimator based on all the samples, it may be very close to the parameter. To be more specific, if we take a representative sample of size two out of a population having three sampling units, this will provide an average that will be an unbiased estimate of the population parameter. This estimate will be closer to the average of three averages obtained from three possible samples of size two (i.e. first and second; first and third; and second and third).

Consistent estimator: An estimator of a population parameter that provides closer estimates of the parameter with increasing sample size is called a consistent estimator. For example, the value of an estimator of haemoglobin level based on a sample size of 30 out of 100 healthy persons is 11.5–16.5 g%. If we increase the sample size (say to 60), the value of the estimator for that variable may now be 13.5–14.5 g%, which is narrower than the estimate obtained from the earlier sample size of 30.

Estimate (sample statistic): This refers to a particular value of an estimator related to a given sample. In other words, based on a sample, the substitution of the values of a variable in the estimator provides a particular value that is known as the estimate of the corresponding parameter. Therefore, the use of an unbiased and consistent estimator will provide an unbiased and consistent estimate.

Sampling error: This is an error in the estimation of any population characteristic (e.g., mean, proportion) based on a random sample drawn from the population, which is caused because of random sampling fluctuations (i.e., by chance), and unavoidable in a sample study. For example, if the average haemoglobin level in a healthy population is 14.5 g% and its estimated value from a sample study is 13.5 g%, this difference could be due to the sampling error.

Sampling distribution: If repeated samples of the same size are taken from the same population and estimates of a particular population parameter (e.g. mean, proportion, median, etc.) are obtained and listed, its distribution is known as the sampling distribution of the parameter considered.

Standard error: The standard deviation present in the sampling distribution of a particular population parameter is said to be the standard error (SE) of the estimate of that parameter (discussed in more detail in Chapter 4). For example, three independent samples of the same size from a healthy population may provide the estimated average haemoglobin level to be 12.5, 13.5 and 14.5 g% respectively. The variability present in the repeated results is known as SE.

2.1.3. Sampling Design/Scheme/Plan

Sampling design: The description of various sample sizes in relation to varying probabilities (e.g., level of significance; power of the study) is known as the sampling design. In other words, the reporting of the minimum sample size required for a study at varying levels of significance and /or power of the study may be addressed as the sampling design in research proposal. This type of reporting is very common in the proposals submitted to international agencies, such as the WHO, UNICEF, etc., for financial assistance.

Sampling scheme: The description of the sampling procedure (i.e., the method of selection of a sample from the population) is known as the sampling scheme.

Sampling strategy/plan: The description of a sampling scheme along with an estimator may be called the sampling strategy or sampling plan. To be more specific, the type of estimator for a population parameter may vary from one sampling scheme to another. Accordingly, the method of sampling together with the corresponding estimator is known as the sampling strategy/or plan.[2]

The funding agency for a research project may require a report on the sampling size requirements (i.e., sampling design); method of sampling (i.e., sampling scheme) and also the use of a specific estimator corresponding to the method of sampling (i.e., sampling strategy/plan). One can provide these under the heading 'sampling'. Otherwise, these details are given under the general heading 'statistical methods' or even 'methods'.

Non-sampling error: In addition to the sampling error, described above, non-sampling errors may also be present in the collected data because of various reasons such as defective research tools / instruments (e.g., open-ended questions without guidelines; vaguely phrased questions; questions placed in an illogical order, non-standardized instruments and equipment, untrained personnel used for data collection and recording. One should try to minimize these problems at the time of planning the study (e.g., development of an appropriate questionnaire in the desired language, pilot testing, training at various levels, built-in provision for supervision in data collection, scrutiny of data, etc.). Once data collection is completed, there is no way to overcome these problems. The considerable presence of non-sampling errors in the collected data can not only nullify all the efforts related to that particular study but also lead to distorted results. Even if data collection is completed with accuracy, there may be errors in data entry in the records and computers that might also add distortion to the results. To overcome this problem, methods such as double entry and/or the physical verification of the data entered with the original data may be helpful. The use of inappropriate statistical methods in data analysis may also affect the study results. Wrong interpretation of even accurate results is another issue that should be addressed with due care through consultation with experts.

2.2. Methods of Sampling

Sampling methods may broadly be divided into two types: probability/random sampling methods and non-probability/non-random sampling methods. Further, each of these is of various types that are described below.

2.2.1. Probability Sampling Methods (Fig. 2.1)

2.2.1.1. Simple random sampling

This is the basic, most commonly used and easiest method of sampling. In this method, each sampling unit of the population has an equal chance of inclusion in the sample. Further, each subgroup of sampling units in the population also has an equal chance of constituting a sample.

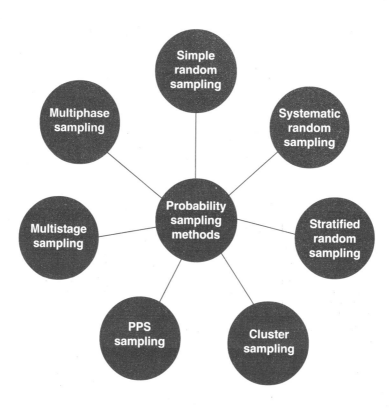

Fig. 2.1: Probability sampling methods

For example, to draw a simple random sample from an outdoor patient registration register of the department of obstetrics and gynaecology, each entry would need to be numbered sequentially. If one wants to draw a sample of size 700 out of 3500, a list of 700 random numbers between 1 and 3500 would need to be prepared using one of the known procedures (described later). The 700 entries made in the registration register corresponding to the 700 random numbers present in the prepared list would make up the sample.

A sample, using simple random sampling, can be drawn with or without replacement. In case of sampling with replacement, there is a possibility that a particular sampled entry in the register may be selected twice or more. Therefore, usually the simple random sampling without replacement is used, which is more convenient and provides more precise samples. Hereafter, the term 'simple random sampling', would mean sampling without replacement.

Mainly, two approaches are used in drawing a simple random sample:

Lottery draw: For the afore-mentioned example, write the number of each and every registered patient on slips (3500) of paper, place them in an empty box and shuffle them. Then, draw out 700 slips for the desired sample size and identity of each of the selected sampling units. This is preferred when the population size is small.

Use of random number table: In this method, a randomly generated numbers' table (Appendix 1) that is generally known as the random number table (appended to most statistical books), is used to draw the desired sample. In the afore-mentioned example, there are four digits in the population size, that is, 3500. Hence, the selected random numbers would need to contain four digits. For the selection to be more precise, the women in the register. If a number recurs, to ensure sampling without replacement, simply ignore it.

The advantages of simple random sampling are: (i) the need for only the complete sampling frame along with information for contact; (ii) no need for additional information on the sampling frame (such as geographic areas); (iii) use of simpler methods to determine the sample size, estimates and other analyses.

The disadvantages are: (i) costly and not feasible in case of large populations because of the need to prepare a complete sampling frame prior to sampling; (ii) further cost if personal interviews are required, since the selected sample may be geographically spread out across the population; and (iii) no use of the supplementary information available on the sampling frame (e.g., rural/urban) that could make the sample design more efficient, since this problem has to be tackled at the time of data analysis through the calculation of appropriate weights and their use in the analysis, which makes the analysis more cumbersome.

2.2.1.2. Systematic random sampling

Systematic sampling literally means that there is an equal interval between each selected sampling unit in the sample. The steps involved in drawing a systematic sample in case of the hypothetical example considered for simple random sample are: (i) numbering each entry in the registration register sequentially, i.e. from 1 to 3500; (ii) calculating the sampling interval, that is, 3500/700 = 5; (iii) selecting a random start that is a random number between 1 and 5, say 3; and (iv) selecting the 3rd sampling unit out of first five women and then every fifth woman, i.e., 3, 8, 13, 18, ..., 3490, 3495. Thus, in this method, there are only five possible samples of size 700 that can be drawn corresponding to the five possible random starts. Each woman of the population belongs to only one of the five samples and each sample has the same chance of being selected. It is thus clear that each woman has a one in five chance of being selected in the sample which is the same as that if a simple random sample of 700 women was selected. The only difference is that with simple random sampling, any combination of 700 women would have a chance of making up the sample, while with systematic sampling, there are only five possible samples depending on the five possible random starts between one and five. This shows the comparative precision of systematic sampling versus simple random sampling. In systematic sampling, the precision will be less compared to that with simple random sampling. The possible samples for systematic sampling are determined in view of the order of the population in the sampling frame.

If the sampling frame has a randomly distributed population, systematic sampling should yield results that are similar to simple random sampling.

In the example considered above, the sampling interval was a whole number. This may not always be true. For example, if a sample of size 700 has to be selected out of a population of size 3400, the sampling interval will be 4.86, which may be rounded off to the nearest whole number five. On the other hand, if a sample size of 700 has to be selected out of a population of size 3100, the sampling interval will be 4.43, which may be rounded off to the nearest whole number four. The remaining steps remain the same. In the first case, one has to continue (even after crossing the sampling frame) in sequence till the desired sample size is achieved. In the latter case, one has to stop after achieving the desired sample size.

As is evident from the above description, systematic sampling has an advantage in the sense that sample selection mainly involves the selection of the random start and the rest of the sample follows automatically. Also, the sample is distributed evenly over the entire sampling frame. But the biggest drawback of this method is that if the sampling frame involves the consideration of some cycle that coincides in some way with the sampling interval, the possible sample may not be representative of the population. For example, if women in a group of five are registered in the outpatient department (OPD) and the first three women in each group are pregnant, then with the sampling interval five, one could end up selecting only pregnant women in the sample. This sample may not provide an appropriate picture of women attending that OPD.

2.2.1.3. Stratified random sampling

When the population is heterogeneous with reference to some major characteristics, applying simple random sampling after stratifying the population with respect to the factor(s) influencing the study variable will enhance the precision of the estimate. In this method, first the population being considered is divided into mutually exclusive categories whose sampling units are heterogeneous between the categories but homogeneous within each category. As the name of this method suggests, these categories are generally called strata. From each stratum, independent samples are selected using any of the known sampling methods. The method of sampling can vary from one stratum to another. If the sample selection is carried out using simple random sampling in each stratum, the sample design is called stratified simple random sampling. Information on the variables used for stratification should be available for all the sampling units present in the sampling frame prior to sampling (e.g., rural/urban; socioeconomic status, etc.).

If the population is heterogeneous, the use of stratified random sampling makes the sampling strategy more efficient. This is because a larger sample size is necessary to get a more accurate estimation of a characteristic that has greater variability from one sampling unit to another than for a characteristic that does not. To be more specific, if every person in the population has the same haemoglobin level, then a sample of even one individual would be enough to get a precise estimate of the average haemoglobin level. Let us clarify it further: under stratified random sampling, sampling units under each stratum have similar characteristics (e.g., haemoglobin levels) but different from those in other strata (e.g., disease status). In such a case, only a small sample from each stratum may provide a precise estimate of the haemoglobin level for that stratum. The estimates obtained for each stratum may be combined to get a precise estimate of haemoglobin levels for the population. A simple random sampling approach to the entire population (without stratification) would require a comparatively larger sample size than the total of stratum-specific samples to obtain an estimate of haemoglobin level with the same level of precision.

Another advantage of this method of sampling is that it may ensure an adequate sample size for the relevant subgroups in a population. After stratification of the population, when each stratum becomes an independent population, one may calculate the sample size required from each stratum. To clarify further, if a study is being carried out based on a sample taken from a population that has only a 1% Christian population, the use of simple random sampling may result in very few Christian being present in the sample, which may not allow analysis for this subgroup. To overcome this problem, stratification with respect to religion may allow the selection of the required Christian population in the sample. However, it is worthwhile to mention here that the use of stratified random sampling may be possible only if the stratifying variables are easy to observe, closely related with the topic under study and operationally simple.

2.2.1.4. Cluster sampling

To cover a study sample that is spread across the population as a whole (e.g., country, state or, district level) may obviously involve a huge additional cost, especially that related to travel. Also, the sampling frame may not be available every time it is necessary to use simple random sampling, systematic random sampling or probability proportional to size (PPS) sampling. In such a situation, one may choose a cluster sampling technique using a list of all the clusters/groups in the population which is either available or easy to create. To ensure the representativeness of the entire population, the clusters are selected randomly followed by complete enumeration (i.e., to cover each and every sampling unit of the selected clusters). This may, however, result in the coverage of a larger or smaller sample size than expected. For example, to conduct a study in a city, each ward of the city may serve as the sampling unit in the form of a cluster. Sometimes, if necessary, clusters may be created with the help of roads, lanes and other landmarks. Accordingly, a list of wards or of created clusters may be used as a sampling frame to randomly select the wards or clusters and enumerate them completely. Thus, this procedure involves the coverage of sampling units (e.g., households, students) in the form of 'pockets of sampled units' (e.g., village, school) instead of spreading the sample over the population. For example, to study the nutrition level among higher secondary students in Delhi, one would like to avoid the costly and lengthy approach of enumerating each and every higher secondary student of Delhi. The selection of a couple of schools followed by their complete enumeration may be advisable. This obviously helps in reducing the cost of the study. However, such studies are less efficient when compared to simple random sampling. To avoid this to some extent, it is advisable not only to increase the sample size in view of the design effect (described later) but also to study a large number of small clusters instead of a small number of large clusters, which may help in incorporating various prevailing conditions of the population in the sample making it more representative. For example, in the afore-mentioned example of a nutritional study, one should prefer considering various sections of higher secondary classes in a school as clusters (e.g., XIA, XIB…and XIIA, XIIB…) instead of classes (e.g., XI and XII) or simply schools, and select more clusters. For doing this, if necessary, one can decide to cover a fixed number of sampling units from the selected large number of clusters instead of complete or partial enumeration of a small number of clusters. This may provide a comparatively more representative sample.

2.2.1.5. Sampling with probability proportional to size (PPS sampling)

As stated earlier, it is essential in case of random or probability sampling that each sampling unit of the population has a chance of being included in the sample. But, it is not necessary that this chance will be the same for every sampling unit. In order to increase efficiency, the information available in the sampling frame about the varying size of each sampling unit (e.g., number of women attending the OPD of each hospital) can be used in the selection of the sample. This is known as PPS sampling. In this method, the bigger the size of the sampling unit, the higher is its chance of being included in the sample. However, the size of the sampling unit needs to be accurate for increased efficiency.

PPS sampling can easily be understood with the help of the hypothetical data presented in Table 2.1. The study involves the following steps:

Step 1: The sampling interval is calculated by dividing the total population by the number of clusters to be selected. In this case, to select, say, 10 clusters, the sampling interval is: 8300/10 = 830.

Step 2: A random number between 1 and the sampling interval (830) is selected using the random number table (Appendix 1). Since maximum number in this interval is 830, a three digit number, the random number may be selected from any row and any three consecutive columns in the Table of random numbers. In the Table of random numbers, the number in the 5th row in columns 10 to 12 (three digits) gives the random number of 677.

Step 3: The first cluster will be from the hospital where the 677th individual is found in the cumulative population column, that is, hospital 'A'.

Step 4: Adding 830 cumulatively selects the remaining clusters. For example, 677+830=1507 indicates the selection of the second cluster from hospital 'C', where the value 1507 is located in Table 2.1; and so on. As is evident from this Table, in hospitals with large populations, more than one cluster will be selected. In such cases, the related hospital has to be divided into sections (with approximately equal populations) equal to the number of clusters to be selected. Depending upon the stipulated sample size, required number of subjects may be selected from each cluster. If the stipulated sample size is 400 and the number of clusters is ten, a sample of 40 subjects may be selected from each cluster to get a sample of 400 subjects for the study.

Table 2.1: Selection of Delhi hospitals using the PPS method

Hospitals	Population of female staff	Cumulative population	Selected clusters
A	700	700	1
B	450	1150	
C	600	1750	2
D	300	2050	
E	1200	3250	3, 4
F	100	3350	
G	200	3550	
H	1500	5050	5, 6
I	500	5550	
J	250	5800	7
K	2500	8300	8, 9, 10

2.2.1.6. Multistage sampling

To adopt sampling at only one stage through cluster sampling, we may completely enumerate the selected clusters. For example, to study the nutrition level among higher secondary students in Delhi, a sample of 10 schools may be considered to cover a sample size of about 1200. Accordingly, it is assumed that each school has almost 120 higher secondary students, enumerating all of them. But, in reality, the number of higher secondary students may vary from school to school, which may affect the desired sample size. To avoid this, a multistage sampling may be used that requires at least two stages. In the first stage, the identification and selection of larger sampling units (e.g., schools) may be carried out. In the second stage, a fixed number of population sampling units may be enumerated from each of the selected large groups or clusters. For example, to study the nutrition level among higher secondary students in Delhi, one may choose a larger number of schools (e.g., 20 schools instead of 10 in the first stage). At the second stage, contrary to complete enumeration, a list of all higher secondary students from the selected schools may be used to select a random sample of 60 students out of the total number of children from each school, which may provide a sample coverage of 1200 children (Fig. 2.2). Likewise, if necessary, more than two stages may be involved. At the second stage in the above example, classes instead of a list of all higher secondary students in the 20 selected schools (say, 65 with an assumption that there are at least three classes in each school) may be used to make random selection of two classes within each school. Accordingly, at the third stage, a list of all higher secondary students for each of the selected 40 classes may be used to select a random sample of 30 students from each class. Thus, this would be a three-stage sampling scheme. Each time we add a stage, the sample may be more spread over the population and representative than that selected earlier. This will still have the benefit of a more concentrated sample leading to cost reduction but unlike cluster sampling which involves only single-stage sampling. This procedure needs a bigger sample size than that in the simple random sampling method and requires more information than cluster sampling. But, much less time and effort are required in this method, e.g., a list of all the higher secondary students in Delhi is not required in the given example.

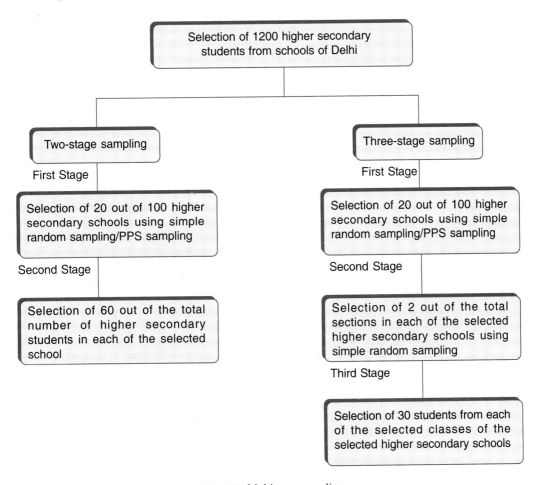

Fig. 2.2: Multistage sampling

2.2.1.7. Multiphase sampling

This method involves collection of basic information on a larger sample size followed by successive collection of more specific information for successive sub-samples out of the earlier sample. However, the consideration of more phases results in a more complex sample design as well as estimation procedure. Contrary to multistage sampling, the sampling units at each phase are structurally the same. This sampling method may be useful when the auxiliary information necessary for stratification or screening is not available. For example, suppose the Indian Council of Medical Research (ICMR) needs specific health information about persons exposed to toxic gas on the nights of 2nd and 3rd December 1984 in Bhopal, and exposure status is not available. In this case, a screening survey involving only a couple of questions, which should obviously incur a low cost per interview, could help assess the exposure status. Once the first sample has been drawn, a smaller sample can be extracted from the persons exposed to the toxic gas and they may be asked for specific health information. This method could help avoid the expenses of surveying persons who were not exposed to the toxic gas.

Multiphase sampling may also be used when: (i) not enough money is available to collect complete information from each unit of the entire sample; or (ii) cost of collection varies from one aspect (e.g., symptomatic data collection) to another (e.g., clinical data collection); or (iii) collection of information on all aspects would create an excessive burden on the respondent. For example, a symptomatic survey may be conducted on n_1 persons; respiratory data collection may be carried out only on n_2 out of n_1; radiological data collection may be carried out only on n_3 out of n_2; and pathological data collection may be carried out only on n_4 out of n_3 persons.

2.2.2. Non-probability Sampling Methods

Non-probability sampling methods are summarized in Fig. 2.3.

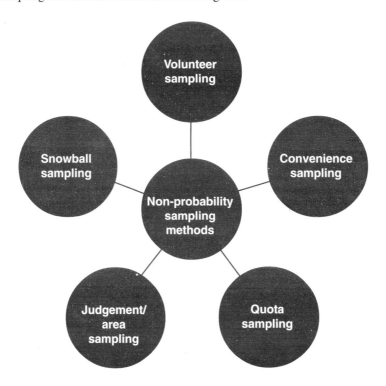

Fig. 2.3: Non-probability sampling methods

2.2.2.1. Volunteer sampling

In this method, a person or sampling unit volunteers to be included in the study. For example, for the testing of a newly developed drug, it may not be appropriate or ethical to randomly enlist patients. In such cases, the patients are requested (with or without offering payments) to volunteer for the study after understanding all the pros and cons of the new drug. The inclusion of volunteers as opposed to probability sampling may obviously introduce serious biases. In an opinion poll on an existing system through television/mobiles/internet, only a selected group of people who have access to these facilities and are concerned about that system may respond resulting in a large selection bias. The respondents might have views different from those who did not respond. Further, there is generally no limit to the number of times one person can respond, so that one person can respond repeatedly.

2.2.2.2. Convenience sampling

This method includes those sampling units which are accessible easily and conveniently. For example, to determine the views of people on a public issue, television reporters conduct street interviews without following probability sampling. An example of this method is consideration of the first 50 persons who enter a temple/mosque/church/gurudwara. This method is easy to use but may add strong biases. This may be useful to conduct an exploratory or preliminary research for a gross idea about the subject. However, it can yield accurate results when the population is homogeneous or well mixed. For example, to assess the water pollution in a pond, any sample may yield a similar result under the assumption that the pond water is well mixed.

2.2.2.3. Quota sampling

This procedure allows the inclusion of sampling units in a study till a specific number of sampling units (quotas) for various subpopulations has been achieved. For example, to select 50 persons, one may decide to include 25 males and 25 females. After satisfying the fixed quotas of sample size from various subpopulations, the selection stops haphazardly. Contrary to stratified random sampling, in this method no probability sampling is considered in selecting sampling units from various subpopulations. This method is often used in market research since it is comparatively inexpensive and easy to administer, and has the property of satisfying population proportions. The assumption that selected persons are similar to those not selected may however, rarely be acceptable. Hence, it may be difficult to overcome the problem of selection bias.

2.2.2.4. Judgement sampling/area sampling

This method is an extension of convenience sampling and involves the selection of the sample based on certain judgements of the researcher. For example, one may decide to draw the entire sample of higher secondary students from one school. Since the preconceptions of the researcher about the representativeness of one school for all the schools may not be accurate, large biases may be introduced. This method is generally used in pre-testing of questionnaires and focus-group discussion. To some extent, the choice of experimental subjects (e.g., animals, humans) also reflects the researcher's pre-existing beliefs about the population.

2.2.2.5. Snowball sampling

This method involves referrals from initial known subjects (of our interest) in reaching additional subjects. It is supposed to be used in special circumstances in which subjects are rare. For example, a family with maternal mortality may have information about other families with the same experience. However, apart from being costly and time consuming, this method may also not provide a representative sample, for example, in cases of maternal mortality, due to obvious selection bias.

2.2.3. Use of Some Other Sampling Methods

2.2.3.1. Sequential sampling

This method does not involve a fixed sample size and is generally used in the field of clinical trials (described in Chapter 9). The selection of persons/patients in various treatment/intervention groups continues until one achieves a predetermined level of significance. This method may be useful when the availability of cases is rare and/or the drug is very costly. However, the use of this method requires expertise in the area.

2.2.3.2. Double sampling

This is another method that is useful in cases of costly enquiry. For example, if it is costly to enumerate one variable (say X_1) and there is another variable (say X_2) that may be enumerated cheaply and easily, with X_1 and X_2 being highly correlated, then, enumeration can be carried out on both, X_1 and X_2 in a smaller sample size to work out the dependence of X_1 on X_2. Later, enumeration on X_2 can be carried out with a desired sample size and X_1 can be estimated using its relationship with X_2. However, this method is rarely used.

2.2.3.4. Interpenetrating subsampling (replicated sampling)

In this method, independent sub-samples are drawn from the population according to simple random sampling without replacement. As a result, some sampling units may be common to the two sub -samples. Thus, coverage (i.e., size of the sub-sample and its number) has to be planned in such a way that distinct sampling units provide the required sample size. This may, however, cause inter-observer variation if each sub-sample is being covered by independent investigators. The National Sample Survey Organization (NSSO) in India is successfully utilizing this procedure. However, its use in clinical studies is rare, because of problems with feasibility and/or for ethical reasons.

2.3. Methods of Data Collection

Basically, there are two types of data which can be used for research purposes. The data collected by an investigator on a set of variables for individual persons/ patients, in a selected sample using any study design, is generally known as primary data. On the other hand, those available through various reports/ publications are addressed as secondary data. While in case of primary data collection the investigator has full control over all aspects of the study right from the definition of the problem through the design and data collection and analysis of data, he /she may not have any control over these aspects in case of secondary data since the data used is from already collected and analyzed data and published reports .When it is difficult to collect primary data, secondary data may be used. For example, if one wants to study the fertility & mortality pattern in the population of a country over a period of time, it would be difficult to collect primary data and, hence, the required information may be collected from already published reports. In case of secondary data, the reliability of the data may be questioned unless the source of the data is well ascertained.

Policy-oriented observations are possible to obtain through an appropriate analysis of quality data. The quality of data is totally dependent on the methods and systems of data collection, which consist of various components (e.g., designing instruments for data collection, translation in desired language, etc.) briefly described in successive sections in this chapter. In addition, the chapter also introduces various terminologies. However, many more steps may be required to ensure the collection of quality data than those described here.

2.3.1. Survey Instruments

This refers to a device used in a survey, e.g., interview schedule, questionnaire, medical examination record form, etc.

2.3.1.1. Designing of survey instruments

To develop an appropriate survey instrument for data collection, the following issues need to be considered:
1. What exactly is to be determined in view of the objectives of the study?
2. What information (e.g., variables and their scales of measurements) may be desired to determine the required answer?

3. Who should be the respondent? What if the respondent is not available?
4. What is the right technique to obtain all the answers, such as questioning/interviewing/ observing, or analysis of existing records?
5. Are the respondents literate? If not, the use of self-administered questionnaires is not an option.
6. What is the sample size? A study with a larger sample size may ideally need shorter and highly structured questionnaires. However, a small study may have the flexibility of using questionnaires with a number of open-ended questions.

2.3.1.2. Interview schedule

This is the precisely designed set of questions used in an interview. This term generally indicates a survey instrument that is used to record responses by an interviewer.

2.3.2. Questionnaire

It refers to a predetermined set of questions used to collect data on various aspects such as clinical, socioeconomic and occupational groups, etc. This term often refers to a self-completed survey instrument, in contrast to an interview schedule.

2.3.2.1. Open-ended questions

These questions allow the recording of free responses in the respondent's own words. For such questions, the respondent is not provided possible answers to choose from. Such questions may help in obtaining information on aspects with which the researcher is not very familiar, especially those involving opinion and attitudes, and suggestions of respondents, or sensitive issues. For example, what would you do if you notice that one of your family members is suffering from AIDS?

2.3.2.2. Closed questions

For these questions, out of listed possible answers that are generally exhaustive and mutually exclusive, the respondent chooses the answer(s) he thinks is most appropriate. Preferably, the number of options should be as few as possible. Closed questions are used to cover the full range of possible responses. For example, have you ever visited the Anganwadi Centre? (1. Yes; 2. No). If only certain aspects of an issue are of interest, the use of closed questions may help avoid wasting the time of both the respondent and interviewer by obtaining only as much information as one needs. For example, to determine the protein content of a family diet, consumption on the previous day of each of the selected items (e.g., cereals; meat/fish; eggs; milk) may be recorded in the form of 'yes' or 'no'. The opinions of respondents may also be recorded by choosing rating points on a scale. For example, how useful would you rate the activities of the *Anganwadis* in the development of the village? (e.g., 1. extremely useful; 2. very useful; 3. useful; 4. not very useful; 5. not useful at all).

2.3.2.3. Advantages and disadvantages of open-ended and closed questions

Open-ended questions help in exploring unknown issues. Replies to these questions are in general spontaneous and are expected to be valid. Including some examples in the respondents' own words enhance the merits of reports. Answers to closed questions may be recorded quickly and analysed easily. However, open-ended questions not only need skilled interviewers but also experienced analysts, and their analysis is time-consuming.

Both types of questions need trained interviewers along with necessary supervision. Pre-testing of even closed questions in the form of open-ended questions may be helpful in assessing whether the categories considered cover all the possibilities. If possible, most common answers to open-ended questions should also be categorized, leaving space for other possible answers. Likewise, closed questions may also be used in combination with open-ended questions. There should be a natural flow between the questions. Detailed guidelines for the interviewers may be an integral part of the questionnaire/interview schedule. An example of a combination of closed and open-ended multiple answers to a question is: What are the reasons for not going to a health facility for delivery?

Not necessary	A
Not customary	B
Cost too much	C
Too far/no transport	D
Poor quality service	E
No time to go	F
Family did not allow	G
Lack of knowledge	H
No health worker visited	I
Others (specify)	J

Such questions need the proper attention of the interviewers/respondents for accuracy of data collection. If necessary, responses to such questions may be recorded both with and without probing.

2.3.2.4. Steps in designing a questionnaire

The major steps in designing a questionnaire, which obviously requires a number of drafts, are:

Step I: Consideration of content: This requires the consideration of objective-specific variables. In view of the objectives, the questions have to be formulated to get information on the desired variables. While developing the questionnaire, if necessary, some variables may be reconsidered and a decision may be taken to add, drop or change them. Also, if necessary, some of the objectives may be changed at this stage.

Step II: Formulation of questions: Questions are required to provide the information needed for each variable. To ensure that different respondents may not interpret the questions differently, they should be specific and precise. If necessary, questions may be broken up into different parts so that each part focuses on only one thing. For example, instead of asking "Where do your family members usually seek treatment when they are sick?" focus on illnesses that have occurred in the family over the week/fortnight and ask what they did to treat each of them. One should try to avoid a leading question that is suggestive of a certain answer, for example: "Do you agree that one should visit a health centre in case of any health problem?" Attempts should also be made to avoid a question that presupposes a certain condition, for example: "What action did you take when your child had fever the last time?"

Step III. Flow of questions: One should prepare the interview schedule or questionnaire so that it is logical and respondent-friendly. This may be possible by keeping the questionnaire as short as possible. If necessary, the interviews may be conducted in two or more parts, e.g., a household questionnaire; a women's questionnaire (background characteristics, antenatal case [ANC] and birth preparedness, contraception, knowledge, opinion and attitude towards sexually transmitted infection/reproductive tract infection [STI/RTI] and AIDS, and anatomy and health); and a youth questionnaire (male/female).

Step IV. Formatting the questionnaire: Each part of the questionnaire should not only be friendly to the respondent but also to the interviewers. The final version of each part of the questionnaire should ideally have the date of the interview, particulars of the respondent (name [sometimes optional]; address, etc.); and particulars of the interviewer (e.g., age). To clarify further, headings, subheadings, sections, etc., may be used within each part. Boxes for pre-assigned answers may be listed on the right side of the page. Sufficient space may be provided for answers to open-ended questions. Provision may be made so that computerized handling of the data, including entry, etc., is easier.

Step V: Translation into local dialects: The interviews have generally to be conducted in the local languages of the study areas. Accordingly, the translation of the questionnaire from English to one or more than one local languages may be necessary to ensure the accuracy of the data collected. Further, re-translation into English is necessary to ensure the accuracy of the translated questionnaires.

2.3.2.5. Guide for interview

Before data collection starts, a detailed and specific instruction manual for every item of each part of the questionnaire may be prepared. If possible, some of these instructions may be accommodated in the questionnaire itself. Special mention should be made about reading/not reading the alternatives-answers; required probing etc. The procedures to deal with various anticipated problems and their solutions should be explained (e.g., non-availability of respondents and their substitutes).

The methods described on the development of survey instruments (Questionnaires, Proformae) may also be useful in developing instruments to be used under other study designs (e.g., case-control, cohort and experimental studies). Further, the developed instruments need to be standardized to be suitably used in a given set up/region. For example, an instrument developed in western countries needs to be modified or updated, so that it can be used in the Indian system to collect data having appropriate reliability and validity. Also, a newly developed instrument needs to be assessed on its reliability and validity before its final use.

2.4. Systems of Data Collection

There are broadly two systems of data collection: regular and ad hoc systems.

2.4.1. Regular Systems

Such a system involves a routine system of data collection through a mechanism for collecting data as they become available. For example, a vital statistics registration system, a disease notification system, a reporting system for cancer cases and registration systems in healthcare facilities. This system of data collection mainly requires: (i) the establishment of rules and regulations instituting the system and giving legal backing to it (e.g., a national/state level system); (ii) decision on items of information to be collected; (iii) design of forms and registers to be used for recording information; (iv) physical establishment of office facilities; (v) recruitment of personnel and their training; (vi) specification of the recording procedure (e.g., who will supply the information, when the information has to be registered, etc.); and (vii) specification and design of registration receipts.

2.4.2. Ad Hoc Systems

Such a system involves planning of an ad hoc survey to collect information that is not available on a regular basis. This may include a totally new study or an elaboration of aspects of data that have been collected on a regular basis. For example, a survey to estimate the proportion of children with malnutrition in a defined population or an investigation of breast-feeding practices among women who registered a birth in the previous year. The data collected may be for administrative or research purposes. This system of data collection mainly requires consideration of: (i) specific objectives of the study; (ii) type of information to be collected; (iii) definition of the population for which the information is required; (iv) need for sampling; (v) sample size; (vi) sampling method; (vii) design of survey instruments (questionnaires, etc.) to be used for recording data; (viii) selection and training of personnel to record the information; and (ix) data collection-identification of selected sampling units and respondents, filling of forms, etc.

2.4.3. Instruments for Measuring Data

These may be of the following types:

Human. This is an instrument with which the collection of data on some variables may mainly involve a person, with little or no involvement of apparatus (e.g., grading spleen enlargement; taking a patient's history).

Apparatus. This is an instrument with which measurement is done using a purely mechanical device (e.g., weighing scales, thermometers).

Combination of human and apparatus. This is an instrument for which the recording of data involves using both humans and apparatus (e.g., reading of X-ray films; reading of blood films).

2.4.3.1. Reliability and validity of data measuring instruments

The instruments for measuring data must have two major characteristics: reasonable reliability and validity

Reliability: Reliability measures the inherent performance of the instrument. A reliable instrument may provide consistent results when it is applied more than once on the same unit under similar conditions. The major factors affecting consistency are variation of the instrument itself (e.g., fluctuating zero mark in a weighing scale), fluctuations in the substance being measured (e.g., respondents' answers depending on their understanding of the questions), intra-observer error, and inter-observer error.

Validity: A valid instrument indicates the condition that it is supposed to measure. For example, fever may be a valid indicator for malaria in areas with high malaria transmission levels, while childlessness may not be a valid index of infertility.

2.4.4. Major Data Collection Techniques

Data collection may involve one or more than one of the following techniques:

Using available information: Using information already available with the respondents may be an inexpensive choice. But there are problems in the easy availability of such information. Most of the time, the methodology used in the collection of such data is not known. Also, there may be problems in obtaining the data in a complete manner.

Observation method: This procedure may provide additional and more accurate information, especially on those aspects that may not be so easy collect (e.g., behaviour-related measures). However, this may sometimes be very time consuming.

Face-to-face interview: This is a commonly used procedure for data collection, especially in public health and socioeconomic surveys, wherein an interviewer contacts the respondent and fills the pro-forma after interviewing him/her. This however requires good planning in terms of the preparation of structured questionnaires and the training of interviewers as detailed earlier.

Administering written questionnaires (self-administered questionnaires): There are many ways of using this procedure for data collection. It may involve the hand-delivery of questionnaires to respondents and their collection after some time. As an alternative, all or some of the respondents may be gathered in one place at one time, and oral or written instructions given to them. The respondents may fill the questionnaires then and there. Sometimes the questionnaires may be sent to the respondents by mail with clear instructions requesting them to complete and mail them within a specified time.

2.4.5. Ethical Considerations

Data collection techniques may possibly cause physical or emotional harm to the respondents. For example, violating the respondents' right to privacy by questioning on sensitive issues, need to access personal data, observing the respondents without their knowledge, or failing to follow certain cultural values, traditions, or taboos. To avoid this, one may obtain informed consent before the interview begins, ensure the confidentiality of the data obtained, not explore sensitive issues before a good relationship has been established, and put up the questions in desired and cordial manner.

2.4.6. Reporting Population and Samples

This is basic to the propagation of research and a study is of little importance if it is not reported adequately. The points that must be borne in mind, apart from sampling design and scheme, are:

1. Due emphasis must be given in reporting to how the sample was chosen. Were the sample units patients who happened to be around? Were they consecutively registered patient in a hospital, who satisfied certain criteria?
2. Differences in defining demographics between the sample and the remaining population must be reported.
3. Reasons for exclusion must be listed, and responders and non-responders must be compared for key variables.
4. In questionnaire surveys, method of choice of the target population should be described and the number of people who refused to complete the questionnaire or were 'not available' should be reported.

Multiple Choice Questions

Choose the correct answers in the following multiple choice questions. The correct answers are listed on p. 342.

Q.1. As compared to the complete enumeration, sample survey helps in reducing:
a. Costs of the study
b. Time required for the study
c. Both costs and time
d. Neither costs nor time

Q.2. Which of the following is a non-random sampling procedure?
a. Stratified sampling
b. Quota sampling
c. Cluster sampling
d. Multistage sampling

Q.3. The major advantage of a probability sample compared with a non-probability sample is that:
a. It saves time
b. It costs less
c. It enables to compute average value
d. Sampling error can be estimated

Q.4. A simple random sample is one where:
a. Each study element in the population has an equal probability of being included in the sample
b. Each study element in the population has got varying probabilities of being included in the sample
c. Each study element in the population has got a probability of 1 for being included in the sample
d. Sample selected without any probability

Q.5. Stratified sampling method is advised when:
a. There is homogeneity in the population with respect to the study variable
b. There is heterogeneity in the population with respect to the study variable
c. More variables have to be studied
d. The distribution of the study variable is normal

Q.6. In a survey of household expenditure on health, if every 4th household in each census block was studied, the sampling plan is called:
a. Simple random sampling
b. Cluster sampling
c. Stratified sampling
d. Systematic sampling

Q.7. Non-response in any survey is:
a. A type of non-sampling error only
b. A type of sampling error only
c. It can be both a sampling and a non-sampling error
d. Neither a sampling nor a non-sampling error

Q.8. **The sampling plan to economize the costs in large national studies is:**
    a. Quota sampling   b. Multistage sampling
    c. Simple random sampling   d. Stratified sampling

Q.9. **The data collected directly by the investigator or his/her team is called:**
    a. Secondary data   b. Primary data
    c. Population data   d. Sample data

Q.10. **The data collected from already published material is called:**
    a. Secondary data   b. Primary data
    c. Population data   d. Sample data

3 | Descriptive Statistical Methods

- Tabulation of data: Tabular presentation of qualitative data, tabular presentation of quantitative data
- Presentation of data by diagrams: Pie chart, bar diagram, adjacent bar diagram, component bar diagram, histogram, frequency polygon, line graph, stem and leaf plot, ogive curves & cumulative frequency polygon, general comments on graphs & diagrams, shape of the frequency distribution
- Measures of central tendency & location: Arithmetic mean, median, mode, geometric mean, harmonic mean, general comments on the measures of central tendency
- Measures of dispersion: Range, interquartile range, mean deviation, standard deviation, coefficient of variation
- Correlation: Scatter diagram, correlation coefficient, interpretation of r, correlation coefficient based on rankings
- Regression: Linear regression, least squares method of estimation, numerical examples of calculation of regression, interpretation of slope and intercept of the regression line, relationship between correlation and regression, uses of regression, limitations of regression analysis, what to use: correlation or regression

3.1. Tabulation of Data

In this chapter, we shall discuss some descriptive analytical methods, which form the first level of analysis of any data. For any given investigation, (i) the target population, (ii) the sample and (iii) the variables should be very clearly identified. Once we have clearly defined variables and a scientifically collected sample from a well-defined population, we get the data for further investigation; but the data (in the form in which they were originally collected) look like a mass of numbers. For example, the ages (in years) of 10 women at their first childbirth can appear as: 22, 25, 18, 21, 29, 26, 24, 22, 24 and 26. These data are called the raw data as they are in the form in which they have been collected. Our idea of collecting this sample information is to determine the age of a woman at her first childbirth, in general. From the sample data, we see that it can range from 18 to 29 years. If our sample size is large (say 1000 women instead of 10), we will be almost lost in the mass of numbers. Useful information is usually not immediately evident from such a mass of data. Therefore, we need to rearrange the mass of numbers (raw data) so that the information they contain clearly reveals the patterns of variation.

Precise methods of analysis can be decided upon only when the data structure and characteristics are understood. The process of reorganizing or summarizing the mass of raw data involves preparation of a frequency distribution or tabular presentation of data. It is also known as reducing the data dimension. This is the first step in the description and analysis of any statistical data.

3.1.1. Tabular Presentation of Qualitative Data

It is often simpler to make a frequency distribution of qualitative data for obvious reasons. Take for example the data set of the smoking status of 20 individuals, collected as yes (y) or no (n). The raw data appears as n, y, n, n, n, y, n, y, n, n, n, y, n, n, y, n, y, n, n and y. To find out the number of smokers and non-smokers, we simply count the number of 'y_s' and 'n_s' in the raw data set, which are 7 and 13 respectively. Thus, data reduction or reducing the dimension of the raw data is only simple counting in the case of qualitative data. The results of the example discussed are shown in Table 3.1 below.

Table 3.1: Smoking status of lung cancer patients attending Hospital A

Smoking status	Number of patients
Yes	7
No	13
Total	20

Suppose in addition to the smoking status, we also have the gender of the 10 lung cancer cases studied. We now have two variables—the smoking status (yes or no) and gender (male or female). This information can be arranged in a tabular form, counting the different combinations that can be formed with the two variables, namely, male smokers, male non-smokers, female smokers and female non-smokers. Such a presentation is called a two-way table as the row forms one way (one variable) and the column forms the other way (other variable). Table 3.2 below shows one such arrangement of the above data. Theoretically, we can extend this concept into a 3-way or multi-way table.

Table 3.2: Two-way table showing the distribution of lung cancer patients according to smoking status and gender

Smoking Status	Gender		Total
	Male	Female	
Yes	5	2	7
No	1	3	4
Total	6	5	11

3.1.2. Tabular Presentation of Quantitative Data

Tabular presentation of quantitative data is not as simple as that of qualitative data. Nowadays, many computer software packages are available and with their help one can tabulate any amount of data for any number of quantitative variables within a fraction of a second. Nevertheless, to understand the methodology and the issues involved, we will discuss them in more detail.

First, we should have an idea of the range of the values. Eyeballing the data will give us an idea of the minimum and maximum values. Then the total range is divided into some arbitrary intervals called class intervals. While choosing class intervals, we should keep in mind the fact that there should not be too many or too few intervals. Too many intervals imply there is not much reduction in the bulkiness of the data, an extreme case being each observation forming an interval in itself. On the other hand, too few intervals may oversimplify the presentation, an extreme case being the total data falling in one interval between the minimum and maximum values. Some authors suggest that six to twelve intervals are optimum. But certainly, a large number, say more than fifteen intervals, will not be advisable.

Sturges[1] (1926) suggested that if we have n observations, the number of intervals k should be equal to the integer nearest to the quantity $1+3.322 \log_{10}(n)$. Once the number of intervals, k, is fixed, dividing the range by k will yield k intervals of fixed width. For example, if we have 50 observations in the sample, we should have $1+3.322 \log_{10}(50) = 6.64$ or 7 intervals. Now supposing that the range of values in the sample is 10 to 100, each of the 7 intervals should have a width of $(100-10)\div7 = 13$ units. Thus, the first interval will be

10–23, second 23–36 and so on. Note that Sturges's rule may lead to class intervals with unconventional lower and upper limits as seen in the example.

It helps further computations if all the class intervals have an equal width, but not necessarily. The class intervals should be defined in such a way that they are mutually exclusive, non-overlapping and exhaustive. In other words, given any observation, it should fall in only one class interval. Also, avoid open-ended intervals such as less than 10 or more than 100, etc., as with these class intervals, one cannot calculate measures such as arithmetic mean or average. If such an interval is made, it should ideally have only a few observations and a footnote may indicate as to the exact values of such observations, to clarify the nature of the observations in such interval.

After forming a set of suitable class intervals, we draw a grid or table on a piece of paper with the first column indicating the class intervals. This column should have an appropriate label along with units of measurement, for example height in cm. The next column is labeled 'tally marks'. Looking at the data, cross ('/') each observation and put a tally mark 'I' against the interval in which that observation falls. Continue with the other observations, indicating every fifth tally mark in an interval by crossing the previous four tally marks as shown 'HH', so that it will be easy to count multiples of five. After placing the tally marks for all the observations in the appropriate groups, count the tally marks and indicate the number as the frequency of that class interval in the next column. The frequency indicates the number of observations falling in that interval. The total of frequencies of all the class intervals will add up to the total number of observations in the data set. Finally, give a suitable heading or title to the table. Indicate if any observations have been excluded due to any reason in the footnote.

As an example of making a frequency distribution for quantitative data, let us consider the systolic blood pressure (BP) values of 68 patients attending a clinic. The data are shown in Table 3.3 and the frequency distribution from these raw data is shown in Table 3.4.

Table 3.3: Systolic blood pressure (mmHg) values of 68 patients attending a clinic

99	110	96	160	106	144	109	156	110	128	118	168	132
140	160	159	102	148	150	156	154	143	108	146	145	148
110	116	116	164	122	122	149	125	154	129	176	124	125
120	130	135	104	174	152	166	139	130	136	118	136	147
162	142	132	128	90	136	155	138	139	131	149	126	134
158	130	136										

Table 3.4: Frequency distribution of systolic blood pressure in patients attending a clinic

Systolic BP (mmHg)	Tally marks	Frequency f_i	Cumulative frequency	Relative cumulative frequency
90 – 100	III	3	3	(3 /68) *100 = 4.4%
100 – 110	HH	5	8	(8/68) * 100 = 11.8%
110 – 120	HH II	7	15	22.1%
120 – 130	HH HH	10	25	36.8%
130 – 140	HH HH HH	15	40	58.8%
140 – 150	HH HH I	11	51	75.0%
150 – 160	HH IIII	9	60	88.2%
160 – 170	HH I	6	66	97.1%
170 – 180	II	2	68	100%
Total		68		

*Multiplication sign

We mentioned that given any observation, it should fall in only one interval. In the class intervals above, the upper limit of each class interval is the same as the lower limit of the next class interval. So the question arises, where should an observation of 100 mm be placed? The limits defined are in tune with the fact that the nature of the variable under consideration is quantitative or continuous. Though the variable could take any value within the range, we could measure it up to the units of millimeters. If we had measured the variable in further smaller and smaller units, the concept of continuity would be clear. Coming back to the specific value of 100 mm, conventionally the upper limit of each class interval is not included in that interval. Thus, values ranging from 90 to 99.99 or more but less than 100 mm will be placed in the interval 90–100, but the value of exactly 100 mm will be placed in the interval 100–110 mm. Similarly, the values 110 mm, 120 mm, etc., will be placed in the intervals 110–120 and 120–130, respectively. We could also show the intervals as 90–99, 100–109 and so on, keeping in mind that the upper limits are actually 99.9 or more but less than 100 and 190.9 or more but less than 110, etc.

The presentation of data in a tabular format enables us to understand the structure of the data distribution. It also helps us make some simple statements about the variable under study. In the example above, we now know that the systolic BP of the maximum number of subjects in our sample was between 130 and 140 mmHg, and very few patients had a BP of more than 170 mmHg. The columns showing the cumulative frequency and the relative frequency help interpret the data more easily. They are also useful for comparing two or more distributions. Table 3.4 reveals that 60 persons of a total of 68 (88.2%) have BP less than 160 mmHg, about 12% have BP less than 110 mmHg and so on. This type of understanding of BP distribution in the sampled study subjects was not easily possible from the raw data.

In practice, it is very cumbersome to give a tally mark to each observation one by one and finally count the total in each category of the variable. This process needs to be checked and re-checked, as there is scope for missing an observation or putting a tally mark in a wrong cell, leading to an incorrect frequency distribution. To overcome this, Hill[2] (1977) suggested that each observation value be written on a piece of paper or a card and then all the cards belonging to a specific category or range be separated and counted for the frequency. The advantage of this method is that it overcomes the mistakes that can occur in the tally mark system. Another method is to arrange all the observations in ascending order and count the number of observations at the desired cut-points or intervals. It should be noted that all these methods could be practicable if the data set had only a limited number of observations. Recourse to a computer is a necessity for quick and correct frequency distribution, especially with bigger data sets.

3.2. Presentation of Data by Diagrams

Frequency tables provide a concise or compact view of the data and its principal characteristics. Diagrams, on the other hand, provide a visual method of examining the data. They make a quick and lasting impression and convey ideas forcefully. Diagrams help us to get a real grasp of the overall picture rather than specific details. Many types of diagrams and graphs are used to represent different types of data.

3.2.1. Pie Chart

Pie (π) is a mathematical constant defined as the ratio of the circumference of a circle to its diameter and is equal to 22/7. In the pie chart, a circle (total 360°) is divided into sectors with areas proportional to the frequencies or the relative frequencies of the categories of a variable. The pie diagram is generally used to represent qualitative or categorical data. Before beginning to represent the data by a pie diagram, we should have the frequencies of different categories at hand. For each category find the proportionate degrees of the total of 360 in the circle. For example, if a category has a 25% frequency of the total, it should be allotted 25% of 360 or 90°. So, a sector with 90° to represents this category of the variable. Similarly, draw sectors for all the categories of the variable under study.

Consider the example of the frequencies of different blood groups in a population, which are shown in Table 3.5 below.

Table 3.5: Frequency distribution of subjects according to blood group

Blood group	A	B	AB	O	Total
Frequency	15	25	20	30	90
Percentage	16.7	27.8	22.2	33.3	100

For the category of blood group A, we have to allot $(15/90) \times 360 = 60°$. Similarly, for group B, $(25/90) \times 360 = 100°$ and so on for the other two categories. Now draw a circle and beginning from any point make a sector with 60° representing blood group A, another of 100° representing blood group B, etc. Note that the area of each sector is proportional to the frequency of the category it represents. Therefore, the higher the frequency, the bigger the sector will be. The pie diagram drawn for this data set is shown in Fig 3.1.

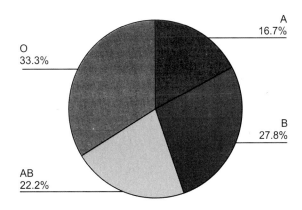

Fig. 3.1: Pie diagram showing the distribution of blood groups among 90 subjects

3.2.2. Bar Diagram

Qualitative or categorical data can also be represented by another diagram called the bar diagram. In this diagram, we show the category of the variable on the X-axis and the frequencies on the Y-axis on a graph paper. A bar for each category of the variable is erected and the height of the bar is proportional to the frequency of that category. Each bar should have an equal width. Since the data is of a qualitative nature (discrete), bars should not be next to each other and there should be an equal gap between two successive bars.

As an example of a bar diagram, consider the three types of lung carcinoma observed in a sample of 100 histologically proven cases. Seventy cases were of squamous cell carcinoma, 22 of adenocarcinoma and the remaining 8 of small-cell carcinoma. The bar diagram representing this information is shown in Fig. 3.2 below. The bar diagram conveys quickly and clearly that an overwhelming number of lung cancers are squamous cell carcinomas and a few are small-cell carcinomas.

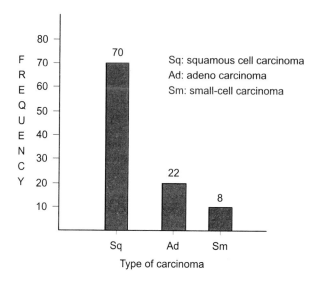

Fig. 3.2: Distribution of lung cancer patients by type of carcinoma

Simple bar diagrams can also be used to depict the relationship between a quantitative variable and another which is either quantitative or qualitative. For example, the monthly occurrence of malaria cases in a village can be shown as a simple bar diagram.

3.2.2.1. Adjacent bar diagram

Bar diagrams can be extended to compare two or more data sets (of a qualitative nature) with regard to the same variable. The bars of each category of the variable for the different data sets are drawn adjacent to each other. The principles of bar width and the gap between the bars will remain similar to those in the simple bar diagram. As an example, consider the comparison of the distribution of lung cancer patients by type of carcinoma in two clinics during a particular year. The data are shown in the Table 3.6 and the adjacent bar diagram in Fig. 3.3.

Table 3.6: Distribution of lung cancer cases in two hospitals according to type of carcinoma

Type of carcinoma	Frequency	
	Hospital A	Hospital B
Squamous cell carcinoma	180	260
Adenocarcinoma	72	140
Small-cell carcinoma	18	20
Total	270	420

3.2.2.2. Component bar diagram

The adjacent bar diagram in Fig. 3.3 shows the general pattern of the type of lung cancers in the two cancer centers studied. In both the centres, the majority of cases were of squamous cell type followed by adenocarcinomas and small-cell carcinomas. Beyond this, the diagram does not convey anything about the similarity of the relative proportions of each type in the two centres being compared. To depict this aspect, we can

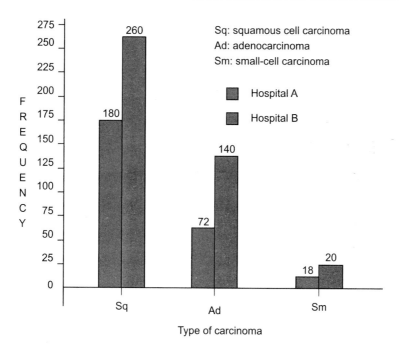

Fig. 3.3: Adjacent bar diagram showing the type of lung cancer cases in the two cancer hospitals studied

present the data in another form of the bar diagram called the component bar diagram. As the name indicates, all the components of data form the bars being compared. As two cancer centres are being compared, there will be two bars, one for each centre. Since the focus is on the relative frequencies of each type of cancer in the two centres, we will work on the relative frequencies or percentages, the length of each bar being the total frequency or 100%. The data set for preparing a component bar diagram of the lung cancer data is shown in Table 3.7 and the component bar diagram for the same data is shown in Fig. 3.4.

Table 3.7: Distribution of lung cancer cases in two hospitals

Type of carcinoma	Frequency			
	Hospital A		Hospital B	
	No.	%	No.	%
Squamous cell carcinoma	180	66.7	260	61.9
Adenocarcinoma	72	26.7	140	33.3
Small-cell carcinoma	18	6.6	20	4.8
Total	270	100.0	420	100.0

From Fig. 3.4, we can see that though the pattern is the same in both the centres, relatively more Adeno-carcinomas and less squamous cell carcinomas were seen at centre B compared to centre A. This additional information could be conveyed by the component bar diagram.

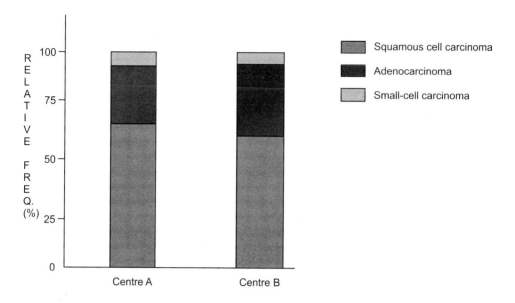

Fig. 3.4: Component bar diagram of the type of lung cancers in two cancer centers. Freq.: frequency

3.2.3. Histogram

The most popular of all diagrams is the histogram, which is used to depict the frequency distribution of a quantitative variable. The class intervals are shown on the horizontal axis (X-axis) and the corresponding frequencies in the form of vertical bars on the vertical axis (Y-axis). The width of each bar need not be the same as it depends on the width of the class intervals. If the width of a class interval is 20 units while the width of the rest is 10 units, it will be misleading to erect a bar with a base of 20 units and height equal to the frequency of that interval. Instead, we have to erect a bar with a base of 20 units and a height of the average frequency per unit width. In the present context, the standard width being 10 units, we have to divide the frequency of the interval whose width is 20 by 2 to fix the height of the bar to be shown for this class interval. The basic idea is that the area of each bar is proportional to the frequency of that class interval. Since the class intervals form a continuum, the bars are kept adjacent to each other. Sometimes in a frequency distribution, there can be open-ended classes, such as birth, weight <1000 g or blood sugar >200 mg, etc. Frequencies for such class intervals are shown separately from the rest, with a break in the X-axis.

A histogram is different from a simple bar diagram in three ways: (i) all the bars are of equal width in a simple bar diagram as against the fact that this may or may not be the case (depending on the width of the class intervals) in a histogram; (ii) in a simple bar diagram two adjacent bars have some gap between them as against no gap between the bars in the histogram; and (iii) the length of each bar is proportional to the frequency in a bar diagram as compared to the area in a histogram.

Table 3.8 gives the age-wise number of incident cancers of the uterine cervix among females of a rural area–Barshi–during the years 1990–96 [Indian Council of Medical Research (ICMR)[3], 2001] and the histogram representing these data is shown in Fig. 3.5. It is clear from the diagram that the occurrence of uterine cervical cancer increases with increasing age up to the age of 65 years, and decreases at higher ages. Very few cases occurred below 30 years of age.

Table 3.8: Age distribution of new cases of cancer of the uterine cervix, Barshi 1990-96

	Age (years)										
	25–29	30–34	35–39	40–44	45–49	50–54	55–59	60–64	65–69	70+	Total
Frequency	3	19	39	47	55	61	47	67	27	23	388

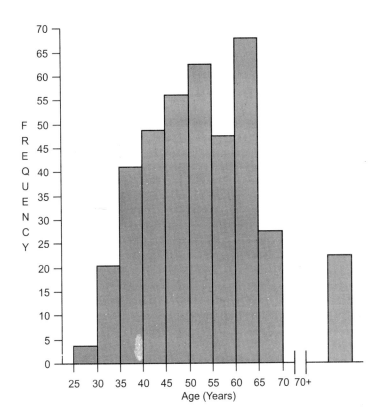

Fig. 3.5: Histogram of the age distribution of uterine cervical cancer, Barshi 1990–96 [Drawn from the data of Table 3.8]

3.2.4. Frequency Polygon

We have seen how a frequency distribution of a quantitative variable is represented in a diagram. What if we wish to compare two frequency distributions? Superimposing one histogram on another will produce a diagram which will be of little help in understanding the similarities and dissimilarities between the two distributions. To facilitate comparison, another diagram called the frequency polygon is used. This diagram is made by simply joining the mid-points of the tops of all the bars with a straight line, and then removing the bars. It is fairly easy to draw, and useful in comparing two or more distributions, as each can be represented on the same graph.

As an example of the frequency polygon, consider the incidence data of cancer of the female breast in two cities, Mumbai and Delhi. The data (ICMR[3] 2001) are shown in Table 3.9.

Table 3.9: Age distribution of new female breast cancers in Mumbai and Delhi 1990-96

Age (years)	Frequency	
	Mumbai	*Delhi*
20 – 24	35	48
25 – 29	146	168
30 – 34	334	358
35 – 39	631	635
40 – 44	844	803
45 – 49	909	773
50 – 54	939	845
55 – 59	772	617
60 – 64	766	587
65 – 69	510	302
70 – 74	392	162
75 – 79	403	186

From the frequency polygon (Fig. 3.6), it can be seen that the age pattern in the number of incident cases is similar in Mumbai and Delhi. In both the cities, the number of breast cancer cases is almost the same up to the age of 45 years and thereafter more cases are seen in Mumbai as compared to Delhi. These differences are absolute differences in the number of cases and need not reflect differences in the incidence rates, as we have not considered the denominators, i.e., the number of women at risk at different ages in both the cities. We can also draw a histogram or frequency polygon based on the rates instead of the absolute number of cases.

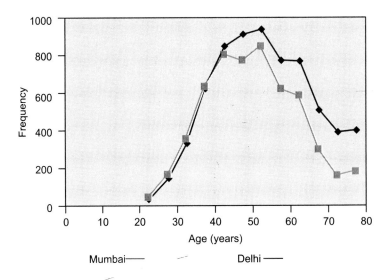

Fig. 3.6: Frequency polygon showing the age distribution of incident female breast cancer cases, Mumbai and Delhi, 1990-96 [Drawn from data of Table 3.9]

3.2.5. Line Graphs or Line Diagrams

Data having some order such as the year-wise immunization coverage or age-wise incidence of a disease can be represented by a line diagram. Technically speaking, we could also present this type of data using simple bar diagrams, erecting one bar for the frequency at each time-point of observation. Since the data are on a continuum in some respect, we could join the observations by a line so that the trend in the frequencies can be easily seen.

As an example of a line diagram, data on the age-specific incidence of cancers in the city of Delhi during 1990-96 (ICMR[3] 2001) are shown in the Table 3.10.

Table 3.10: Age-specific incidence of cancer among males, Delhi 1990–96

Age (years)	Number of cases	Mid-period population	Annual incidence rate (per 100, 000)
0 – 9	1200	11 40 275	15.0
10 – 19	1094	10 27 844	15.2
20 – 29	1440	10 33 609	19.9
30 – 39	2233	8 23 825	38.7
40 – 49	3949	5 06 396	111.4
50 – 59	6225	2 85 816	311.1
60 – 69	5949	1 57 804	538.6
70 – 80	4128	84 200	700.4
Total	26218	50 59 769	74.0

Figure 3.7 shows the line diagram of the average annual incidence rates of cancers among males in the city of Delhi during 1990-96. As can be seen from the line diagram, the incidence is very low and almost constant till the age of 30 years and then gradually rises with increasing age.

One advantage of these diagrams is that we can interpolate to guess the incidence rate for any given age, within the observed range. For example, if one wants to know the probable incidence at the age of say, exactly 50 years, a vertical line can be extended from the horizontal axis at 50 years to the vertical axis where it intersects the line diagram. The point on where this line intersects the Y axis will give us an idea of the incidence at exactly 50 years of age.

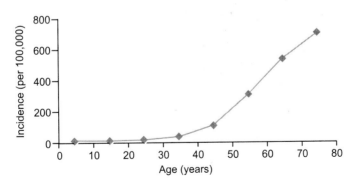

Fig. 3.7: Annual age-specific incidence (per 100 000) of cancer among males, Delhi, 1990-96 [Drawn from data from table 3.10]

3.2.6. Stem and Leaf Plot

Another useful way of representing data is by a stem and leaf display, which is a different version of the histogram. The advantages of this diagram are that it can be drawn using the raw data, it depicts the general shape or structure of the frequency distribution and reveals whether there is any digital preference in the data.

It is also less prone to errors compared to the tally mark system used for the preparation of a frequency distribution. We will explain the construction of a stem and leaf plot using the systolic BP data shown in Table 3.3.

The first digit (from the left) or the first two digits in the value of each observation will form a row, called the 'stem' while the last (right-most) digit will form the 'leaf'. For example, the observation 99 has the stem 9 and the leaf 9. Similarly, the second observation of 110 has the stem 11 and the leaf 0. The leaves for each stem are shown in a row (Table 3.11 a). The leaves are arranged in ascending order within a stem (Table 3.11 b), so that we can easily count the number of observations taking specific values and also know whether there is any digital preference within the stem.

If the observations include decimals like 4.65, 8.90, etc., the stems will be 46 and 89, and the leaves will be 5 and 0, respectively.

Table 3.11a: Leaves for each stem from the data of systolic BP of 68 patients

Stem	Leaf
9	9 6 0
10	6 9 2 8 4
11	0 0 8 0 6 6 8
12	8 2 2 5 9 4 5 0 8 6
13	2 0 5 9 0 6 6 2 6 8 9 1 4 0 6
14	4 0 8 3 6 5 8 9 7 2 9
15	6 9 0 6 4 4 2 5 8
16	0 8 0 4 6 2
17	6 4

Table 3.11 b: Stem and leaf (placed in ascending order) display for the distribution of systolic blood pressure

Stem	Leaf	Cumulative frequencies
9	069	3
10	24689	8
11	0006688	15
12	0224556889	25
13	000122456666899	40
14	02345678899	51
15	024456689	60
16	002468	66
17	46	68

From Table 3.11 b we can see that the stem 13 has the maximum number of leaves, implying that the maximum number of observations are between 130 and 139 (15 to be precise) and of these 15 observations, three are 130, one 131, two 132, one each 134 and 135, four 136, one 138 and two 139. The distribution is almost bell-shaped. Tukey[4] (1977) gives more details and other variants of this plot.

3.2.7. Ogive Curves and Cumulative Frequency Polygons

If the frequency polygon is drawn for the cumulative rather than the absolute frequencies of class intervals, it is called a cumulative polygon. Further, if the points of the cumulative polygon are joined with a smooth curve instead of straight lines, it is called an ogive curve. Though they do not convey the general shape of the distribution, the advantage of the cumulative polygon or ogive curve lies in that they enable us to answer queries related to the frequency distribution of the variable under consideration.

Consider the systolic BP data shown in Table 3.4. The two ogive curves for these data, namely, the one indicating the frequency of observations less than or equal to a particular limit and the second indicating the frequency of observations more than or equal to a particular limit, are shown in Fig. 3.8. The ogive curve indicating the cumulative frequency less than a particular limit is sigmoid-shaped. As mentioned earlier, for any given value on the horizontal axis, we can determine the frequency of observations that are less than or equal to that value by extending a line vertically from that given value on the X-axis to the ogive curve and then extending it to the vertical axis from the point where the vertical line intersects the ogive curve. From Fig. 3.8, we can guess that there are about 62 observations whose value is less than or equal to 160 mmHg, which incidentally is equal to the actual observations satisfying this condition, as can be verified from the raw data given in Table 3.3.

Similarly, we can have cumulative frequencies beginning from the bottom of the table, and these frequencies convey the number of observations falling above the lower limit of the respective class intervals. The ogive curve drawn from these cumulative frequencies will also be sigmoid-shaped, starting with the total frequency with all the observations falling above the lower limit of the first class interval, and of a smaller and smaller number above the lower limit of subsequent class intervals. This diagram is helpful in determining the number of observations above a specific value, within the range of the observed data. From Fig. 3.8, we can see that there are about 56 observations whose value is above 120 mmHg.

When we draw both the ogive curves on the same graph sheet, they intersect at some point and the corresponding value of the variable as indicated on the X-axis will be the middle position of the entire data, when arranged in ascending or descending order. This value is referred to as the positional average or median of the distribution. Note that both the ogive curves intersect at about 135 mmHg. We will discuss this intersection point further in the **section on median value** (3.3.2).

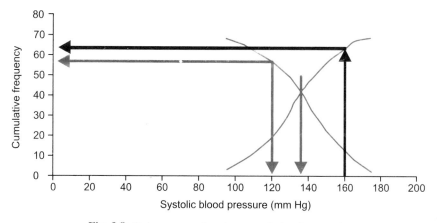

Fig. 3.8: Ogive curves showing cumulative frequencies

3.2.8. General Comments on Graphs and Diagrams

The main purpose of any diagrammatic presentation of data is to convey information quickly. This very purpose is defeated if the diagrammatic presentation is poor or does not clearly convey the intended message(s). Crowded graphs or those conveying too much information in one diagram should be avoided. Every diagram should be suitably labeled with an appropriate title, so that it can stand on its own.

In addition, one should be circumspect in interpreting various diagrams as they are prone to some errors and may mislead the viewer. We shall mention some common pitfalls of diagrams that one should guard against.

- The most common misleading graphs or diagrams are those with the Y-axis starting from non-zero values. Since the vertical scale starts with a non-zero value, it may introduce an artificially apparent increase or decrease in the frequencies, compared to the gradual rise or decrease in the data. In other words, even small changes in the frequencies are inflated and shown as substantial changes in the diagram. The effect of this phenomenon is more dramatic if, in addition, the X-axis is also compressed and starts with a non-zero value.

- Diagrams with equal intervals on the horizontal axis for unequal data intervals are not appropriate. Similarly, for unequal data intervals, showing the corresponding frequencies as observed on the vertical axis is also not appropriate. As mentioned earlier, we need to convert the frequency of intervals of unequal width to a frequency for the standard width and then plot the converted frequency on the vertical axis.

- Sometimes, due to enthusiasm and with easy access to powerful personal computers, there is a tendency to decorate diagrams. In this process, the accuracy of the diagram may be compromised. For example, a pie diagram, though it looks simple, may convey numbers accurately. But the same may not be true if we add three-dimensional features to it. Similarly, in a simple bar diagram, the bars can be replaced by columns of pictures to make the diagram more appealing. These diagrams, called pictograms, can be misleading as it might seem that the volume represents the frequency when in fact the height of the bar of pictures represents the frequency.

We should remember that all diagrams are only approximate, as exact numerical accuracy cannot be translated completely into the diagram. Further, diagrams only supplement the tabular presentation of data and are not substitutes for tables.

3.2.8.1. Shape of the frequency distribution

The histogram and stem and leaf plot give an idea about the shape of the frequency distribution. For example, the data of Tables 3.4 or Table 3.11 indicate that the distribution of systolic BP values has a symmetric shape, with the majority of observations concentrated around a central or middle point, and fewer and fewer observations as we move away from the central point in either direction. Further, the deviations from the central point are approximately equal in both the directions. A distribution with these properties is called a symmetric distribution. Most often, quantitative variables such as height, weight, blood sugar, etc., follow this pattern. The central point we refer to is called the most frequent value or mode of the distribution. In our example, we see that maximum (15) observations are between 130 and 140, and so the interval 130-140 is the most frequent interval. As we move towards the left from the most frequent interval, the frequencies are 10, 7, 5 and 3. Similarly, as we move towards the right, the frequencies are 11, 9, 6 and 2.

In the example discussed above, the maximum frequency occurred in only one place in the entire distribution and the other frequencies tapered off in both directions. That is, there is only one mode and so the distribution is called unimodal. In some situations, like the one seen in Fig. 3.5, there can be more than one mode. In such cases, we have two modes or the distribution is **bimodal**, one in the interval 50-55 years and the other in the interval 60-65 years. Before we conclude that the frequency distribution is bimodal, it is necessary to distinguish whether it is a real phenomenon or a result of the small number of observations that have been studied. Most often, distributions are unimodal.

In some situations, the frequency distribution may be unimodal, but may not be symmetric. Such distributions are called asymmetric or skewed distributions. Fig. 3.9a shows a frequency distribution which is unimodal but asymmetric. It has a long tail towards the right of the most frequent group. Fig. 3.9b, on the other hand, has a long tail towards the left of the most frequent group. Both these distributions are unimodal and asymmetric, but the asymmetricity is in different directions. Distributions with a long right-sided tail are called positively skewed and those with a long tail towards the left are called negatively skewed. If a distribution is perfectly symmetric and unimodal, it will be bell-shaped and its skewness is said to be zero.

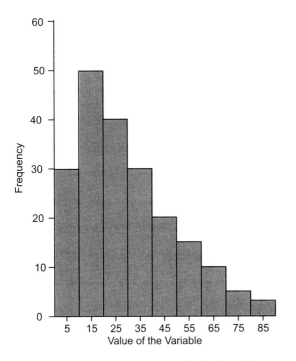

Fig. 3.9a: Histogram showing a positively skewed distribution

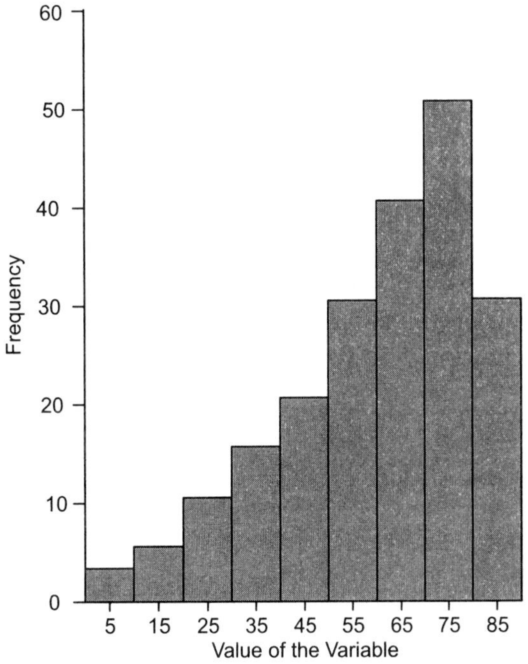

Fig. 3.9b: Histogram showing a negatively skewed distribution

3.3. Measures of Central Tendency and Location

It has already been mentioned the main purpose of the statistical treatment of any data is to summarize and describe the data meaningfully and adequately. Sets of observations cannot be meaningfully described by the values of all the individual measurements. Thus, we have seen how to summarize a set of observations or measurements by using frequency tables. Though we could reduce the mass of numbers into a few meaningful categories, frequency distributions do not give us a single index or one value which is typical for the entire data set. Such measures are necessary for summarizing or for comparison with other similar data sets. Appropriate summary indices must, therefore, be obtained. Certain summary indices tell about the centre or middle of the data set around which the other observations are lying and some others indicate different locations in the data set, which divide the total data into certain proportions. For example, we might summarize the data by saying 50% of the observations are above a certain value (location) and 50% below that. These indices are called measures of central tendency and location, and we shall discuss them in this section.

3.3.1. Arithmetic Mean

The arithmetic mean, or simply the mean, is the average value of the variable and is obtained by taking the sum of all the observations and dividing it by the number of observations. For example, if the gestational ages (weeks) of 10 newborns are 36, 38, 40, 37, 42, 35, 39, 32, 40 and 41, the mean gestational age of these 10 newborns will be the sum of the 10 observations divided by 10. Thus, the mean will be $380 \div 10 = 38$ weeks.

To indicate this mathematically, we introduce some algebraic notation. The individual observations are denoted by,

$$X_1, X_2, X_3, ..., X_i, ..., X_n \qquad \qquad 3.1$$

We have n observations and the first one is denoted as X_1, the ith one as X_i and the nth one as X_n. In the example above, we have $n = 10$ observations and the first observation $X_1 = 36$, second observation $X_2 = 38$ and the last observation $X_{10} = 41$. The sum of all these observations is denoted as

$$\sum_{i=1}^{n} X_i \qquad \qquad 3.2$$

The symbol Σ is the upper case Greek letter sigma and it denotes summation. We read the above notation as the summation of X_i values, i ranging from 1 to n. The mean of the n values of X is denoted by $\bar{X}$. Therefore,

$$\text{Mean } \bar{X} = \frac{1}{n}\left[\sum_{i=1}^{n} X_i\right] \qquad \qquad 3.3$$

Using the raw data, as seen in the example of gestational ages given above, we can compute the average or mean by simply summing up all the values and dividing the sum by the number of observations. This is quite easy with small data sets but will not be as easy with a large number of observations. In such situations, we have the frequency distributions or grouped data to work with. The computation of the mean for grouped data is also based on the same principle as for ungrouped or raw data.

We will explain the calculation of the mean for grouped data using the systolic BP data shown in Table 3.4. The table shows the frequencies for some well defined ranges of the observed variable. We assume that the frequency in any class interval is uniformly distributed within that interval and so all the values within that interval can be represented by the mid-point of that interval.

Table 3.12a: Calculation of mean for grouped data

Systolic BP (mmHg)	Frequency f_i	Mid-point of interval X_i	$f_i * X_i$	$X_i(x_i - 90)$	$f_i * X_i'$
90 – 100	3	95	3 * 95 = 285	95 – 90 = 5	15
100 – 110	5	105	5 * 105 = 525	105 – 90 = 15	75
110 – 120	7	115	7*115 = 805	25	175
120 – 130	10	125	10*125 = 1250	35	350
130 – 140	15	135	15*135 = 2025	45	675
140 – 150	11	145	11*145 = 1595	55	605
150 – 160	9	155	9*155 = 1395	65	585
160 – 170	6	165	6*165 = 990	75	450
170 – 180	2	175	2*175 = 350	85	170
Total	68		9220		3100

To get the mid-point of the interval, simply add the lower limit and the upper limit of any interval, and divide the sum by two. This value is representative of all the observations falling in that specific interval, assuming that the observations in the interval are uniformly distributed. Most often, this condition is met, unless there is some sort of serious digital preference and, hence, we can safely assume that the mid-value of the interval is representative of all the observations lying in the interval. Once we have the representative value within each interval (denoted as X_i in Table 3.12a), multiplying the mid-point of the interval with the respective frequency (shown as f_i in Table 3.12a), we get the sum of all the observations within that interval. Adding up the sums for each interval will give us the total for all the observations in the sample. Dividing the total by the total frequency or the number of observations will give us the mean for the frequency distribution. Thus, the mean systolic BP in the example is $9220 \div 68 = 135.6$ mmHg.

The notation for the mean value in grouped data will be

$$\text{Mean} \quad \overline{X} = \frac{1}{n}\left[\sum_{i=1}^{k} f_i X_i\right] = 9220 \div 68 = 135.6 \text{ mmHg} \tag{3.4}$$

Note that the summation here is over the k intervals and not over the n observations as was the case with raw data. The denominator in both cases is n, i.e., the total number of observations.

To avoid the manipulation of big numbers, we can subtract a constant, say 90, from the mid-point of each interval and proceed in exactly the same way. The resultant mean will be the mean of all the observations, each subtracted by 90. We add back this constant value to the obtained value of the mean to get the mean of the original observations in the sample. We can see from our example that both yield exactly the same mean values.

$$\overline{X} = 90 + \frac{1}{n}\left[\sum_{i=1}^{k} f_i X_i{}'\right] = 90 + (3100 / 68) = 90 + 45.6 = 135.6 \text{ mm/Hg}$$

Nowadays, with the advent of computers, one need not bother about the magnitude of the numbers one has to work with.

Clearly, the sample mean cannot be computed for nominal scale data or for non-numerical ordinal scale data. Further, for the sake of discussion, if we add up all the values of systolic BP of all 68 patients (Table 3.3) and divide the sum by 68, we get a mean value $9200 \div 68 = 135.3$ mmHg. Notice that the mean estimated earlier from the grouped data is fairly close to the exact mean of the sample, the difference being 0.3 mm/Hg. This difference between the exact estimate and that from grouped data is the price we pay for simplifying the data structure or arranging the raw data into a frequency distribution. The greater the number of intervals in the frequency distribution, the closer will be the mean value calculated from the raw data and the frequency distribution.

In the example of the gestational ages of newborns, if the first observation was 26 weeks instead of 36 weeks, the mean of the sample will be $370 \div 10 = 37$ weeks. Notice that the extreme observation of 26 weeks has pulled the mean towards it. Thus, in general, the sample mean is sensitive to extreme values in the data set. When some extreme observations are present, one must check whether there is any recording or measuring error. Another limitation with mean is that we cannot compute it from a grouped distribution with open-ended class intervals. In the frequency distribution of systolic BP, if the last interval was ≥ 170 mmHg instead of 170–180 mmHg, it would not have been possible for us to guess the representative value in this open-ended interval. The mid-value for this interval will depend on the upper limit of the interval, which is not given in the frequency distribution. However, the advantages of arithmetic mean include the fact that it uses all the observations and is amenable to further mathematical treatment. We can also easily guess the behaviour of the sample mean over repeated samples.

3.3.2. Median

Another way of summarizing a frequency distribution is by way of quantiles, which are values of the variable that divide the distribution in such a way that there is a given percentage or proportion of observations below them and the remaining above. Median is a quantile and it is the central value of the distribution. Half the values will lie below the median and half above it. In case of a raw data set, the median will be the middle value after arranging the observations in ascending or descending order. Since it is the middle-most value by position, the median is also referred to as the positional average.

Consider the ungrouped data on gestational ages. The 10 observations arranged in ascending order will be:

$$\underbrace{32,35,36,37,\ 38,39}_{\text{4 observations}}\quad\underbrace{40,41,42}_{\text{4 observations}}$$

If we had an odd number of observations, identifying the middle most value would have been simple. Since we have an even number of observations (10) in this case, there will be two middle-most observations. Technically speaking, any value between these two middle-most observations will be the median. For convenience, the average of the two middle-most observations is taken as the median. Thus, in this example, 38.5 weeks is the median gestational age of the 10 newborns. It is easy to verify that half the total observations are below the median and hence, half will be above it. Thus, if we have n observations arranged in ascending order, the median M will be:

1. Equal to the value of the observation occupying the position number $(n+1)\div 2$, if n is odd;
2. Equal to the average of the observations occupying the position numbers $n\div 2$ and $(n\div 2)+1$, if n is even.

We can obtain any quantile in a similar fashion. If we want a quantile such that one-fourth or 25% of the observations lie below it, pick the observation number $n/4$ when all the observations are arranged in an ascending order. Quantiles that divide the total distribution into four equal parts are called quartiles. There will be three quartiles; 25% of observations will lie below the first quartile, 25% will fall between the first and second quartiles, and another quarter will lie between the second and third quartile. The remaining 25% of observations will lie above the third quartile. In other words 25% of the observations fall below the first quartile, 50% below the second quartile (which is the median) and 75% lie below the third quartile. Similarly, the nine deciles that divide the total distribution into 10 equal parts and the 99 percentiles that divide it into 100 equal parts or any other quantiles can be defined and obtained.

For a grouped data given as a frequency distribution, the computation of the value of the median follows the same logic as with raw data. The frequency distribution in itself is a sort of arrangement of observations in the ascending order, the first interval containing the smallest set of observations and the last interval containing the largest set of observations within the sample data. We use the cumulative frequency in each interval to locate the probable interval where the middle point of the data set lies and this interval is called the median class interval. Considering the distance between the middle point of the data (observation number $n\div 2$) and the cumulative frequency of the interval before the median class interval, we interpolate the value of the variable within the median interval proportionately to arrive at the median value of the distribution.

Again, we consider the grouped data of systolic BP shown in Table 3.4. We have a total of 68 observations and, therefore, the middle-most observation will be the observation number $n\div 2$ or the 34th observation. In a frequency distribution, we are not much concerned whether the total number of observations is even or odd, as the total frequency in a frequency distribution is generally not too small, and so it does not matter practically. As mentioned earlier, the frequency distribution in itself is an arrangement of observations in ascending order. Looking at the cumulative frequencies of each interval, we note that there are 25 observations with a BP value less than 130 mmHg, while 40 observations are below 140 mmHg (Table 3.12b). Therefore, the 34th or middle-most observation required falls in the interval 130–140 mmHg. In other words, 130–140 mmHg is our median class interval.

Table 3.12b: Calculation of median for grouped data

Systolic BP (mmHg)	Frequency f_i	Cumulative frequency
90 – 100	3	3
100 – 110	5	8
110 – 120	7	15
120 – 130	10	25
130 – 140	15	40
140 – 150	11	51
150 – 160	9	60
160 – 170	6	66
170 – 180	2	68
Total	68	

The cumulative frequency up to the class interval preceding the median class interval is 25, and the difference between this cumulative frequency and the mid-point we are looking for is $(n \div 2) - 25 = 9$. There are 15 observations in the median interval spread from 140 to 150mmHg and we have to find where the 9th observation in this interval (which will be the middle-most observation in the total distribution) falls.

The width of the median class interval is 10 mm and in this width, 15 observations lie uniformly distributed. For each observation in this interval, the width will be $10 \div 15$ mmHg and for 9 observations, it will be $10 \div 15 \times 9$ or 6 mmHg of width. We add this 6 mmHg to the lower limit of the median class interval to get the median or mid-point of the data set. The above concept can be translated into a notation as,

$$\text{Median } M = L_M + \left[\left(\frac{W}{f} \right) \times \left(\frac{n}{2} - CF \right) \right]$$

3.5

where L_M is the lower limit of the median class, n is the total frequency or number of observations, CF is the cumulative frequency of the interval before the median class interval, f and W are the frequency and width, respectively, of the median class interval and n is the total frequency. In the example we discussed, $L = 130$, $n \div 2 = 34$, $CF = 25$, $f = 15$ and $W = 10$. Using these values in the equation given above, we get the median value 136 mmHg, which is also the median value based on the raw data. As shown for the arithmetic mean, generally the median computed from the frequency distribution will also be quite close to the one computed from raw data.

The median for a frequency distribution can be obtained graphically as can be recalled from the discussion on ogive curves. When we draw two ogive curves based on two types of cumulative frequencies for the same frequency distribution, the abscissa or the point on the X-axis corresponding to the point where the two ogive curves intersect indicates the median of the distribution. Recall Fig. 3.8, wherein we saw that the two ogive curves drawn on the systolic BP data of Table 3.4 intersect at about 135 mmHg. The value of the median calculated by the equation just defined is very close to that obtained graphically.

The equation 3.5 above for calculating the median can also be used to obtain any quantile. If we wish to find the first quartile that divides the distribution into two parts of 25% and 75% of the observations, we replace $n \div 2$ by $n \div 4$ in the equation. The median class will be replaced by the first quartile class and accordingly, the cumulative frequency up to the interval before the quartile class, its frequency and width will be used in the calculation. Similarly, a third quartile or a decile or a percentile can be obtained.

Note that median, like arithmetic mean, can be computed for data on a ratio or interval scale. In addition, the median may also be determined for ordinal scale data. For example, if 20 oral cancer patients are classified according to the stage of the disease at diagnosis, with 3 diagnosed to be in stage I, 4 in stage II, 7 in stage III and the remaining 6 in stage IV, the median stage of the disease is stage III.

The median is an intuitively appealing estimate of the central tendency of a frequency distribution, as it is easy to compute and comprehend. It is not influenced by extreme observations. As an example, in the raw data of 10 gestational ages discussed in the section on arithmetic mean (3.3.1), the median will remain the same whether the smallest observation is 32 or 22 weeks. The median is also a fairly stable estimate of the central tendency, as it does not vary much in repeated sampling from the same population. However, the median has certain disadvantages or limitations. It does not take into account the precise magnitude of most of the observations. In other words, it does not utilize all the information available in the sample and, therefore, it is usually less efficient than the arithmetic mean. When we pool two groups of observations, the median for the pooled data cannot be expressed in terms of the two medians of the component groups that have been pooled. The median is also not amenable to further mathematical manipulation and so is not much used in more analytical work as compared to the arithmetic mean.

3.3.3. Mode

Another index for the central tendency is mode, defined as the most frequently occurring value of the variable. Because the value of the variable is the most frequent one, it is a natural choice to represent the typical value of the distribution. In a raw data set, it is very straightforward to identify the mode. In the data of the gestational ages (weeks) of 10 newborns discussed earlier, the 10 observations are 36, 38, 40, 37, 42, 35, 39, 32, 40 and 41. We notice that there are two observations with a gestation age of 40 weeks, with the rest of the values occurring only once. Thus, the mode of the sample data is 40 weeks. If two distinct values occur the same number of times, then there will be two modes. If no value is repeated, no mode is defined.

In a grouped data, the mode of the distribution is obtained from the following expression:

$$\text{Mode} = L_{Md} + \left[\left(\frac{d_1}{d_1 + d_2} \right) \times W \right] \qquad 3.6$$

where L_{Md} is the lower limit of the modal class, i.e., the interval for which the frequency is maximum, d_1 is the difference between the frequencies of the modal class interval and the preceding class interval, d_2 is the difference between the frequencies of the modal and succeeding class intervals, and W is the width of the modal class interval. Let us work out the mode for the systolic BP data of Table 3.3, reproduced in Table 3.13

Table 3.13: Calculation of mode for a grouped data

Systolic BP (mmHg)	Frequency f_i
90 – 100	3
100 – 110	5
110 – 120	7
120 – 130	10
130 – 140	15
140 – 150	11
150 – 160	9
160 – 170	6
170 – 180	2
Total	68

We see that the maximum frequency is in the interval 130–139 mmHg. Therefore, this is the modal class interval and L_M is 130. The difference between the frequencies of the modal class and the preceding class, i.e., d_1 is 15–10 = 5. Similarly, d_2, the difference between the frequencies of the modal class interval and the succeeding class interval, is 4. The width W of the modal class is 10.

Substituting these values in the equation 3.6, we get,

$$\text{Mode} = 130 + \left[\left(\frac{5}{9}\right) \times 10\right] = 130 + 5.6 = 135.6 \text{ mmHg}.$$

The mode is highly dependent on the way the class intervals have been formed while preparing the frequency distribution. For instance, in the example above, if we had an interval 140–160 mmHg with a frequency of 20, the mode for the distribution would have been obtained as 145.3 mmHg, while the mean and median would have had little effect. Thus, one should be cautious while interpreting the mode of the distribution when there are intervals of unequal width in a frequency distribution. Also, the mode is not much used in analytical work as fluctuations in the frequencies of observations when the sample size is small can lead to spurious modes.

3.3.4. Geometric Mean

In certain situations, we come across a variable that can take only non-zero, positive values that vary over a wide range. Because of this, the distribution of the variable will be skewed and variation will be high. Therefore, the arithmetic mean would not be an appropriate measure to convey the central tendency of the data. We can overcome this problem by transforming the observations into logarithms (log) and calculating the arithmetic mean of these transformed values. Logarithmic transformation reduces the skewness in the data distribution and makes it closer to the normal distribution. On a log scale, the distance between any pair of observations will be the same if their ratios are equal and not the differences. Thus, the distance between 10 and 100 will be same as that between 1 and 10 or 2 and 20, though the differences between these pairs are not same.

This measure of the central tendency is called the geometric mean (GM) and is defined as the arithmetic mean of the values taken on a log scale. The GM can also be interpreted as the nth root of the product of n observations. For example, if 20, 25 and 15 are weights (kg) of 3 children, the GM of these 3 observations will be the cube root of the product $20 \times 25 \times 15$.

$$\text{GM} = (20 \times 25 \times 15)^{1/3} = (7500)^{1/3} = 19.57 \text{ kg}$$

Alternatively, the same value can be obtained as the arithmetic mean of the 3 observations taken on the log scale. We have log 20 = 1.3010, log 25 = 1.3979 and log 15 = 1.1761, the sum of which will be 3.8750. Dividing the sum by 3, we get 1.2917. Since we have worked on log values, we use antilog to get back into the original units. The antilog of 1.2917 is 19.57 kg and so the GM of the observations is 19.57 kg. Note here that we have to take a sufficient number of decimal places to be accurate.

For grouped data, the calculation of GM is similar to that of arithmetic mean, except that the mid-point of class intervals x_i will be replaced by the log values of x_i. After calculating the mean of log values, we take the antilog of the mean of log values to get the mean in the observed units.

$$GM = antilog \left[\frac{1}{n} \sum_{i=1}^{k} f_i \log X_i \right]$$

3.7

GM is used more in microbiological or serological research. One major limitation of GM is that it cannot be obtained if any observation is zero or negative, as the log values of such observations are not defined.

As an example, let us consider the CD4 counts in subjects who are at high risk for HIV infection. The data and the details of calculation are shown in Table 3.14.

Table 3.14: Distribution of CD4 counts in high-risk persons screened for HIV

CD4 count	Number of subjects (f_i)	Midpoint (X_i)	log (X_i)	f_i *log(X_i)
0 – 99	42	50	1.6990	71.3580
100 – 199	38	150	2.1761	82.6918
200 – 299	38	250	2.3979	91.1202
300 – 399	45	350	2.5441	114.4845
400 – 499	31	450	2.6532	82.2492
500 – 599	30	550	2.7404	82.2120
600 – 699	22	650	2.8129	61.8838
700 – 799	21	750	2.8751	60.3771
800 – 899	10	850	2.9294	29.2940
900 – 999	17	950	2.9777	50.6209
1000 – 1099	11	1050	3.0212	33.2332
1100 – 1199	10	1150	3.0607	30.6070
1200 – 1299	5	1250	3.0969	15.4845
Total	320			805.6162

*Multiplication symbol

$$GM = antilog \left[\frac{1}{n} \sum_{i=1}^{k} f_i \log X_i \right]$$

= antilog [805.6162/320]

= 329.3

Had we ignored the skewed nature of the data and computed the arithmetic mean, the central representative value would be 449.1.

3.3.5. Harmonic Mean

Another measure of the central tendency of a frequency distribution, called harmonic mean (HM), is based on the reciprocals of the actual observations. It is defined as the reciprocal of the arithmetic mean of the reciprocals of the observations. Thus, when we have the observations $X_1, X_2, X_3, ..., X_i, ..., X_n$, HM will be

$$HM = \left[\frac{1}{\left(\frac{1}{n} \sum_{i=1}^{n} \frac{1}{X_i} \right)} \right] \qquad 3.8$$

The calculation of HM for grouped data involves taking the reciprocals of the mid-points of the class intervals and proceeding as though we are calculating the mean of the reciprocals of the observations. After the mean of the reciprocals is obtained, take the reciprocal of the mean of the reciprocals to obtain the HM of the grouped data.

$$HM = \left[\frac{1}{\left(\frac{1}{n} \sum_{i=1}^{K} f_i \frac{1}{X_i} \right)} \right] \qquad 3.9$$

The use of HM is appropriate when the reciprocals of the observations seem more useful for determining the central tendency. HM may be used to compute the average of rates, say, typing speed (number of words per minute), speed of the car (kilometers per hour), etc. It is used very rarely in medical or biological applications.

3.3.6. General Comments on the Measures of Central Tendency

We have discussed five types of measures of central tendency in the preceding sections, and each has its own advantages and disadvantages. The arithmetic mean is the most often used measure of central tendency followed by median and mode. The other two measures are not used much.

If the distribution is symmetric or even approximately symmetric, and is also unimodal, then the mean, median and mode are the same, and any of these three measures conveys the central tendency equally well. Note that if the distribution is symmetric and bimodal, this will not be the case. In such a distribution, the median and mean may be the same and the two modes are different from the mean and median, as in the hypothetical distribution shown in Fig. 3.10.

What if the distribution is asymmetric? Recall the discussion in the section on the shape of frequency distributions (3.2.8.1). In a positively skewed distribution, maximum observations lie on the left side of the distribution and a few on the right side, forming a longer tail on the right side. Therefore, the mode is towards the left side of the distribution. We also saw earlier that the arithmetic mean is always pulled towards the extreme observations. So if the distribution is positively skewed, the mean will be pulled towards the right side. The median, the middle value of the distribution, will fall in between. In contrast, in a negatively skewed distribution, the mode will be more (lies on the right side), the mean will be least of the three (lies on the left side) and, again, the median falls in between.

Given the values of any two of these three measures of central tendency, we should be able to guess the likely shape of the distribution. For example, if in a distribution, the mean is 25 and the mode 30, we can guess that the distribution is negatively skewed or the left tail is longer than the right tail with the median lying between 25 and 30 units. Similarly, if the median is 40 and the mode 35, such a distribution is positively skewed with a longer right tail and the mean is likely to be more than 40 units.

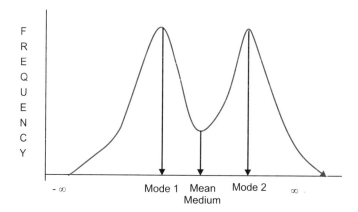

Fig. 3.10: A hypothetical bimodal and symmetric distribution

Having discussed the various measures of central tendency, we might ask ourselves which measure is appropriate for a given set of data. The answer will depend on the nature of the distribution of the observations and also on what we want the data to convey. There are no hard and fast rules, but some broad guidelines can be suggested.

When the distribution is symmetric or approximately symmetric, the mean, median and mode coincide, and any of these three values will suffice .If the distribution is asymmetric or skewed, the mean is generally not appropriate for conveying the central tendency. As we have seen, if the skewness is positive, the mean will be the highest of the three measures (mean, median and mode) and if the skewness is negative, the mean will be the least of the three. In such situations, the median is preferable for conveying the middle point of the distribution or the mode is preferable for conveying the most frequent observation. When there are certain observations that are different from the rest or the homogeneity of the data is doubtful, the median will be a better measure for conveying the middle or central value and the mode will be appropriate for conveying the typical observation. When the relative standing of individual observations is of interest, the median is the better-suited measure.

Because of the advantages and disadvantages of each of the measures, it may be advisable to use two or three measures so that the reader can better understand the distribution of the observations.

3.4. Measures of Dispersion

In any investigation, the mass of raw data is unwieldy and difficult to comprehend and draw any conclusions. Therefore, there is a need to reduce the data into some meaningful indices that indicate the typicalness or central tendency of the total data. The entire data are represented by one value, which is the 'typical' value of the population. We have seen different measures of central tendency in earlier sections. Though these measures are very useful, they do not convey the total picture of the mass of data. Consider the following three sets of data:

Data set	Observations	Mean
A	1, 4, 7	4
B	4, 4, 4	4
C	3, 4, 5	4

In all the data sets, mean is 4. But, while there is no variation in Data set B, variation in Data set C is small and that in Data set A is high.

Take the example of intraocular pressure (IOP) measurements (mm) of glaucoma patients taken in two ophthalmic clinics, as shown in Fig. 3.11.

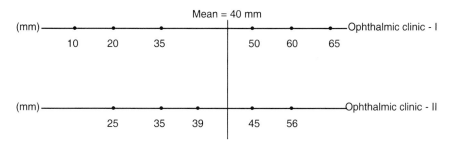

Fig. 3.11: Two sets of observations of intraocular pressure

Though the average IOP (central tendency) is the same in both sets of patients, they vary differently around the central value of 40 mm. In the first set, the values are more spread than in the second set. Such information, which tells us how dense or compact the data are, is not conveyed by the measures of central tendency. In other words, the measures of central tendency alone cannot summarize the data. Other measures that indicate the spread of the data points or how they vary are also needed. These measures are called the measures of dispersion. Terms such as deviation, spread, scatter and variability are also used synonymously with dispersion.

The entire concept of statistics revolves around variation. If there is no variation and all individuals are alike, there is no need for any sample and the observation of any one subject will tell us everything about the phenomenon being studied. Health workers need to classify individuals as healthy or sick, needing treatment or not, etc., based on the 'normal' values of certain clinical, laboratory and other measurements. The word 'normal' here is a statistical concept and depends on the distribution of the characteristic in the population. Also, since variation in any phenomenon is inherent, statistical techniques help us to explain the variation in one phenomenon due to other factors. Thus, understanding of dispersion or variation is essential for understanding, using and interpreting the concept of 'normal' values. There are many indices on the dispersion of data. We shall present them in the next section.

3.4.1. Range

One of the simplest measures that indicate the dispersion of data is the range. It is defined as the difference between the lowest and highest values in the data. For the data on gestational ages discussed in the section on arithmetic mean (3.3.1), the range is 32 weeks to 42 weeks. Note that we should not subtract the lowest value from the highest and quote the range as 10 weeks, as it does not convey the values in the sample. If we take the difference and say, the range is 10 weeks, whether the sample values lie between 25 and 35 or 30 to 40 or 34 to 44 weeks, the range of all is 10 weeks. Therefore, the range should be presented as an interval with the lowest and highest observations in the sample. The narrower the range, the less is the variability in the data, and the wider the range, the more is the spread or scatter in the data.

Though the range is a simple and useful measure to indicate the spread or scatter in the data, its main drawback lies in the fact that it is dependent on the two extreme observations, which may vary from sample to sample. Further, the size of the sample also influences the range of the data. Larger samples will give rise to more extreme values as compared to smaller samples.

3.4.1.1. Interquartile range

As the name indicates, the interquartile range is defined as the difference between the lower and the upper quartiles of the data. We calculated different quantiles in the section on median (3.3.2). The upper quartile (or the third quartile) divides the distribution in such a way that 75% of the observations lie below and 25% above the value. Similarly, 25% will lie below the lower quartile or the first quartile and 75% will lie above it. Therefore, the interquartile range gives us the two limits of the distribution, between which the central or middle 50% of the observations lie. If these two quartiles are close, it implies that the middle-most 50% of the observations are very tightly placed and thus, the variation is small. The converse is indicated if they are widely apart.

Calculation of the interquartile range from the leaf and stem plot of systolic BP in Table 3.11b, which is reproduced here, will be as follows.

Table 3.11b: Stem and leaf display from the distribution of systolic BP (mmHg)

Stem	Leaf	Cumulative frequencies
9	0 6 9	3
10	2 4 6 8 9	8
11	0 0 0 6 6 8 8	15
12	0 2 2 4 5 5 6 8 8 9	25
13	0 0 0 1 2 2 4 5 6 6 6 6 8 9 9	40
14	0 2 3 4 5 6 7 8 8 9 9	51
15	0 2 4 4 5 6 6 8 9	60
16	0 0 2 4 6 8	66
17	4 6	68

Since the sample size is 68, the first and fourth quartiles are at the 17th and 51st position, i.e., 122 mmHg and 149 mmHg. Hence, the interquartile range is 122–149 mmHg.

To give another example of the calculation of interquartile range, we reproduce Table 3.12b, used earlier for obtaining the median.

Table 3.12b: Calculation of median for grouped data

Systolic BP (mmHg)	Frequency f_i	Cumulative frequency
90 – 100	3	3
100 – 110	5	8
110 – 120	7	15
120 – 130	10	25
130 – 140	15	40
140 – 150	11	51
150 – 160	9	60
160 – 170	6	66
170 – 180	2	68
Total	68	

$$\text{Lower quartile } Q_1 = L_{Q_1} + \left[\left(\frac{W}{f} \right) \times \left(\frac{n}{4} - CF \right) \right] \qquad 3.10$$

We calculate $n \div 4 = 17$, lower quartile class interval = 120–130 mmHg, $\therefore L_{QI} = 120$

CF, the cumulative frequency up to the lower quartile class = 15; *f*, the frequency of lower quartile class = 10; and *W*, the width of the lower quartile class = 10.

Substituting these values in the equation 3.10:

$$Q_1 = 120 + \left[\left(\frac{10}{10}\right) \times (17 - 15)\right] = 120 + 2 = 122 \text{ mmHg}$$

Similarly, the upper quartile $Q_3 = L_{Q_3} + \left[\left(\frac{W}{f}\right) \times \left(\frac{3n}{4} - CF\right)\right]$ 3.11

After substituting the relevant quantities in the equation 3.11, we get Q_3:

$$\text{Upper quartile } Q_3 = 140 + \left[\left(\frac{10}{11}\right) \times (51 - 40)\right] = 140 + 10 = 150 \text{ mmHg}$$

Therefore, the distribution of systolic BP values in our sample of 68 observations has an interquartile range from 122 to 150 mmHg. In other words, the middle-most 50% of the data lie in the interval 122–150 mm and 25% of the observations lie below 122 mmHg while the remaining 25% lie above 150 mmHg. This gives us an idea of the variability in the sample data.

The interquartile range is a useful descriptive measure of variability in the data and it is unaffected by the presence of extreme observations. It can also be computed if we have open-ended class intervals. However, it is quite variable from sample to sample and is also not amenable to further mathematical manipulations.

3.4.2. Mean Deviation

We have seen that the arithmetic mean is a measure of the central tendency and it provides the typical value of the observations in the sample. A measure of the variability in the data can be obtained as the average deviation of observations from the arithmetic mean. This is called mean deviation.

Let us consider the birth weight (g) of 10 newborns. The values are 2850, 2650, 2340, 1925, 2810, 2475, 3100, 2975, 2315 and 2480g.

The mean birth weight is (2850+2650+...+2315+2480), 10 = 25920 ÷ 10 = 2592 g. Now consider the deviation of each observation from the arithmetic mean. The deviations are 258, 58, –252, –667, 218, –117, 508, 383, –277 and –112. To find the average deviation, we have to sum up all these deviations and divide the sum by the number of observations. Notice that the sum of all positive deviations (observations more than the mean) is 1425 and so is the sum of negative deviations (observations less than the mean); therefore, the net sum is zero. This is the property of the arithmetic mean and the total deviation of observations from their mean is always zero. Thus, we cannot calculate the mean deviation, as it will always be zero.

To overcome this problem, it has been suggested that the sign of the deviation be ignored and the absolute deviations be taken. Thus, we have a total of 10 deviations equal to 1425+1425=2850 and the average deviation will be 285 g. This implies that, on an average, each observation is 285 g away from the central value of 2592 g. The less the value of mean deviation, the more closely are the data packed.

Algebraically, the mean deviation for an ungrouped data will be,

$$\text{Mean deviation} = \frac{1}{n} \sum_{i=1}^{n} \left| X_i - \overline{X} \right|,$$ 3.12

where $\left| X_i - \overline{X} \right|$ indicates the absolute difference between the *i*th observation and the arithmetic mean.

For grouped data, we have to calculate each deviation as the difference between the mid-point of the class interval and the arithmetic mean, weigh each deviation with the corresponding frequency of the interval and then sum up deviations in each of the k intervals. Dividing the total deviation by the total number of observations, we obtain the mean deviation for the grouped data. This can be shown in a notation as,

$$\text{Mean deviation} = \frac{1}{n} \sum_{i=1}^{k} f_i \left| X_i - \overline{X} \right| \qquad\qquad 3.13$$

As an example, we will use the frequency distribution of systolic BP shown in Table 3.13. The data are reproduced in Table 3.15.

Table 3.15: Calculation of the mean deviation of data of systolic BP

Systolic BP (mmHg)	Frequency f_i	Mid-point X_i	Deviation $|X_i - X|$	$f_i * |X_i - X|$
90 – 100	3	95	40.6	121.8
100 – 110	5	105	30.6	153.0
110 – 120	7	115	20.6	144.2
120 – 130	10	125	10.6	106.0
130 – 140	15	135	0.6	9.0
140 – 150	11	145	9.4	103.4
150 – 160	9	155	19.4	174.6
160 – 170	6	165	29.4	176.4
170 – 180	2	175	39.4	78.8
Total	68			1067.2

In the section on arithmetic mean (3.3.1) we calculated the arithmetic mean to be 135.6 mmHg. From the last column of Table 3.15, we get the total deviation to be 1067.2 mmHg. Thus, the average deviation or mean deviation will be $1067.2 \div 68 = 15.7$ mmHg.

Mean deviation is easy to compute as well as to comprehend. It utilizes all the observations. However, taking absolute deviations introduces a sort of artificiality in the computation; it is not much used in practice.

3.4.3. Standard Deviation

To overcome the problem of calculating absolute deviations, we can calculate the square of the deviations and, finally, the square root of the average of squared deviations. This is called the standard deviation (SD) and is the most important measure of dispersion in the data set. The sum of squared deviations of observations taken from their mean divided by the number of observations is called variance and the SD is the square root of variance.

To compute variation, subtract the mean from each observation; square the difference; sum up the squared differences for all the observations and divide the sum by the number of observations. Taking the square root of this quantity will give us the SD. For easy remembrance, one can say that SD is the root mean square error. Starting in reverse order, find the error, i.e., the deviation between the observation and the mean, square it, find the mean of the squared errors and then calculate the square root.

Algebraically standard deviation is,

$$\text{SD} = \sqrt{\frac{1}{n} \sum_{i=1}^{n} \left(X - \overline{X} \right)^2} \qquad\qquad 3.14$$

In the example on birth-weights discussed in the section on mean deviation (3.4.2), the errors or deviations are 258, 58, –252, –667, 218, –117, 508, 383, –277 and –112. The sum of the squares of these deviations will be $258^2 + 58^2 + (-252)^2 + ... + (-112)^2 = 1133560$. The average of the squared deviations, i.e., the variance = 113356. Thus, the SD will be = $\sqrt{113356}$ = 336.7 g.

For grouped data, as in the case of other measures, each x_i is replaced by the mid-point of the class interval; the deviation between the mean and the mid-point of the class interval is squared and weighted with the respective frequency of the class interval to arrive at the total of squared deviations in the k intervals. The average of the squared deviations will be the variance and the square root of that will be the SD. In algebraic notation, SD for grouped data can be shown as

$$SD = \sqrt{\frac{1}{n}\sum_{i=1}^{k} f_i (X_i - \overline{X})^2} \qquad ... 3.15$$

We shall work out the SD for the grouped data on systolic BP, used for finding the mean deviation in the previous section. The data are shown in Table 3.16. In the section on arithmetic mean (3.3.1) we calculated the value of the arithmetic mean to be 135.6 mmHg. Using this value, we will obtain the deviation in each interval by calculating the difference between the mid-point of the interval and the mean.

Table 3.16: Calculation of standard deviation

Systolic BP (mmHg)	Frequency f_i	Mid-point X_i	Deviation $(X_i - \overline{X})$	Deviation^2	$f_i (X_i - \overline{X})^2$
90 – 100	3	95	– 40.6	1648.36	4945.08
100 – 110	5	105	– 30.6	936.36	4681.80
110 – 120	7	115	– 20.6	424.36	2970.52
120 – 130	10	125	– 10.6	112.36	1123.60
130 – 140	15	135	– 0.6	0.36	5.40
140 – 150	11	145	9.4	88.36	971.96
150 – 160	9	155	19.4	376.36	3387.24
160 – 170	6	165	29.4	864.36	5186.16
170 – 180	2	175	39.4	1552.36	3104.72
Total	68				26376.48

From Table 3.16, the sum of the squared deviations is equal to 26376.48 and when divided by 68, the variance comes out to be 387.8894. SD, the square root of variance = 19.69 mmHg.

Variance is usually denoted as s^2 and SD as s. The quantity $\sum_{i=1}^{n}(X_i - \overline{X})^2$ in equations 3.14 and 3.15 is also called the corrected sum of squares and the denominator n is called the degrees of freedom of the sum of squares. The SD is more appropriate when calculated with $n-1$ degrees of freedom rather than n, because it gives the estimate of SD of some optimum properties. Also, in a way, it is desirable, as we have seen that the sum of deviations is always zero and so for any given data set, there are only $n-1$ deviations that are independent, since the last or nth deviation has to be 0 minus the sum of the deviations of the remaining $n-1$ observations. Thus, the better way of estimating SD will be,

$$s = \sqrt{\frac{1}{n-1}\sum_{i=1}^{n}(X_i - \overline{X})^2} \text{ in case of raw or ungrouped data} \qquad 3.16$$

and

$$s = \sqrt{\frac{1}{n-1}\sum_{i=1}^{k} f_i (X_i - \overline{X})^2} \quad \text{in case of grouped data} \qquad 3.17$$

When the sample size is large, the impact of using n or n-1 in the denominator is negligible, but in data sets of a small size, using n instead of n-1 considerably underestimates the SD. So it is always advisable to use n–1 in the denominator while calculating the estimate of variability in the sample, as it is a virtue to be conservative.

Accordingly in the ungrouped data on birth-weights considered above, the variance will be 1133560 ÷ 9 = 125951.1 and the SD will be 354.90 g, as against 336.7 g obtained with the denominator equal to n. Similarly, in the grouped data on systolic BP, the corrected sum of squares is 26376.48 and the estimate of variance will be 26376.48 ÷ (68 –1) = 393.68. The SD will be 19.84 mmHg, as compared to 19.69 mmHg when the denominator is equal to n. Notice the effect of using n–1 in the denominator in the two instances. In the ungrouped data of 10 observations, the estimate of SD has increased by approximately 18 units while in the grouped data with 68 observations, the estimate of SD has gone up by 0.15 units.

Though the concept of variation and SD are easy to comprehend, the numerators in the equations 3.16 and 3.17 are tedious to compute as is evident in the example. The numerators can be simplified without losing any accuracy. Mathematically, they can be changed into quantities that are easy to compute and are already available:

$$\sum_{i=1}^{n} f_i (X_i - \overline{X})^2 = \sum_{i=1}^{n} (X_i^2) - n\overline{X}^2 \qquad 3.18$$

and

$$\sum_{i=1}^{k} f_i (X_i - \overline{X})^2 = \sum_{i=1}^{k} f_i (X_i^2) - n\overline{X}^2 \qquad 3.19$$

In these two expressions, we avoided taking the difference or deviations, which are quite cumbersome, especially if the mean is to be considered with sufficient decimals for accuracy. Further, the mean is already available before we attempt to obtain the SD. The right-hand side quantities of equations 3.18 and 3.19 above divided by the number of total observations minus one will give us the variance for ungrouped and grouped data, respectively. Taking the square root, we can obtain the respective SD estimates. Continuing with the same example, we re-calculate the SD using equation 3.19 for the data in Table 3.17.

Table 3.17: Calculation of standard deviation using simplified expressions

Systolic BP (mmHg)	Frequency f_i	Mid-point X_i	X_i^2	$f_i \times X_i^2$	$X_i'(X_i -135)$	$X_i'^2$	$f_i \times X_i'^2$
90 – 100	3	95	9025	27075	–40	1600	4800
100 – 110	5	105	11025	55125	–30	900	4500
110 – 120	7	115	13225	92575	–20	400	2800
120 – 130	10	125	15625	156250	–10	100	1000
130 – 140	15	135	18225	273375	0	0	0
140 – 150	11	145	21025	231275	10	100	1100
150 – 160	9	155	24025	216225	20	400	3600
160 – 170	6	165	27225	163350	30	900	5400
170 – 180	2	175	30625	61250	40	1600	3200
Total	68			1276500			26400

$$s^2 = \frac{1}{n-1}\left[\sum_{i=1}^{k} f_i (X_i^2) - n\overline{X}^2\right]$$

$$= [1276500 - 68 \ (135.5882)^2] \div 67$$

$$= [1276500 - (68 \times 18384.16)] \div 67$$

$$= 26377.12 \div 67$$

$$= 393.69$$

$\therefore s = 19.84$ mmHg, which is the same as the value obtained earlier.

The computation of SD can be further simplified by subtracting a constant value from all the raw observations or from the mid-point of each class interval in a grouped data. This will lead to the manipulation of smaller numbers. The value of s^2 and s are unaffected by this approach, as can be verified from Table 3.17. The sum of squared deviations after subtracting 135 from each X_i is 26 400 and the mean with the modified X_is will be 0.5882 mmHg. Using the equation 3.19 with these quantities leads to an estimate of $s^2 = 393.68$ and $s = 19.84$ mmHg, the same as that obtained earlier.

3.4.4. Coefficient of Variation

Sometimes we are interested in the comparison of the variability of two or more variables, say blood sugar measured in mg and weight measured in kg. Alternatively, one can come across a parameter, say birth weight, measured in grams in one investigation and in kilograms in another investigation. Notice that these two have been measured in different units and so the comparison of the respective SD or any other measure of dispersion will not convey which of the two is relatively more varying than the other. In such situations, a measure called the coefficient of variation (CV) is used.

CV is defined as the SD expressed as a percentage of the arithmetic mean. Thus, to obtain CV, one should already have the estimates of the mean and SD of the data. Unlike mean and SD, CV does not have any units.

Coefficient of variation CV$= \dfrac{\sigma}{\overline{X}} \times 100$; where s is the estimated SD $\qquad\qquad$ 3.20

In the example using the data of birth-weights (section on mean deviation (**3.4.2**)) the mean birth-weight = 2592 g and SD = 354.90 g. Therefore, the CV is

CV = (354.90 ÷ 2592) × 100 = 13.69%

Similarly, for the grouped data on systolic BP, the CV will be (19.84 ÷ 135.6) × 100 = 14.63%. Comparing the CV in the 2 variables, we realize that both are almost equally varying, and systolic BP has slightly more variation.

CV can also be used for the comparison of variability in the same variable measured in two different heterogeneous populations. For example, let us suppose that the mean and SD of the weight of children are 20.7 kg and 4.2 kg, respectively, and the corresponding values among adults are 62.5 kg and 10.5 kg, respectively. We cannot directly compare the SD values in both the populations since the magnitude of the values (weight) is very different in the two groups. The coefficient of variation is 20.3% among children and 16.9% among adults, which indicates that the percentage of variation in the weight of children is higher than that in adults. Comparison of the SD values would have led us to the opposite conclusion.

We have seen two types of measures, namely, the measure of central tendency and the measure of dispersion. Both these measures provide us the information about the data completely. After these two measures are available, we do not really need the raw data or the grouped data to comment on the type of values that can be expected in the population with a certain probability or how probable a specific value is in the population. Of course, this requires the assumption that the distribution of data follows a certain law or a mathematical rule such as Normal distribution. Most often, the assumption about the distribution is not grossly violated and more details about the type of distributions and their properties will be given in Chapter 4.

3.5. Correlation

In the sections on measures of central tendency and location (3.3) and measures of dispersion (3.4), we have seen how to summarize a single quantitative variable in terms of its central tendency and dispersion. In practice, we have to work on more than one variable at a time to understand their relationship or the dependence of one variable on another variable or a set of variables. For example, a neonatologist may want to know the relationship or association between the birth-weight of newborns and their gestational ages, parity, and maternal factors such as anaemia, hypertension, etc. Similarly, a cardiologist might be interested in knowing the relationship between a person's cardiac output and his/her age, smoking habit, physical activity, etc.

Many medical decisions depend on the idea of causal relationships and much of the evidence in medical science is of a statistical nature. Therefore, understanding the concept of relationships between two or more variables is important not only to appreciate the limitations of the conclusions one reads about in the literature, but also to evaluate one's own experience more rationally, quantitatively and objectively. There are methods to describe the association or interrelationship among many variables, but in this section we shall discuss how to assess an association or relationship between two quantitative variables.

3.5.1. Scatter Diagram

When we have to assess the relationship between two variables, each observation has a pair of values. The first value indicates the level of the first variable, while the second indicates that of the second variable on the same individual or subject. For instance, let us consider the gestational age and birth-weight of 20 newborns. The data are shown in Table 3.18.

Table 3.18: Gestational age and birth weight of 20 newborns

Baby no.	Gestation (weeks)	Birth weight (g)	Baby no.	Gestation (weeks)	Birth weight (g)
1.	36	2475	11	35	2390
2.	38	2625	12	39	2630
3.	40	2810	13	40	2750
4.	37	1435	14	38	2550
5.	39	2570	15	31	1910
6.	34	2220	16	38	2480
7.	32	1865	17	39	2650
8.	41	2615	18	36	2360
9.	40	2640	19	42	2750
10.	38	2700	20	30	1900

The first step in understanding the relationship between two variables is to plot the data, one variable against the other, taking the pair of values in each observation. In our example, taking the gestational age on the horizontal axis (X-axis) and birth-weight on the vertical axis (Y-axis), we show the birth-weight corresponding to each gestational age as a point. After plotting all the observations, we can see how the values on the vertical axis (birth-weight) are scattered for a given value on the X-axis (gestation) and similarly, how the values on the X-axis are scattered for a given value on the Y-axis. Because this diagram shows the scatter of the two variables with respect to each other, it is called the scatter diagram (Fig. 3.12).

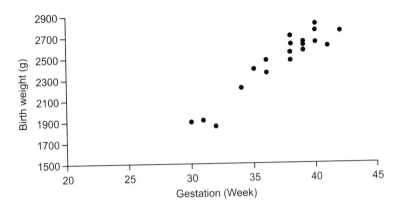

Fig. 3.12: Scatter diagram of gestation and birth-weight

We can see from the scatter diagram in Fig. 3.12 that the band of dots forms the shape of an ellipse with the major axis showing upwards towards the right side. As the gestation increases, the birth-weigh tends to increase, thereby showing a relationship or association between the two variables, gestation and birth-weight. Since the relationship is like a line, it is called a linear relationship. Two variables may also be related or associated in such way that the form of the relationship may not be linear. These types of associations are called non-linear associations, and are more complicated to study and quantify as compared to linear relationships.

In the example we considered, if there is no association between gestation and birth-weight, we would expect the points plotted in Fig. 3.12 to scatter randomly without revealing any pattern, as shown in Fig. 3.13(a). Similarly, there could be a linear relationship, which is different from the one seen in Fig. 3.12. Instead of one variable increasing with an increase in the second, one variable could be decreasing while the other is increasing, as shown in Fig. 3.13(b). The type of association shown in Fig. 3.12 is referred to as a positive association as the change in both the variables is in the same direction (either both increase or both decrease together) and the type shown in Fig. 3.13(b) is referred to as a negative association because the direction of change in one variable is opposite to that in the second.

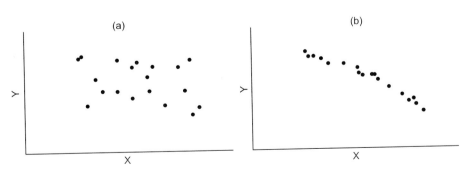

Fig. 3.13: Scatter diagrams showing no association (a) and a negative association (b)

Examples of negative correlation: Socio-economic score and the incidence of malnutrition in children from different localities/regions/countries (higher the socio-economic score, lower will be the incidence of malnutrition.)

Examples of no correlation: Correlation between height of the individual and the number of cigarettes smoked per day; correlation between IQ and the height of the individuals.

3.5.2. Correlation Coefficient

The scatter diagram no doubt helps us to visualize the type of relationship or association between the two variables, but it does not help to quantify the association between the two. If the relationship appears linear or near-linear, it can be quantified by a measure called the correlation coefficient proposed by Karl Pearson[5] (1902-3).

The correlation coefficient is defined as the measure of the linear association between two quantitative variables. We have to take note of the word linear here, as the measure is specific only to line-type associations, which are shown in Fig 3.12 and 3.13(b). It implies that if a non-linear relationship exists, the measure of correlation coefficient is of little value.

Mathematically, the correlation coefficient is defined as the ratio of covariance between two variables to the product of the SD of the two. If we denote our two variables as X and Y, the correlation coefficient between them is defined as,

$$\text{Correlation coefficient} = \frac{\text{Covariance}\,(X,Y)}{s(X)s(Y)} \qquad 3.21$$

To calculate the correlation coefficient, we use covariance, which is a measure that quantifies how two (or more) variables vary together. In case of the two variables X and Y, it is defined as,

$$Cov,\,(X,\,Y) = \text{average value of } (X - \bar{X})\,(Y - \bar{Y}) \qquad 3.22$$

which can also be expressed as,

$$Cov\,(X,\,Y) = \frac{1}{n-1}\left[\sum\left(X_i Y_i - \overline{XY}\right)\right] \qquad 3.23$$

Covariance is nothing but the average deviation between the product of the pair of values of the two variables and the product of the arithmetic means of the same two variables. Notice that the sign of each deviation is to be considered while summing up the total deviation. Therefore, covariance between two variables can be positive or negative, depending on the total of deviations between the product of the two values and the product of the two arithmetic means. If covariance is equal to zero or small, the two variables are said to be not related or not associated or not dependent on each other.

Covariance is also a measure of the linear association between the two quantitative variables being considered. Since it is an absolute measure of the linear association between the two variables, we make it a relative measure, relative to the SD in each variable by dividing the covariance with the product of the SD in each variable.

Translating these concepts into algebraic expressions, the correlation coefficient, denoted by r, is

$$r = \frac{\frac{1}{n-1}\left[\sum_{i=1}^{n}\left(X_i Y_i - \overline{XY}\right)\right]}{\sqrt{\frac{1}{n-1}\sum_{i=1}^{n}\left(X_i - \overline{X}\right)^2 \frac{1}{n-1}\sum_{i=1}^{n}\left(Y_i - \overline{Y}\right)^2}} \qquad 3.24$$

Simplification of this equation 3.24 will yield

$$r = \frac{\left[\sum_{i=1}^{n}\left(X_i Y - \overline{X}\,\overline{Y}\right)\right]}{\sqrt{\sum_{i=1}^{n}\left(X_i - \overline{X}\right)^2 \sum_{i=1}^{n}\left(Y_i - \overline{Y}\right)^2}} \qquad 3.25$$

For easier computation, we can re-write the equation 3.25 as,

$$r = \frac{[\text{sum } XY - \{(\text{sum } X)(\text{sum } Y)/n\}]}{\text{sqrt}[\{(\text{sum } X^2) - (\text{sum } X)^2/n)\}\{(\text{sum } Y^2) - (\text{sum } Y)^2/n)\}]} \qquad 3.26$$

$$r = \frac{\left[\sum_{i=1}^{n} X_i Y_i - \left(\sum_{i=1}^{n} X_i\right)\left(\sum_{i=1}^{n} Y_i\right)/n\right]}{\sqrt{\left[\sum_{i=1}^{n} X_i^2 - \left(\sum_{i=1}^{n} X_i\right)^2/n\right]\left[\sum_{i=1}^{n} Y_i^2 - \left(\sum_{i=1}^{n} Y_i\right)^2/n\right]}} \qquad 3.27$$

Table 3.19 shows the details of the calculation of r using the data shown in Table 3.18.

Table 3.19: Calculation of the correlation coefficient between gestation and birth-weight of newborns

Serial no.	Gestation (weeks)X_i	X_i^2	Birth weight (g)Y_i	Y_i^2	$X_i \times Y_i$
1.	36	1296	2475	6125625	89100
2.	38	1444	2625	6890625	99750
3.	40	1600	2810	7896100	112400
4.	37	1369	1435	2059225	53095
5.	39	1521	2570	6604900	100230
6.	34	1156	2220	4928400	75480
7.	32	1024	1865	3478225	59680
8.	41	1681	2615	6838225	107215
9.	40	1600	2640	6969600	105600
10.	38	1558	2700	7290000	102600
11.	35	1225	2390	5712100	83650
12.	39	1521	2630	6916900	102570
13.	40	1600	2750	7562500	110000
14.	38	1558	2550	6502500	96900
15.	31	961	1910	3648100	59210
16.	38	1558	2480	6150400	94240
17.	39	1521	2650	7022500	103350
18.	36	1296	2360	5569600	84960
19.	42	1764	2750	7562500	115500
20.	30	900	1900	3610000	57000
Total	743	27811	48325	119338025	1812530

We have n = 20,

$$\sum_{i=1}^{n} X_i = 743 \quad \sum_{i=1}^{n} Y_i = 48325 \quad \sum_{i=1}^{n} X_i Y_i = 1812530 \quad \sum_{i=1}^{n} X_i^{\,2} = 27811 \quad \sum_{i=1}^{n} Y_i^{\,2} = 119338025$$

Substituting these values in equation 3.26, correlation coefficient r will be,

$$r = \frac{\left[\sum_{i=1}^{n} X_i Y_i - \left(\sum_{i=1}^{n} X_i\right)\left(\sum_{i=1}^{n} Y_i\right)/n\right]}{\sqrt{\left[\sum_{i=1}^{n} X_i^2 - \left(\sum_{i=1}^{n} X_i\right)^2 / n\right]\left[\sum_{i=1}^{n} Y_i^2 - \left(\sum_{i=1}^{n} Y_i\right)^2 / n\right]}}$$

$$r = \frac{\left[1812530 - (743)(48325)/20\right]}{\sqrt{\left[27811 - (743)^2 / 20\right]\left[119338025 - (48325)^2 / 20\right]}}$$

$= [17256.25] \div \text{Sqrt}[(208.55)(2572743.75)]$

$= 17256.25 \div 23163.46 = 0.745$

Therefore, the two variables, gestational age and birth-weight of newborns, are highly positively correlated (Fig. 3.12), the correlation coefficient being 0.745.

3.5.2.1. Interpretation of r

From the above description, we realize that the sign of the correlation coefficient depends on the sign of the covariance. Further, the correlation coefficient can never be more than 1 and can also never be less than –1. A value close to +1 indicates a perfect or near-perfect positive relationship between the two quantitative variables considered and a value close to –1 indicates a perfect negative relationship between them. A value close to zero indicates that the two variables are not linearly related. Again, we stress here that there could be a relationship of another type between the two, but definitely not a linear one. A correlation coefficient close to +1 or –1 indicates a high degree of linear relationship and both such variables are said to be highly correlated. It may be mentioned here that perfect correlation can be obtained only if a law-like relationship holds, such as in mathematical or physical principles. For example, the relationship between the pressure and volume of a gas at normal temperature are perfectly correlated. Generally, biological or physiological variables do not exhibit perfect linear relationships and have at most a close-to-perfect correlation.

Examples of positive correlation include the height and weight of children, age and height of children, age and weight of children, systolic BP and age, etc. Negative correlation can be expected between age and peak expiratory flow rate in adults aged above 45 years, glomerular filtration rate and plasma creatinine, etc. Examples of no correlation could be height and Intelligence Quotient, height of smokers and the number of cigarettes smoked per day, etc.

We discussed in the section on measures of dispersion (3.4), that statistical techniques help us to explain the variation in a phenomenon due to other factors. In this context, another useful interpretation of the correlation coefficient r is that the square of the correlation coefficient (r^2) is the proportion of variance in one variable that can be explained by the other. If r^2 is close to one, it implies that the total variation in one variable can be explained by the other. By taking the square of r in the example data on the gestation and birth-weight of newborns, we get $r^2 = 0.555$ or 55.5%, which implies that 55.5% of variation in birth weights can be explained by the gestational ages of newborns or 55.5% of variation in gestational ages can be explained by the birth-weights (though an unlikely proposition).

Pitfalls in the interpretation of correlation coefficient: The correlation coefficient r is a pure number without any units, which takes values between –1 and +1 and always lies within these limits Again, it should be emphasized that the presence of a high correlation implies the existence of a linear relationship. The absence of correlation or poor correlation may not mean that the two variables are unrelated or not associated in any way. It only means that no linear relationship exists. In that sense, a scatter diagram will tell us more than the correlation coefficient, because if the scatter is random, there is no association at all (linear or non-linear) between the two variables. Therefore, computation of the correlation coefficient is logical only when the scatter diagram indicates a linear relationship. Also, there should be biological or physiological plausibility for the presence of an association, so that one can try to quantify it. Otherwise, we can compute the correlation coefficient between any two variables, say for example the daily number of eggs laid by a fish in the Indian Ocean and the daily number of road accidents in the city of Delhi. Such correlations are meaningless.

The presence of high correlation should also be not interpreted as the two variables being related directly, because it may be due to the presence or absence of other common factor(s). For example, a high correlation between the heights of brothers and sisters should not be interpreted as the greater height of a girl being due to the greater height of her brother or vice versa. The result may be due to a common set of factors, such as the heights and nutritional status of their parents, etc.

Some investigators often tend to interpret high correlation as an indication of high agreement between the values of the two variables. This is highly erroneous. The presence of a relationship does not mean agreement, but the presence of an agreement implies the existence of a good correlation. Two sets of measurements can be highly correlated even if there is a constant difference between them or one is a multiple of the other. For example, consider two physicians measuring the systolic BP of a group of persons. Suppose one physician measures the BP accurately and the second always measures the same by 10 mmHg more than the first. If we calculate the correlation coefficient of the two BP measurements of same group of individuals, we get a perfect correlation due to the fact that one measurement is exactly related to the other measurement of BP of a given person. But there is a difference of 10 mmHg between the measurements taken by the two physicians. Therefore, the presence of the correlation coefficient is not related to the presence or absence of agreement.

In case of grouped data, the calculation of r proceeds on similar lines. First, the data should be arranged in a two-way frequency distribution, in which both the variables are categorized into certain ranges or class intervals, as we have done in the case of a single variable in the section on tabulation of data (3.1). The frequencies of one variable in different class intervals are then shown for each class interval of the other variable. For instance, for the data in gestation and birth-weight of newborns, the total frequency of babies with a gestation age of say 30–31 weeks can be shown as the frequency in the birth-weight groups 1800–2000 g, 2000–2200 g and so on as a row. Similarly, for other babies with gestational ages 33–34 weeks, 35–36 weeks, etc. The mid-point of each interval of one variable can be taken as X_i and the same of each interval of the other variable as Y_i proceeding in the usual manner with f_{ij} representing the frequency in the ith category of variable X and jth category of variable Y.

The Pearson correlation coefficient is also called the product–moment correlation coefficient. After quantifying the amount of linear dependence or association between two quantitative variables, it is natural to ask how such an estimate is likely to vary from sample to sample or whether such a magnitude of association can happen by chance. We shall present these aspects in Chapter 5.

3.5.2.2. Correlation coefficient based on rankings

The calculation of Pearson's product–moment correlation coefficient requires the condition that both the variables together follow a distribution called a bivariate normal distribution. The properties of such distributions are presented in Chapter 4. While this assumption may not be seriously violated, often a bivariate population can be far from normal. If so, the computation of r as an estimate of the population correlation coefficient is not valid. In such situations, we can try with the transformed data, so that the joint distribution of the two transformed variables will become at least approximately bivariate-normal and then compute the correlation coefficient in the new scale of measurements.

If any transformation also fails to bring normality to the data, the correlation coefficient can be calculated on the ranks of the measurements of the two variables. In this method, there is no requirement for a bivariate normal distribution of the two variables being considered. This method, proposed by Spearman[6] (1904) is called rank correlation and is computed in exactly the same way as with a bivariate normal data, presented in the section on correlation coefficient (3.5.2). Instead of the actual measurements, we use the ranks. Intuitively, if the ranks of X_s and Y_s are close for each pair, then there appears to be a positive association between the ranks of the two variables X and Y. On the other hand, if the ranks of X_s and Y_s tend to be far apart in each pair of values, a negative association is indicated. If there is absolutely no rank order relationship between X and Y, then the ranks of X_s will appear to be randomly assigned for a given rank of Y. Assuming no ties in the ranks, correlation coefficient r_s can be computed as,

$$r_s = 1 - \frac{6\sum_{i=1}^{n} d_i^2}{n(n^2 - 1)}$$

3.28

where d_i is the difference in the two ranks of the ith observation in the data and n is the total number of observations.

We will use the data on gestation and birth-weight, reproduced in Table 3.20 that we used to calculate the Pearson correlation for calculating Spearman's rank correlation coefficient.

Table 3.20: Calculation of Spearman's rank correlation coefficient

Serial no.	Gestation (weeks) X_i	Gestation rank	Birth-weight (g) Y_i	Birth-weight rank	Difference in ranks d_i	d_i^2
1.	36	6.5	2475	8	1.5	2.25
2.	38	10.5	2625	13	2.5	6.25
3.	40	17	2810	20	3	9
4.	37	8	1435	1	7	49
5.	39	14	2570	11	3	9
6.	34	4	2220	5	1	1
7.	32	3	1865	2	1	1
8.	41	19	2615	12	7	49
9.	40	17	2640	15	2	4
10.	38	10.5	2700	17	6.5	42.25
11.	35	5	2390	7	2	4
12.	39	14	2630	14	0	0
13.	40	17	2750	18.5	1.5	2.25
14.	38	10.5	2550	10	0.5	0.25
15.	31	2	1910	4	2	4
16.	38	10.5	2480	9	1.5	2.25
17.	39	14	2650	16	2	4
18.	36	6.5	2360	6	0.5	0.25
19.	42	20	2750	18.5	1.5	2.25
20.	30	1	1900	3	2	4
Total	743		48325			196

The third and fifth columns of Table 3.20 indicate the ranks given to the actual values of gestation and birth-weight, respectively. We have given the ranks in the ascending order, but it does not matter whether they are in ascending or descending order. Notice that when a value is repeated, an average rank is given for the repeated observations. For example, the baby with a gestation of 35 weeks is given a rank of 5. There are two babies with a gestation of 36 weeks; since these two would be the 6th and 7th observations in the ascending order, we give them both an average rank of 6.5 and continue with next higher observation with a rank of 8 onwards. A similar approach is also adopted for the birth-weight. After appropriate ranks have been assigned to the two variables, we obtain the difference between the ranks of the two variables for each child. These differences in ranks, called d_i, are shown in the 6th column and the square of d_i in the last column of Table 3.20. Now we have,

$$\sum_{i=1}^{n} d_i^2 = 196 \qquad n = 20$$

Substituting these values in equation 3.27,

$$r_s = 1 - \frac{6(196)}{20(20^2 - 1)} = 1 - \frac{1176}{7980} = 1 - 0.1474 = 0.8526$$

The rank correlation coefficient between the gestational age and birth-weight of newborns also indicates a high degree of association. Like the Pearson correlation coefficient, Spearman's rank correlation also ranges from −1 (complete discordance between the rankings) to +1 (complete concordance). A value close to zero indicates that the two variables are independent. Rank correlation can also be used to evaluate the agreement between the rankings given by two raters or judges to a group of observations. Because the calculation of Spearman's rank correlation does not require any assumption of the distribution of the data, it is also referred to as a non-parametric method.

3.6. Regression

In the sections on measures of dispersion (3.4) and correlation (3.5) we saw how to quantify the association between two variables. During this process, we did not take into account prior knowledge on whether one variable is dependent on the other or one causes the other since our aim was only to quantify the association between the two variables. In practical applications in medical science, we often know that one variable is dependent or caused by another variable. For example, in the example of data in gestation and birth-weight, it is logical to consider that the birth-weight of the newborn is dependent on its gestation rather than gestation on birth-weight. Similarly, it is reasonable to postulate that high levels of low-density lipoproteins tend to lead to high levels of coronary heart disease than vice versa. Thus, the occurrence of coronary heart disease is 'dependent' on the levels of low-density lipoproteins. The variable coronary heart disease status is the 'dependent variable' and the level of low-density lipoproteins is an 'independent variable'. We can also call them the 'predicted variable' and the 'predictor variable' respectively.

In this section, we see how to predict the dependent variable for a given value of the predictor variable or independent variable, based on a sample of measurements on both the dependent and independent variables. That is, we observe a set of values on both the dependent and independent variables and using a mathematical relationship between these measurements, we calculate back or 'regress' the dependent variable based on the values of the independent variable. Thus, this technique is called regression analysis.

3.6.1. Linear Regression

For easier understanding, we denote the independent variable as X and the dependent variable as Y. The first step in regression is to draw a scatter diagram for X and Y. If there is any association between X and Y, a trend can be seen in the scatter diagram of the values of the dependent variable Y for given values of X. The regression technique applied to situations where the trend happens to be like a line or linear is called a linear regression. It is one of the simplest types of regression analysis.

The concept of regression lies in identifying a line called the regression line, that is nearest to the data points marked on the scatter diagram, so that for a given value of X, we can make a close prediction of the value of Y. Towards this objective, using the observed data, we find the mathematical quantities of the equation of a straight line, so that the regression line achieves the desired properties. The identified line also passes through the point whose coordinates are the means of X and Y. Mathematically, the equation for any straight line is,

$$Y = a + bX \hspace{8em} 3.29$$

where Y is the value of the dependent variable Y shown on the vertical axis, x is the value of the independent variable X shown on the horizontal axis, b is the slope of the line and a is the point where the line intercepts the vertical axis, *i.e.*, the value of Y when X is zero. The slope is also called the regression coefficient. Our aim in fitting a regression line to the data is then to obtain the values of a and b in the equation 3.29. The method of estimating the slope and the intercept of a linear regression is called the least squares method.

Before giving more details of regression analysis, we state here that for the regression analysis to be applicable, we assume that: (i) for each value of the independent variable X, the dependent variable Y can take more than one value and the distribution of such values will follow a normal distribution with a certain mean and variance; (ii) the mean of the distributions of Y at different values of X fall on the regression line; (iii) the variance of the distributions of Y at different values of X is same (also called constant variance or homoscedasticity and (iv) the distribution of the errors (the difference between the observed and predicted values of the dependent variable) follows a normal distribution with mean zero and some variance.

3.6.2. Least Squares Method of Estimation

To explain this method, we draw a plot of data as shown in Fig. 3.14. Three data points as well as the regression line are shown in the scatter diagram. Notice that the three data points are not falling on the regression line. But the method of least squares ensures that the vertical distance between the fitted regression line and the data points is minimum in totality. To be precise, the sum of squares of these vertical distances or deviations will be the least of all possible regression lines on this data. The value on the Y-axis coinciding with the point on the regression line where the vertical line drawn from the observed point intersects the regression line is called the predicted or expected value of the dependent variable Y for a given value of the predictor or independent variable X.

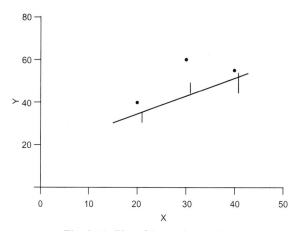

Fig. 3.14: Plot of three observations

In statistical terminology, the difference between the observed value of the dependent variable Y and its expected value by the regression model is called the residual. Thus, the length of each of the vertical lines from the observed data point to the regression line is a residual. For the data points falling above the regression line, the residual is positive and for those falling below the line, the residuals will be negative.

The expressions for the least square estimates of the slope $(\hat{b})$ and the intercept $(\hat{a})$ (leaving the details of derivations) are obtained as,

$$\hat{b} = \frac{sum \ of \ XY - \{(sum \ X)(sum \ Y)/n\}}{sum \ X^2 - (sum \ X)^2/n} \quad \text{and} \quad \hat{a} = [(sum \ Y)/n] - [b(sum \ X)/n] \qquad \text{3.30, 3.31}$$

Using the notations for summation:

$$\hat{b} = \frac{\left[\sum_{i=1}^{n} X_i Y_i - \left(\sum_{j=1}^{n} X_i\right)\left(\sum_{j=1}^{n} Y_i\right)/n \right]}{\left[\sum_{i=1}^{n} X_i^2 - \left(\sum_{j=1}^{n} X_i\right)^2 /n \right]} \qquad \text{3.32}$$

3.6.3. Numerical Example of the Calculation of Regression

Let us work out the estimates of a and b for the example of data on gestation and birth-weights. In this example, gestation is the independent variable or predictor variable or regressor X, and the birth-weight is the dependent or predicted variable or the regressed variable Y.

Accordingly from the section on correlation coefficient, (3.5.2) we have,

$$n = 20 \quad \sum_{i=1}^{n} X_i = 743 \quad \sum_{i=1}^{n} Y_i = 48325 \quad \sum_{i=1}^{n} X_i Y_i = 1812530 \quad \sum_{i=1}^{n} X_i^2 = 27811 \quad \sum_{i=1}^{n} Y_i^2 = 119338025$$

$$\hat{b} = \frac{\left[\sum_{i=1}^{n} X_i Y_i - \left(\sum_{j=1}^{n} X_i\right)\left(\sum_{j=1}^{n} Y_i\right)/n \right]}{\left[\sum_{i=1}^{n} X_i^2 - \left(\sum_{j=1}^{n} X_i\right)^2 /n \right]}$$

= [1812530 – (743)(48325)/20)] ÷ [27811 – (743)²/20]

= [1812530 – 1795273.75] ÷ [27811 – 27602.45]

= 17256.25 ÷ 208.55 = 82.744

$\hat{a}$ = [(*sum Y*)/n] – [b(*sum X*)/n]

= [48325 / 20] – [(82.744)(743)/20]

= 2416.25 – 3073.94

= – 657.69

3.6.3.1. Interpretation of the slope and intercept of the regression line

In the regression of birth-weight on gestation, we obtained the slope of the regression line as 82.74 and the intercept as –657.69. It is important to know what these quantities convey, so that we can really appreciate the technique of regression.

Let us consider the form of the linear regression line shown in equation 3.29. We have,

$Y = a + bX$

,

in which Y is the value of birth-weight and X is the value of gestation for a newborn. The equation implies that the birth-weight of a newborn is the sum of two components—a constant component irrespective of the gestation and a component that varies with the level of gestation.

The variable component will be high for high values of gestation and low for lower values of gestation. Thus, the slope or regression coefficient b can be viewed as the change in the value of the birth-weight if the value of the gestation is changed. In particular, b conveys the average change in the dependent variable for a unit change in the independent variable. Therefore, naturally, the units of b will be that of the dependent variable and to report it requires that both units be stated. Coming back to our example, the slope or b is 82.74 g, implying that for an increase of one week in gestation, the birth-weight of the newborn goes up by nearly 83 g.

The intercept is a constant value that is unrelated to the value the independent variable takes. As mentioned earlier, a is the point where the regression line intercepts the vertical axis. To put it another way, even if the independent variable takes the value of zero, there can be a certain value for the dependent variable and this is equal to the intercept term a in the model. The intercept has a practical meaning of its own, only when zero is a plausible value for the independent variable. Otherwise, it is useful to find the expected value of the dependent variable as the sum of the two quantities that have been described already. Since the intercept also indicates the value of the dependent variable, its units are also those of the dependent variable. Thus, in our example, the regression line is,

Birth-weight = - 657.69 + 82.74(gestation)   ... 3.32

The fitted regression on the sample data indicates that for a baby with a gestation of 40 weeks, we can expect the birth-weight to be –657.69+82.74(40) = 3309.6–657.54=2651.9 g. Thus, the regression technique provides more insight into the relationship between the two variables. The type of inferences that can be drawn through the regression analysis, as shown above, are very useful in studying the aetiology of a disease or the factors associated with a clinical condition as they convey the impact of one variable on the other. Therefore, the regression technique is a powerful tool in the armour of an epidemiologists or a biostatistician.

The expected birth-weight for a given value of gestation is called the expected value and is denoted by $\hat{y}_i$. The difference between the observed and expected values is called the residual.

$Y_i - \hat{Y}_i$ = residual   3.33

We may recall here that the method of least squares used to determine the regression line ensures that the sum of squares of all the residuals is the least for the regression line fitted to the data. If any other line is fitted, this quantity will be more than what is obtained by the least squares method.

3.6.4. Relationship between Correlation and Regression

Notice that the covariance between the two variables is the numerator for the slope b of the linear regression line (equation 3.30) as well as for the correlation coefficient between the two variables (equation 3.27). In the denominator, we consider only the standard deviation of the independent variable for obtaining the slope of the regression line, and as the product of the standard deviations of X and Y for correlation coefficient r. Thus, there is a close relationship between b and r. If the two variables are positively correlated, the slope or regression coefficient will also be positive. If the correlation is negative, so will be the regression coefficient.

Further, as we have seen the regression of Y on X, we can also consider the regression of X on Y. If we denote the two regression coefficients as $b_{y.x}$ and $b_{x.y}$, simple algebra will indicate that their product will be equivalent to the square of correlation coefficient.

Thus, linear regression and correlation coefficient are closely interrelated.

3.6.5. Uses of Regression

We have seen in the previous sections how regression analysis enables us to describe the relationship between two variables. In practical applications of health and medical research, it can be used in a variety of ways. Some of the common applications are:

1. To describe or summarize the level of one variable with the level of another variable that is associated with the first one.

2. Sometimes we are interested in finding the association of one variable with another, after adjusting or accounting for the differences with respect to one or more other variables. For example, we might be interested in knowing the association between the birth-weight and gestation, adjusting for maternal factors such as antenatal visits to the physician, anaemia, etc. In such situations, regression analysis can help assess the association between the dependent and independent variables, after adjusting for the effect of maternal anaemia and health check-ups, etc.

3. Regression analysis can also be used to identify the variables that influence a particular variable so that the mechanisms of action among different variables can be understood. This aspect of regression analysis is very useful in identifying the causative factors for a particular condition. It must be noted that evidence by a regression analysis in itself can never be proof of causality, but a careful and well-planned analysis may lead to the formulation of a hypothesis or confirm the same.

4. Regression can also aid in predicting or forecasting a level of the dependent variable for a given value(s) of the independent variable(s). For example, if a regression model has been developed for the hospital mortality associated with acute liver failure (ALF) on the age, serum bilirubin, encephalopathy and prothrombin time of patients attending a liver clinic, using this model, we can predict the mortality for a new patient by knowing his/her age, bilirubin, encephalopathy and prothrombin time. This can help to triage patients seeking liver transplant.

    Regression analysis can also be used to identify the abnormal values or outliers, so that we can re-examine them for their accuracy in measurement, recording or in transcription. If no errors are found, such outlier observations may merit a detailed individual study.

3.6.6. Limitations of Regression Analysis

As already mentioned, evidence by regression in itself can never be a proof of causality between the dependent and independent variable(s). It can only be of a supportive nature to the biological or physiological plausibility of the relationship between the dependent variable and the independent variable(s) that have been studied.

Similarly, when we use regression to predict or forecast, we should keep in mind the fact that the values of the predictors should be within the range of values that have been used to develop the model. In our example of data on birth-weight and gestation, the value of gestation is between 30 and 42 weeks. Based on the model of this data set, we should try to predict the birth-weight of a newborn whose gestation ranges between 30 and 42 weeks. Predicting the birth-weight of a newborn with gestation outside these limits will be hazardous.

3.6.7. What to Use: Correlation or Regression?

Correlation coefficient measures the closeness of a linear relationship between two variables. When we are not aware of which one of the two causes the other, correlation is a useful measure to summarize the relation. For example, if we want to quantify the association of a trait (e.g., height, body mass index, bone mineral density, etc.) among members of the same family, correlation coefficient is appropriate summary of the association. Here we are interested in knowing whether the trait is familial or random and not interested in the influence of the value of the trait in one member on that of the other member(s).

Even if we are aware of the causal mechanism, correlation helps to summarize the association between the two variables under consideration. But it cannot quantify the change that can be effected in a variable by changing the other variable that causes the change. If the interest lies in quantifying the change in one phenomenon when we change the other, regression analysis is preferred. In other words, regression analysis requires prior knowledge on the cause-effect relation. Linear regression is related to correlation coefficient and it provides two parameters that are directly related to the data. So, it is more informative to use regression analysis when there is at least a reasonable knowledge on the causal pathway, though it helps to quote the correlation coefficient as a measure of the strength of a relationship. However, when one is interested only in the strength of a relationship as in some epidemiological surveys, then the correlation coefficient is preferable.

Multiple Choice Questions

Choose the correct answers in the following multiple choice questions. The correct answers are listed on p. 342.

Q.1. **To represent the data of the distribution of systolic blood pressure in a population, the appropriate diagram would be:**
a. Pie diagram
b. Bar diagram
c. Histogram
d. Scatter plot

Q.2. **The appropriate diagram to represent the distribution of patients admitted in a hospital according to their disease and sex would be:**
a. Simple bar diagram
b. Pie diagram
c. Histogram
d. Adjacent bar diagram

Q.3. **To see whether any correlation exists between HDL and LDL graphically the appropriate diagram would be:**
a. Histogram
b. Line
c. Scatter diagram
d. Bar

Q.4. **Number of malaria cases reported in a town from 1990 to 1995 were as follows:**

Year	1990	1991	1992	1993	1994	1995
No. of Cases	100	200	5000	150	300	120

The most appropriate average for this data is:
a. Geometric mean
b. Median
c. Arithmetic Average
d. Mode

Q.5. **For comparing the relative variation in height (cm) and weight (kg) of children, the statistic to be calculated is:**
a. Mean
b. Range
c. Standard error
d. Coefficient of variation (CV)

Q.6. **Arranging the sample values in ascending or descending order is essential to calculate:**
a. Arithmetic mean
b. Mode
c. Standard deviation
d. Median

Q.7. **Mean and standard deviations of hemoglobin in 25 sick children are 8 mg% and 2 mg% respectively. Coefficient of variation of this sample is:**
a. 16%
b. 25%
c. 4%
d. 2%

Q.8. **Median of a sample of values is defined as:**
a. The values which is repeated most often in the sample
b. The value, which is obtained by adding up all the sample values and dividing it by the sample size
c. The difference between highest and lowest values in the sample
d. None of the above

Q.9. **The value of correlation coefficient between the variables X and Y lies between:**

  a. -1 and +1   b. 0 and 1
  c. 1 and 2   d. None of the above

Q.10. **To find out the degree of linear association between age and systolic blood pressure of a sample of factory workers, the parameter to be estimated is:**

  a. Standard deviation   b. Standard error
  c. Median   d. Correlation coefficient

References

1. Sturges HA. The choice of a class interval. *J Am Statist Assocn.* 1926; 1: 65-66.
2. Hill AB. *A Short Textbook of Medical Statistics.* London: Hodder and Stoughton; 1977.
3. Indian Council of Medical Research. *Consolidated Report of the Population Based Cancer Registries, 1990-1996.* New Delhi: ICMR: National Cancer Registry Programme; 2001.
4. Tukey JW. *Exploratory Data Analysis.* Reading, Massachusetts: Addison-Wesley; 1977.
5. Pearson K, Lee A. *Biometrika.* 1902-3; 2:357.
6. Spearman C. The proof and measurement of association between two things. *American Journal of Psychology.* 1904; 15:72-101.

4 | Logic of Statistical Inference

4.1. Statistical Methods

We have seen earlier that there are two branches of statistical methods: (a) descriptive methods and (b) inference methods. Let us recollect their definitions as:

Descriptive methods: Statistical methods used for describing (summarizing) the collected data are included in this category, e.g., preparation of statistical tables, drawing diagrams & graphs, computation of averages, location parameters, proportions & percentages, deviation measures and correlation measures and regression analysis.

Inference methods: Statistical methods used for drawing inferences (generalizations), from the results obtained from the sample, about the population from where the sample was selected are included in this category.

Most of the problems faced in the world must be solved inductively. The state of human knowledge concerning life is such that we are unable to make true general statements and deduce the answers to the questions logically. It is, however, possible to stipulate a set of assumptions and deduce logically a set of conclusions. However, the conclusions thus drawn will be true only within the framework of these assumptions used for deduction. If we are unwilling to take the risk of setting assumptions that are not true in order to deduce logically, we are forced to draw conclusions inductively. Almost every decision we take in this world is made inductively and in the face of uncertainty on the basis of previous experiences drawn. In this process, there is a risk of being wrong in our conclusions. The knowledge gained from experiments, even conducted very well, is really applicable only to those subjects in the experiment under the same conditions as those that existed during the experiment. In classical statistics, two types of inferences can be made about a target population on the basis of sample of observations – a universal value (parameter) can be estimated or a hypothesis (a declarative statement) about the target population can be tested.

In any scientific study the scientist would like to know the reliability of the results and also to see whether the differences between the observed and the expected results, based on an anticipated statistical hypothesis, would have occurred only because of chance or it could be real, due to any external, internal or interventional factor. The reliability of the results is studied by computing the Confidence interval for the estimate and the chance /reality of the hypothesis is studied by testing the statistical significance of the hypothesis where the chance element is computed and compared with certain stipulated figure and a decision is taken whether the difference is just by chance alone or it is real. Inference statistical methods are discussed in the next Chapter. In this Chapter the important terms and concepts concerned with statistical inference methods are discussed.

Important terms/concepts concerned with the statistical inference: Probability and probability distributions or statistical distributions (normal, binomial and Poisson), standard error, statistical hypothesis, null hypothesis, alternate hypothesis and Type-I and Type-II errors.

4.2. Probability

Probability may be defined as the probable chance of occurrence with which a defined event is expected to occur out of the total possible occurrences. It is the relative frequency of the number of occurrences of a favorable event to the total number of occurrences of all possible events. If an event can occur in N mutually exclusive and equally likely ways and if m of them possess a specific characteristic E, then,

$$P(E) = \frac{n}{N}$$

Many statements are made with certain elements of uncertainty — it may probably rain tomorrow; he may probably be selected for the post for which he has applied; the new drug tested may be effective, etc. No conclusion can be drawn with 100 % certainty (confidence). Probability is the measurement of chance/uncertainty/subjectivity associated with a conclusion. Or, in other words, statistical probability is concerned with the decision making in the face of uncertainty.

Probability ranges from 0 to 1. If the happening of an event is impossible, P =0 and if the happening of an event is sure, P =1. Historically, gambling situations led the mathematicians to study and develop the probability theory. The mathematicians/statisticians who have contributed substantially to the development of the theory of probability are: Galileo (1564-1643), Pascal (1623-1662), Fermat (1601-1665), James Bernoulli (1654-1705), Abraham De Moivre (1667-1754), Thomas Bayes (1702-1761), Feller and Simon Denis Poisson (1781-1840).

4.2.1. Uses of Probability

Probability theory is used (1) to take decisions in case of uncertainty and (2) to derive inferences about the population regarding a parameter or a hypothesis.

1. Taking decisions in case of uncertainty: There are two types of probability (a) mathematical and (b) statistical.

(a) Mathematical probability: An experiment or a trial where the probabilities of occurrences of various events/possibilities are already established mathematically.
Examples:
  (1) Prob. of getting a head when a coin is tossed (½)
  (2) Prob. of getting five when a dice is thrown(1/6)
  (3) Prob. of getting spade ace from a deck of cards(1/52)
  These probabilities are also called Classical or a priori

(b) Statistical/empirical probability: An experiment or a trial is required to find out the probabilities of occurrences of various events/possibilities.
Examples:
  (1) Prob. of getting a boy in the first pregnancy

(2) Prob. of getting a twin for a couple

(3) Prob. of improvement after the treatment for a specified period

(4) Prob. of getting lung cancer in smokers

To find out the probability in all the above given problems, evidence based on empirical data is required. For example, if the past experience indicates that out of 1000 first pregnancies resulted in the delivery of 550 boys and 450 girls, probability of getting a boy in the first pregnancy is 550/1000 = 0.55 or 55% and that of a girl is 45% . Similarly, if the past data shows that out of 1000 smokers 50 had cancer, probability of getting cancer in a smoker is equal to 50/1000 = 0.05 or 5%

2. Deriving inferences about the population regarding a parameter or a hypothesis from the sample studied: Theory of probability provides the foundation for statistical Inference regarding a parameter or a hypothesis in the population.

Examples:

(a) To estimate the percentage of people affected by diabetes in a country based on the result obtained from a sample of randomly selected persons from that country, confidence limits of the estimate based on the sample statistic can be computed and it can be stated with a certain amount of confidence (say 95% or 99% or 99.9%) that the population value of the percentage of persons affected by diabetes will lie between certain limits. In other words, probability that the population value may lie outside these limits will be 5% or 1% or 0.1%

(b) In case of a clinical trial, if the percentage of patients who showed improvement after receiving the standard drug is 60% and in those receiving the new treatment is 80%, then to test the statistical hypothesis that this difference could occur due to chance and not due to the better effect of the new treatment, a statistical test of significance is done and the probability that this difference could occur due to chance in repeated trials is computed. If this probability is greater than 5% then it is inferred that the difference is only by chance and not real and if the probability is less than 5%, it is inferred that the additional percentage of patients who showed improvement may be due to the better effect of the new drug compared to that of the standard drug.

There are several basic theorems based on which probability theory has been developed. The most important probability theorems are the Addition Theorem, Multiplication Theorem and the Conditional Probability Theorem.

4.2.2. Definitions of Some Basic Terms

Event of a trial/experiment is the result or outcome of that trial/experiment.

Example: If a coin is tossed, there can be two outcomes (events) – getting a head or a tail.

Two events A_1 & A_2 are called **mutually exclusive** if the occurrence of one event precludes the occurrence of the other event. In other words, both the events cannot occur simultaneously.

If A is an event occurring from one trial and B is an event occurring from a second trial and if both the trials are done simultaneously, these two events are called **independent** if the occurrence of event A does not affect the occurrence of the event B.

4.2.3. Addition Theorem

If A, B, C and D are the possible, exhaustive mutually exclusive events in a trial/experiment, then,

P (A or B or C or D) = P (A) + P (B) + P (C) + P (D) = 1

Examples:

Example 1. A 'die' is thrown. What is the probability of getting: (a) 3 or 4, (b) any number between 1 and 6 (excluding 1 & 6)?

Total number of possibilities = 6

(a) Since the events are equally likely and are mutually exclusive, probability of getting 3 or 4 = P (3) + P (4) = 1/6 + 1/6 = 2/6 = 1/3 = 33.3%

(b) Probability of getting any number between 1 & 6 (excluding 1 & 6) = P (2) + P (3) + P (4) + P (5) = 1/6 + 1/6 + 1/6 + 1/6 = 4/6 = 2/3 = 66.7%

Example 2. From a deck of cards, what is the probability of getting (a) ace of spade and (b) spade ace or diamond ace?

A deck of playing cards has 52 cards. When a card is chosen randomly from the deck, total number of possibilities = 52 and events are mutually exclusive.

(a) Probability that the card picked up is ace of spade = 1/52 =1.9%

(b) Probability that the card picked up is spade ace or diamond ace = 1/52 + 1/52
$$= 2/52 = 1/26 = 3.8\%$$

4.2.4. Multiplication Theorem

If A, B, C and D are independent events in trials/experiments, then,

P (A and B and C and D) = P (A) * P (B) * P (C) * P (D)

Examples:

Example 1. Two dice are thrown simultaneously. Find out the probability of getting:

(a) 1 on the first 'die' and 2 on the second 'die'

(b) 1 or 2 on the first 'die' and 4 or 5 or 6 on the second 'die'

Events in the two trials are independent. Probability of getting 1 on the first die = 1/6. Probability of getting 2 on the second die = 1/6.

(a) P (1 on the first die and 2 on the second die) = 1/6 × 1/6 = 1/36 = 2.8%

(b) P (1 or 2 on the first die) = 1/6 + 1/6 = 2/6 = 1/3

P (4 or 5 or 6 on the second die) = 1/6 + 1/6 + 1/6 = 3/6 = 1/2

P (1 or 2 on the first die and 4 or 5 or 6 on the second die = 1/3 × 1/2 = **1/6 =16.7%.**

Example 2. A problem in epidemiology was given to four students A, B, C and D. Their chances of solving it are 1/2, 1/3, 1/4 and 1/5. What is the probability that the problem will be solved by anybody?

Since computing the probability of solving the problem directly will be laborious, the probability of not solving the problem by each student can be found and from this, the probability of solving the problem can be found.

P (not solving the problem by A) = 1 - (1/2) = 1/2

P (not solving the problem by B) = 1 - (1/3) = 2/3

P (not solving the problem by C) = 1 - (1/4) = 3/4

P (not solving the problem by D) = 1 - (1/5) = 4/5

Since these probabilities are independent of each other, P (not solving the problem by anybody) = (1/2) * (2/3) * (3/4) * (4/5) = 24/120 = 1/5.

P (the problem is solved by any of A, B, C & D) = 1- (1/5) = 4/5 = 80%

Example 3. The probability that a 60-year old man will live up to 70 is 0.73 and the probability that a 50-year old woman will live up to 60 is 0.81. What is the probability that a man who is 60 and his wife who is 50, will:

(a) Both be alive 10 year hence?

(b) Only one of them be alive 10 years hence?

(a) P (both alive 10 years hence) = 0.73 * 0.81
$$= 0.5913 = 59.13\% \text{ (both probabilities are independent)}$$

(b) P (only one of them be alive 10 years hence = 0.73 (1 – 0.81) + 0.81(1-0.73)
   = 0.1387 + 0.2187 = 0.3574 = 35.74%

(Probabilities are independent and only one of them is alive, but, it is not known who will be alive.)

Examples of Addition and Multiplication Theorems Combined:

Example 1. In the Microbiology Department in a hospital, Laboratory A has 6 experts and 4 assistants and Laboratory B has 4 experts and 3 assistants. A Laboratory is chosen randomly and a person (expert or assistant) is chosen randomly. Find out:

(a) The probability that the randomly chosen person is an expert.

(b) The probability that the randomly chosen person is an assistant.

P (an expert from the Lab A) = 6/10

P (an expert from the Lab B) = 4/7

The selected Lab could be either A or B; hence,

(a) P (the randomly chosen is an expert)
   = (1/2) {6/10 + 4/7} = (1/2) * (42 + 40) / 70= (1/2) * (82/70) = 41/70 = 58.6%

(b) P (the randomly chosen is an assistant) = 1-(41/70)
   = 29/70 = 41.4%, since the total probability = 1

Example 2. In a clinical trial, two-thirds of the patients received Drug A and the rest, Drug B. It is known that the probability that a patient receiving Drug A will be cured is 0.3 and the probability that a patient receiving Drug B will be cured is 0.35. Find the probability that:

(a) A patient chosen at random will be cured.

(b) The randomly chosen patient is not cured.

(a) P (a patient chosen at random will be cured) = {(2/3) * (0.3)} + {(1/3) * (0.35)}
   = 0.2 + 0.1167 = 0.3167 = 31.67%

(b) P (the randomly chosen patient is not cured) = 1 – 0.3167 = 0.6833 = 68.33%
   or = P {(2/3) * (0.7) + (1/3) * (0.65)} = 68.33%

4.2.5. Conditional Probability

If A & B are two dependent events, then the probability that a randomly selected individual has A, given that he already has B is obtained using the Multiplication Theorem taking into consideration that the two events are not independent:

P(A|B) = P (A) * P(B|A)

Examples:

Example 1. In a locality consisting of 1000 persons, 200 were attacked by cholera. In the population a total of 700 had been vaccinated against it. Among vaccinated only 50 were attacked. Find out the probability that:

(a) A randomly selected person is attacked given that he is not vaccinated.

(b) A randomly selected person is not attacked and given that he is vaccinated.

The above data can be presented in a 2 * 2 contingency table as follows:

	Attacked	*Not attacked*	*Total*
Vaccinated	50	650	700
Not vaccinated	150	150	300
Total	200	800	1000

P (the randomly selected person is vaccinated)   = 700/1000 = 7/10
P (the randomly selected person is unvaccinated) = 300/1000 = 3/10
P (the randomly selected person is attacked)   = 200/1000 = 2/10
P (the randomly selected person is not attacked) = 800/1000 = 8/10

(a) P (the randomly selected person is attacked given that he is not vaccinated) =
    P (attacked) * P (not vaccinated in attacked) = (2/10) * (150/200) = 3/20 = 15%
    (Conditional probability)

(b) P (the randomly selected person is not attacked given that he is vaccinated)
    = P (not attacked) * P (vaccinated in not attacked) = (8/10) * (650/800)
    = 13/20 = 65%

Example 2. 20% of the patients admitted in a hospital are suffering from heart disease and 30% of the hospital patients are children. 50% of children are having heart disease. Find out probability that:

(a) A randomly selected patient is a child given that he has heart disease.
(b) A randomly selected patient is an adult with heart disease.

	Heart disease	*No heart disease*	*Total*
Adult	5	65	70
Child	15	15	30
Total	20	80	100

P (children) = 30% = 0.3; P (heart patient) = 20% = 0.2
P (Heart disease in children) = 15/30 = 50%

(a) P (Randomly selected patient is a child given that he has heart disease)
    = P (child) * P (heart disease in children) = 0.3 * 0.5 = 0.15 = 15 %

(b) P (Randomly selected patient is an adult given that he has heart disease)
    = P (adult) * P (heart disease in adults) = (7/10) * (5/70) = 35/700=5/100 = 1/20 = 5 %

4.2.6. Bayes Theorem

The concept of conditional probability can be used in medical diagnosis using Bayes Theorem. Bayes Theorem can be stated as follows:

$$P(D+|S+) = \frac{P(D+) * P(S+|D+)}{[P(D+) * P(S+|D+)] + [P(D-) * P(S+|D-)]}$$

D+: Presence of the disease; D-: Absence of the disease
S+: Presence of the symptom, S-: Absence of the symptom

$$P(D+|S+) = \frac{\text{Diseased with symptom}}{\text{Total with symptom}} = \frac{A}{B}$$

Where, A = P(D+) * P (S+|D+) and
B = (With S+ in D+) + (With S+ in D-)
= P(D+|S+) + P(D-|S+)
= [P(D+) * P(S+|D+] + [P(D-) * P(S+|D-)]

$$P(D+|S+) = A \mid B = \frac{P(D+) * P(S+/D+)}{[P(D+) * P(S+/D+)] + [P(D-) * P(S+/D-)]}$$

Examples:

Example 1. In a group of 20 subjects, 6 were found to be having respiratory disease and the remaining normal with respect to this disease. In all the subjects, presence or absence of the symptom 'cough'(S) was noted and the information on this is tabulated below:

Disease Group		Normal Group	
1.	S+	1.	S–
2.	S–	2.	S+
3.	S–	3.	S–
4.	S+	4.	S+
5.	S+	5.	S–
6.	S+	6.	S–
		7.	S+
		8.	S–
		9.	S–
		10.	S–
		11.	S+
		12.	S–
		13.	S–
		14.	S+

Applying Bayes theorem, find the probability that:

(a) A randomly selected person having cough is declared a patient.

(b) A randomly selected person not having cough is declared a patient.

$$P(D+) = \frac{3}{10} \qquad P(D-) = \frac{7}{10}$$

$$P(S+ \text{ in } D+) = \frac{4}{6} \qquad P(S+ \text{ in } D-) = \frac{5}{14}$$

(a) $P(D+|S+) = \dfrac{P(D+) * P(S+|D+)}{\left[P(D+) * P(S+|D+)\right] + \left[P(D-) * P(S+|D-)\right]} = \dfrac{\dfrac{3}{10} * \dfrac{4}{6}}{\dfrac{1}{5} + \left[\dfrac{7}{10} * \dfrac{5}{14}\right]} = \dfrac{\dfrac{1}{5}}{\dfrac{1}{5} + \dfrac{1}{4}} = 4/9$

(b) $P(D+|S-) = \dfrac{P(D+) * \left[1 - P(S+|D+)\right]}{P(D+) * \left[1 - P(S+|D+)\right] + P(D-) * \left[1 - P(S+|D-)\right]} = \dfrac{\dfrac{3}{10} * \dfrac{2}{6}}{\dfrac{1}{10} + \left[\dfrac{7}{10} * \dfrac{9}{14}\right]} = \dfrac{\dfrac{1}{10}}{\dfrac{1}{10} + \dfrac{9}{20}} = 2/11$

Example 2. Records of two symptoms, cough (S_1) and breathlessness (S_2), of 6 patients (D+) of respiratory disease and 4 normal persons (D–) are given below:

Data:

	D+	D–	
1.	$S_1 + S_2 +$	$S_1 + S_2 -$	$(P(D+) = \dfrac{6}{10} = 0.6$
2.	$S_1 - S_2 +$	$S_1 - S_2 -$	$P(D-) = 0.4$

3. $S_1 - S_2 +$ $\qquad$ $S_1 - S_2 +$ $\qquad$ $P(S_1 + inD+) = \dfrac{3}{6} = 0.5$

4. $S_1 + S_2 -$ $\qquad$ $S_1 - S_2 -$ $\qquad$ $P(S_2 + inD+) = \dfrac{4}{6} = \dfrac{2}{3} = 0.67$

5. $S_1 + S_2 +$ $\qquad\qquad\qquad\qquad\qquad$ $P(S_1 + / D-) = \dfrac{1}{4} = 0.25$

6. $S_1 - S_2 -$ $\qquad\qquad\qquad\qquad\qquad$ $P(S_2 + /D-) = \dfrac{1}{4} = 0.25$

Find the probabilities that:

    (a) A randomly selected person having cough, but no breathlessness is taken as a patient.

    (b) A randomly selected person having cough, but no breathlessness is taken as a normal person.

Probability that a randomly selected person having cough but no breathlessness is taken as a patient is given by the Bayes theorem,

$$P(D+|S_1+, S_2-) = \frac{P(D+) * P(S_1+|D+) * [1 - P(S_2+|D+)]}{\{P(D+) * P(S_1+|D+) * [1 - P(S_2+|D)]\} + \{P(D-) * P(S_1+|D-) * [1 - P(S_2+|D-)]\}}$$

(If the symptom is present, the Probability is computed as P (S+|D+) and if the symptom is absent, the probability is computed as 1- P (S+|D+) in case of those diagnosed with the disease and similarly for those without the disease.)

$$P[D+|S_1+, S_2-] = \frac{\dfrac{6}{10} * \dfrac{3}{6} * \dfrac{2}{6}}{\left(\dfrac{6}{10} * \dfrac{3}{6} * \dfrac{2}{6}\right) + \left(\dfrac{4}{10} * \dfrac{1}{4} * \dfrac{3}{4}\right)} = \frac{\dfrac{1}{10}}{\dfrac{1}{10} + \dfrac{3}{40}} = \frac{\dfrac{1}{10}}{\dfrac{7}{40}} = \dfrac{1}{10} * \dfrac{40}{7} = 4/7$$

$$P(D-/S_1+, S_2-) = \frac{P(D-) * P(S_1+|D-) * [1 - P(S_2+|D-)]}{\{P(D+) * P(S_1+|D+) * [1 - P(S_2+|D+)]\} + \{P(D-) * P(S_1|D-) * [1 - P(S_2+|D-)]\}}$$

$$P(D-|S_1+, S_2-) = \frac{\dfrac{4}{10} * \dfrac{1}{4} * \dfrac{3}{4}}{\dfrac{7}{40}} = \frac{\dfrac{3}{40}}{\dfrac{7}{40}} = 3/7$$

or $P(D-|S_1+, S_2-) = 1 - P(D+|S_1+, S_2-) = \left(1 - \dfrac{4}{7}\right) = 3/7$

4.3. Probability Distributions

A series of probabilities associated with various occurrences/outcomes/possibilities of events in an experiment/trial/study will generate a probability distribution. Basically, there are three types of probability distributions: Binomial, Poisson and Normal. Binomial and Poisson distributions are for discrete variables (countable) and Normal distribution is for continuous (measurable) variables.

4.3.1. Permutation and Combination (Fig. 4.1)

Permutation is the process of selecting a group of elements (r) from a total of available elements (n) and arranging them in a certain order (r < = n). It is written as ^nP_r. It is computed as $^nP_r = n! / (n-r)!$.

Where n! = n * (n-1) * (n-2) * (n-3) * ….. * 1; and 0! = 1

Note: ! is a sign called factorial, and * is a sign representing multiplication.

Combination is the process of selecting a group of elements (r) from a total of available elements (n) and arranging them without any regard to the order of arrangement. It is written as $^{n}C_{r}$ and computed as = n! /{r! * (n-r) !}

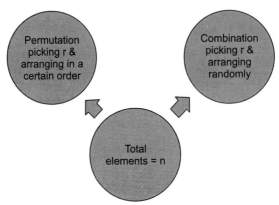

Fig. 4.1: Permutation and combination

Examples:

Example 1. If there are 10 food preparations and three have to be given to a patient, the number of ways these can be selected will be a Combination problem since the order of food preparations does not matter.

$10C_{3}$ = 10 !/{3! * (10-3)!} ! = 10 !/(3! * 7!) = (8 * 9 *10)/6 = **120.** Thus, three dishes can be selected from 10 dishes in 120 ways.

Example 2. In a hospital kitchen, there are 3 categories of food items: vegetarian, non-vegetarian and dessert. There are 5 veg. food items, 4 non-veg. food items and 3 desserts. Out of these, if 1 non-veg. and 2 veg. food items and 1 dessert have to be selected, the number of ways it can be done is a Combination problem since the order of dishes does not matter.

The number of ways it can be done = $4C_{1}$ * $5C_{2}$ * $3C_{1}$
= (4! / 3 !) * 5!/ (3! * 2!) * 3! / (2 !) = (4 * 4 * 5 * 3) / 2 = **120**

Example 3. If there are 6 patients for a surgery on a specific day and the number of operation theatres available is only 2, how many ways these patients can be operated in these two theatres is a Permutation problem, because the order of patients allocated to the 2 operation theatres matters.

The number of ways it can be done = $6P_{2}$ = 6! / (6-2) ! = 6!/4! = 5 * 6 = **30**

4.3.2. Binomial Distribution

It describes the distribution of discrete variables giving probabilities of various outcomes of the trial/experiment. This distribution was developed by the Swiss mathematician James Bernoulli (1654-1705). Assume that an event of a trial can happen in two different ways, say, "favorable" and "unfavorable" (positive and negative; living and dead; cured and not cured, etc.). A favorable result may be called a success and an unfavorable one, a failure. Let 'p' be the probability of a success (neither close to zero nor to one) and q (=1-p), the probability of failure. If the trial is repeated n times under essentially the same conditions, then the probability of getting exactly x successes in the n repeated trials is given by Binomial distribution.

- Probability of getting success in the first x trials = p^{x}
- Probability of getting failures in the remaining (n- x) trials = $q^{(n-x)}$

- Probability of getting success in the first x trials and failure in the remaining (n-x) trials = $p^x q^{(n-x)}$, since all the trials are independent. This is the probability of getting x successes and (n-x) failures in a particular order.

Exactly x successes in n independent trials can occur in ^nC_x ways. Therefore, probability of getting exactly x successes and (n-x) failures in all possible orders is given by $^nC_x p^x q^{(n-x)}$. This expression is known as Binomial distribution or function or Bernoulli function. This can be expressed as,

$$P(x) = {}^nC_x p^x q^{(n-x)} = \frac{n! \, p^x q^{(n-x)}}{x! \, (n-x)!}$$

The whole Binomial distribution probabilities can be written as,

$$(p+q)^n = P \, (x = 0 \text{ to } n) = {}^nC_n \, p^n \, q^0 + {}^nC_{(n-1)} \, p^{(n-1)} q^1 + {}^nC_{(n-2)} \, p^{(n-2)} q^2 + \ldots \ldots$$
$$\ldots \ldots + {}^nC_0 \, p^0 q^n = 1$$

The Binomial distribution has the property called 'additive property'. Thus, probability of getting less than 3 successes in 5 trials can be computed by adding:

$$P(x=2) + P(x=1) + P \, (x=0)$$

Probability of getting more than 2 successes can be computed as:

$$P \, (x=3) + P \, (x=4) + P \, (x=5)$$

Two useful quantities in the practical applications involving binomial distribution are the mean of binomial distribution and standard deviation of binomial distribution. **Mean of a binomial distribution is given by np**. This is also called 'expected value' (expected number of successes). **Standard deviation of the binomial distribution is given by** $\sqrt{npq}$.

Examples:

Example 1. It has been found that probability of getting a male child is equal to the probability of getting a female child (p = q = ½). In a family with a size of 5 children, what is the probability of getting:

    (a) 2 males,   (b) at least 1 male,

    (b) at the most 1 male,   (d) all females

    (a) $P \, (2 \, M) = {}^5C_2 \, (1/2)^2 \, (1/2)^3 = 10 * (1/2)^5 =$ **10/32 = 31.25%**

    (b) $P \, (\text{at least } 1 \, M) = 1 - P \, (0 \, M)$

          $P \, (0 \, M) = {}^5C_0 \, (1/2)^0 \, (1/2)^5 = (1/2)^5 =$ **1/32 = 3.125%**

          $P \, (\text{at least } 1 \, M) = 1 - (1/32) =$ **31/32 = 96.875%**

    (c) $P \, (\text{at the most } 1 \, M) = P \, (0 \, M) + P \, (1 \, M)$

          $= {}^5C_0 \, (½)^5 + {}^5C_1 \, (½)^5 = (1/32) \, \{ {}^5C_0 + {}^5C_1) = (1/32) \times 5$

          = **5/32 = 15.625%**

    (d) $P \, (\text{all } F) = P \, (0 \, M) =$ **1/32 = 3.125%**

Example 2. Suppose that the probability is 0.55 for the birth of a male child and that two successive births are independent. If a woman is to have three children, the possibilities are: 3M, 2M & 1F, 1M & 2F and 3F.

The binomial expression is given by $(p+q)^n = (\, 0.55 + 0.45 \,)^3$

$= {}^3C_3 \, (0.55)^3 (0.45)^0 + {}^3C_2 (0.55)^2 (0.45)^1 + {}^3C_1 (0.55)^1 (0.45)^2 + {}^3C_0 (0.55)^0 (.45)^3$

$= 0.166375 + 0.408375 + 0.334125 + 0.091125 = 1$

For the above given data, find:

    (a) The probability that she will have 1 boy and 2 girls;

    (b) The probability that she will have children of both sexes;

    (c) The probability that she will have son, daughter and son in that order;

    (d) The probability that she will have at least 2 sons.

P (B) = 0.55; P (G) = 0.45

(a) P (1B & 2 G) = $^3C_1$ * 0.55 * 0.45 * 0.45 = 3 * 0.111375 = **0.3341**

(b) P (children of both sexes) = P (1B & 2 G or 2B & 1 G)

   P (1B & 2 G) = 0.3341; P (2B & 1 G) = $3C_2$ * 0.55 * 0.55 * 0.45 = 0.4084

   P (children of both sexes) = 0.3341 + 0.4084 = **0.7425**

(c) P (B, G, B in that order) = 0.55 * 0.45 * 0.55 = **0.1361**

(d) P (at least 2 B) = P (2B & 1 G or 3B & 0 G)

   = $\{^3C_2 (0.55)^2 * 0.45\} + \{^3C_3 (0.55)^3\}$

   = 0.4084 + 0.1664 = **0.5748**

Example 3. Suppose the fatality rate of a certain disease has been observed as 30% in children. If there are 500 children in a small town with the disease, what is the expected number of deaths resulting from this disease? Also find out the SD

p (fatality) = 0.3 ; q = 0.7 n = 500

Expected number of deaths resulting from the disease= 0.3 * 500 = **150**

$$SD = \sqrt{npq} = \sqrt{(500 * 0.3 * 0.7} = \mathbf{10.25}$$

Example 4. From a previous experience on a large series of allergy patients, it had been noted that 60% gave positive reaction to a certain skin test. An allergy clinic tested an average of 10 patients per day. Find out the probability that among the 10 patients:

(a) All gave +ve reactions, (b) 3 gave +ve reaction, (c) at least 1 gave +ve reaction, and (d) at the most 1 gave +ve reaction.

   P (+) = 0.6

(a) P (all the 10 +) = $^{10}C_{10} (0.6)^{10}$ = **0.006**

(b) P (3+) = $^{10}C_3 (0.6)^3 (0.4)^7$ = **0.0425**

(c) P (at least 1 +) = 1- P (0 +) = $1-(0.4)^{10}$ = 1-0.0001 = **0.9999**

(d) P (at most 1 +) = P (1 +) + P (0 +)

   = $(0.4)^{10} + {}^{10}C_1 (0.6) (0.4)^9$ = **0.0017**

Example 5. Case fatality rate previously recorded for a particular disease has been 0.3. What is the probability that three successive cases recently admitted in a hospital could be fatal?

P (fatality) = 0.3, P (3 deaths) = $^3C_3 (0.3)^3 (0.7)^0$ = **0.027**

Example 6. The five-year survival rate of a large series of cancer patients has been 40%. Five patients, with a particular type and stage of cancer, were subjected to a new form of treatment:

(a) If survival under new treatment was really the same as under the old, what is the probability that all 5 patients would be living at the end of 5 years?

(b) What is the probability that at least 4 will be living five years or more with the new treatment?

p = 0.4 q = 0.6

(a) P (all 5 will survive at the end of 5 years) = $5C_5 (0.4)^5 (0.6)^0$ = **0.01024**

(b) P (at least 4 will survive at the end of 5 years) = P (5) + P (4)

   = $^5C_5 (0.4)^5 (0.6)^0 + {}^5C_4 (0.4)^4 (0.6)^1$

   = 0.01024 + 0.0768 = **0.0870**

Example 7. A virus suspension is prepared, and it is found that when a certain quantity is inoculated into eggs, 25% of eggs (p = 0.25) become infected. If a random group of 3 eggs is inoculated, what are the probabilities that (a) none, (b) one and (c) two eggs become infected, (e) if at one time 1,000 eggs are inoculated, find the average number of eggs being infected. Also find the SD.

(a) P (0 infected) = $^3C_0$ (0.25) ^{0}(0.75)^3 = **0.4219**
(b) P (2 infected) = $^3C_2$ (0.25) ^{2}(0.75) = **0.1406**
(c) P (3 infected) = $^3C_3$ (0.25) ^{3}(0.75)^0 = **0.0156**

Average number of eggs infected out of 1000 eggs = Mean = np = 1000 × 0.25 = **250**

$$SD = \sqrt{npq} = \sqrt{1000 * 0.25 * 0.75} = 13.69$$

Example 8. Suppose for a particular disease, the case fatality rate for many years with the standard treatment is 0.8.

(a) What is the probability that 3 patients having the same disease will survive with the treatment? (b) If in a town, there are 500 patients of the same disease, find the average number of survivors with the standard treatment. Also find the SD.

p = 0.2; q = 0.8
(a) P (all 3 will survive) = $^3C_3$(0.2) ^{3} = **0.008**
(b) Average number of survivors out of 500 patients = mean = np
    = 500 × 0.2 = **100**

$$SD = \sqrt{npq} = \sqrt{500 * 0.2 * 0.8} = 8.94$$

Example 9. The incidence of occupational disease in an industry is such that the workers have a 20% chance of suffering from it. What is the probability that out of 6 workers chosen at random:
(a) 5 will suffer from the disease?
(b) 5 or more will suffer from the disease?
    p = 20 % = 0.2
(a) P (5 will suffer from the disease out of 6) = $^6C_5$ (0.2)^5 (0.8)
    = **0.001536**
(b) P (5 or more will suffer from the disease) = P (5 will suffer) + P (6 will suffer)
    P (6 will suffer) = $^6C_6$ (0.2)^6 = 0.000064
    P (5 or more will suffer from the disease = 0.001536 + 0.000064 = **0.0016**

4.3.3. Poisson Distribution

If the probability (p) of a defined event to happen is extremely small (rare event) in a large number of trials (n) done under the same conditions, the distribution of the various occurrences follows Poisson distribution. In other words, when n tends to infinity and p tends to zero, the distribution is Poisson, i. e., Poisson distribution is the limiting form of the Binomial distribution. For all practical purposes, n can be taken as 100 or more and p can be taken as 0.05 or smaller and in such a way that np is less than 5. The Poisson distribution was developed by the French mathematician Simon Poisson (1781-1840). The form of the Poisson distribution is given by:

$$f(x) = \frac{e^{-\lambda}\lambda^x}{x!}$$

where λ is the mean value of the Poisson variable and x is the outcome
(0, 1, 2,...., ∞)

The probabilities of the various outcomes under a Poisson distribution are given by:

$$f(x = 0, 1, 2, \& n) = \sum_{x=0}^{n} \frac{e^{-\lambda}\lambda^x}{x!}$$, where λ is the Mean of the Poisson variate, which is equal to np and stan-

dard deviation = $\sqrt{(np)}$. Value of $e^{-\lambda}$ can be obtained by multiplying $-\lambda$ by 0.4343 (log (e)—log to the base e) and taking its antilogarithm value.

Like the Binomial distribution, Poisson distribution also has the additive property, i.e., P (x less than 3) = P (0) + P (1) + P (2)

P (x = 2 or 3) = P (2) + P (3)

Examples:

Example 1. The mortality rate for a certain disease was found to be 3 per 1000. What is the probability of:

    (a) Just 3 deaths from this disease in a group of 500 persons?

    (b) Getting less than or equal to 5 deaths (probability of getting at the most 5 deaths)?

    (c) Getting at least 1 death?

       (group size is 500 for b & c also)

P = 0.003, q = 0.997, n = 500, np = 1.5 < 5, and, hence, the distribution of deaths from this disease is Poisson. ($e^{-1.5} = 0.2231$: $e^{-1.5}$ = A, Log (A) = $-1.5 \times$ log (e) to the base 10 = -1.5×0.4343 = - 0.65145, A= Antilog of (- 0.64145) = 0.2231). Note the minus sign for 0.64145.

    (a) P (3 deaths) = $\dfrac{e^{-\lambda}\lambda^3}{3!}$

$$= \dfrac{0.2231}{6} * (1.5)^3$$

$$= 0.1255$$

    (b) P ($\leq$ 5 deaths) = P(0) + P(1) + P(2) + P(3) + P(4) + P(5)

$$= e^{-\lambda} + \lambda e^{-\lambda} + \frac{\lambda^2}{2!}e^{-\lambda} + \frac{\lambda^3}{3!}e^{-\lambda} + \frac{\lambda^4}{4!}e^{-\lambda} + \frac{\lambda^5}{5!}e^{-\lambda}$$

$$= e^{-\lambda}\left(1 + \lambda + \frac{\lambda^2}{2} + \frac{\lambda^3}{6} + \frac{\lambda^4}{24} + \frac{\lambda^5}{120}\right)$$

$$= 0.2231\left(1 + 1.5 + \frac{(1.5)^2}{2} + \frac{(1.5)^3}{6} + \frac{(1.5)^4}{24} + \frac{(1.5)^5}{120}\right)$$

$$= 0.2231(1 + 1.5 + 1.125 + 0.5625 + 0.5625 + 0.2109 + 0.0633$$

$$= 0.9954$$

    (c) P (at least 1 death) = 1 - P (no death)

$$= 1 - e^{-\lambda} = 1 - 0.2231$$

$$= 0.7769$$

Example 2. If a particular dose of Phenobarbital produces high giddiness in a receiver with a probability of 0.005,

    (a) What is the probability that exactly 3 patients will have reactions out of 200 who are going to receive this?

    (b) Find out the probability that at the most 1 will get reaction.

    (c) At least one will get reaction (e^{-1}= 0.3679).

       p = 0.005, n = 200, np = 1 < 5 and, hence, the distribution of giddiness of those who received Phenobarbital is Poisson.

    (a) $P(x = 3) = \dfrac{e^{-\lambda}\lambda^3}{3!} = \dfrac{.3679}{6} = 0.0613$

(b) P (at the most 1) = P(x = 0) + P(x = 1)

$$\frac{e^{-\lambda}\lambda^0}{0!} + \frac{e^{-\lambda}\lambda^1}{1!}$$

$$= e^{-\lambda}(1+1) = 2 * 0.3679$$

$$= 0.7358$$

(c) P (at least 1) = 1–P(x = 0)

$$= 1 - \left[\frac{e^{-1}(1)^0}{0!}\right]$$

$$= 1 - e^{-1}$$

$$= 1 - 0.3679 = 0.6321$$

Example 3. It is 1 in 1,000 that a twin birth takes place in a town and on any one day, 100 births occur. Find the probability that one or more twins are born.

$$p = \frac{1}{1000} = 0.001$$

n = 100

$\lambda = 100 * 0.001 = 0.1$

$e^{-\lambda} = 0.9048$

$P(x \geq 1) = 1 - P(x = 0)$

$= 1 - P(x = 0) = 1 - 0.9048 = 0.0952$

Example 4. Red blood cells deficiency may be determined by examining a specimen of the blood under a microscope. Suppose a certain small fixed volume contains, on an average, 5 red cells for normal persons. Using Poisson distribution, obtain the probability that a specimen from a normal person will contain 2 or more cells ($e^{-5} = 0.0067$).

Mean = 5

$P (x >= 2) = 1 - \{P (0) + P (1)\}$

$P (0) = 0.0067$, $P(1) = 0.0067 \times 5 = 0.0335$, $P(0) + P(1) = 0.0402$

$P (x >= 2) = 1 - 0.0402 = 0.9598$

Many a times, problems may be encountered where definition of success and failure can be made, but while it is possible to count the number of successes in the trials, it may not be possible to count the number of failures. For example, one can count the number of times an adult person gets measles, but it is not possible to count the number of time he does not get measles, in a defined period of time. In such a situation also, the distribution of the variable will be Poisson. Here also p (success) is very small and n is very large and np will be a finite number (say, n > 100 and mean is less than 5)

Example 5. The following table gives the distribution of visits to the physician by 100 persons in a locality during a particular year:

No. of visits(x)	No. of persons(f)
0.	10
1.	20
2.	40
3.	15
4.	10
5.	5
	100 (n)

Find out the probability that:
(a) A randomly selected person has not visited the physician at all during the last year ($e^{-2.1}=0.1225$)
(b) He has visited the physician at least once.
(c) At the most once
(d) Visited the physician thrice.

$$\lambda = \text{Mean} = \left\{\sum fx\right\}/n = \frac{210}{100} = 2.1$$

$$e^{-2.1} = 0.1225$$

(a) $P(x = 0) = e^{-\lambda} = 0.1225$

(b) $P(\text{at least once}) = 1 - P(x = 0)$
$$= 1 - 0.1225 = 0.8775$$

(c) $P(\text{at the most one}) = P(x = 0) + P(x = 1)$
$$= e^{\lambda} + \lambda e^{-\lambda}$$
$$= e^{-\lambda}(1 + \lambda) = 0.1225 * 3.1 = 0.3798$$

(d) $P(x = 3) = e^{-\lambda}\dfrac{\lambda^3}{3!} = \dfrac{(2.1)^3(0.1225)}{6} = 0.1891$

4.3.4. Normal Distribution

This distribution describes the distribution of a continuous variable. The most important probability distribution in statistical inference is normal distribution (Gaussian distribution). The person who developed this distribution was Karl F. Gauss (1777-1855) and, hence, it is also called 'Gaussian' distribution. The distribution is called 'normal', not because all other distributions are 'abnormal', but because it was found that many distributions of many continuous variables in biology and other sciences followed this particular distribution. The Belgian mathematician Quetelet (1796-1874) noticed that the distribution of heights of army people approximated to a normal curve. Later it was observed that many other biological variables followed Normal distribution.

Normal distribution is very important in applied statistics since most of the biological variables follow normal distribution. Also, even if the distribution of the values of the variable is not normal, if the sample size studied is large enough, normal distribution can be assumed for all practical purposes based on an important theorem in statistical theory, called Central Limit Theorem. It states that if the sample size is large enough, the sampling distribution of mean follows normal distribution.

The Normal distribution has two parameters – mean & variance (square of SD). The distribution is completely described by these two parameters. The typical normal curve, generated from the normal distribution is shown in Fig. 4.2.

The functional form of the Normal distribution is expressed as:

$$f(x) = \frac{1}{\sqrt{\sigma 2\pi}} e^{\frac{1}{2\sigma^2}(x-\mu)^2}$$ where x ranges from $-\infty$ to $+\infty$, σ is the population standard deviation of the variable,

μ is the population mean of the variable, X is the sample value and $\pi = 22/7$. The total area under the normal curve will be equal to "1".

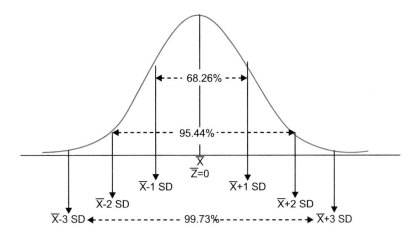

Fig. 4.2: Normal (Gaussian) curve

4.4. Properties of Normal Curve

1. It is bell shaped & symmetric.
2. The three types of averages — the mean, the median & the mode will be equal. But, practically, they will be almost equal.
3. Fifty percent of the sample values will lie on the left of the perpendicular drawn on the middle and the remaining 50% will lie on the right of this line.
4. Mean – 1 SD & mean + 1 SD will include about 68% of the sample values.
5. Mean – 2 SD & Mean + 2 SD will include about 95% of the sample values.
6. Mean – 3 SD & mean + 3 SD will include about 99% of the sample values.
7. Theoretically, the curve touches the horizontal line only at the infinity.
8. **(Sample value – mean)/SD,** which is called **Standard Normal Deviate (SND)** or **Z- score**, is distributed with a mean of "0" and an SD of "1", whatever the variable may be. This is a very important property of the Normal distribution. Inference theory is based on this property.

For every set of mean and standard deviation, there will be separate normal distribution depending upon the values of mean and standard deviation of the different variables. To avoid the inconvenience of comput-ing probabilities from normal distributions using different means and standard deviation values, statisticians adopted a convenient method of converting all normal curves to Unique normal curve having the same mean value (zero) and the same standard deviation (one), irrespective of the variable. Once the original values are converted to their SND values, the mean is zero and standard deviation is one, whatever the variable may be. This is nothing but changing the origin and scale of values by subtracting a constant quantity from each value of the variable and dividing it by a constant. The constant subtracted is the corresponding mean and the constant by which the resultant value is divided is the corresponding standard deviation, i.e., $\dfrac{(X - \bar{X})}{SD}$.

The property of standard normal deviate 'Z' (mean = 0 and SD = 1) is illustrated in the following two examples:

Example 1. The following values are the ages (years) of 5 cancer patients: 60, 55, 65, 72, 48.

Age (yrs.) (X)	X^2	$(X - \bar{X})$	$(X - \bar{X})^2$	$Z = \dfrac{(X - \bar{X})}{SD}$	Z^2
60	3600	0	0	0	0
55	3025	-5	25	−0.5439	0.2958
65	4225	5	25	+0.5439	0.2958
72	5184	12	144	+1.3054	1.7041
48	2304	-12	144	−1.3054	1.7041
Total	300	18338	0	338	0	3.9998

$$\text{Mean}_x = \frac{300}{5} = 60$$

$$SD_x = \sqrt{\frac{18338 - \dfrac{(300)^2}{5}}{4}} = \sqrt{\frac{338}{4}} = 9.1924$$

$$\text{Mean}_z = \frac{\sum z}{n} = \frac{0}{5} = 0$$

$$SD_z = \sqrt{\frac{\sum Z^2 - \dfrac{(\sum Z)^2}{n}}{(n-1)}} = \sqrt{\frac{3.9998 - 0}{4}} = 0.99997 = 1$$

Example 2. The following are the birth weights in kg of 7 babies born in a hospital: 2.8, 2.5, 3.0, 3.2, 2.6, 3.3 and 3.6.

BW (X)	X^2	$(X - \bar{X})$	$(X - \bar{X})^2$	$Z = \dfrac{(X - \bar{X})}{SD}$	Z^2
2.8	7.84	-0.2	0.04	-0.5053	0.2553
2.5	6.25	-0.5	0.25	-1.2633	1.5959
3.0	9.00	0	0.00	0	0
3.2	10.24	0.2	0.04	0.5053	0.2553
2.6	6.76	-0.4	0.16	-1.0106	1.0213
3.3	10.89	0.3	0.09	0.7579	0.5744
3.6	12.96	0.6	0.36	1.5160	2.2982
Total	21.0	63.94	0	0.94	0	6.0004

$$\text{Mean}_x = \frac{21}{7} = 3$$

$$SD_x = \sqrt{\frac{63.94 - \dfrac{(21)^2}{7}}{6}} = \sqrt{\frac{63.94 - 63}{6}} = \sqrt{\frac{0.94}{6}} = 0.3958$$

$$\text{Mean}_z = 0$$

$$SD_z = \sqrt{\frac{6.0004 - 0}{6}} = 1.0$$

In the above examples the mean of the SND is zero and the standard deviation is one in both the variables – age and birth weight. While the unit of measurement of age is years and of birth weight is kg, SND has no unit of measurement. SND ranges from –1 to + 1 depending upon whether the value of the variable is above or below the mean.

4.4.1. Divergence (Deviation) from Normality

There are many variables the values of which may not be following normal distribution, resulting in certain type of deviation from normality. This departure from normality can be of two types: skewness and kurtosis.

4.4.1.1. Skewness

It defines the departure from symmetry of the distribution. In normal distribution, which is symmetric, 50% of the values will be below the mean (which is also the median and the mode) and the remaining 50% will be above the median. Also, the two quartiles Q1 and Q3 will be equidistant from the median. The tendency of the distribution to depart from symmetry is called skewness.

Two types of skewness can be defined depending upon the concentration of values with respect to the median. If more values are concentrated above the mean, it is called negative skewness; and if more values are concentrated below the mean, it is called positive skewness. If the values are symmetrically distributed on either sides of the median, there is no skewness and it is normal curve (Figs. 4.3 to 4.5).

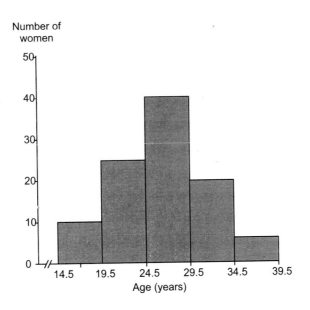

Fig. 4.3: Histogram of the data following normal distribution

The extent of departure from symmetry can be measured statistically. There are many measures of skewness, which are used. Some of them are more accurate, but difficult to compute and some others are simple to compute. One of the simple measures of skewness is in terms of the quartiles.

Since Q_1 and Q_3 are equidistant from the median in case of a normal distribution, any deviation from this is taken as a relative measure of skewness.

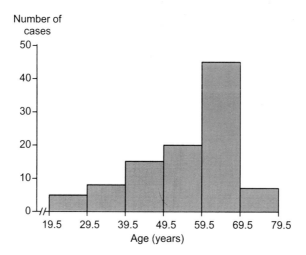

Fig. 4.4: Histogram of data following negatively skewed distribution

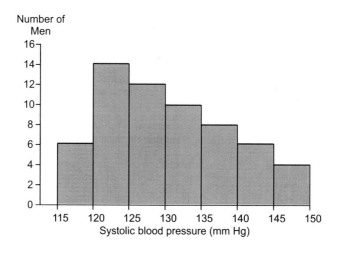

Fig. 4.5: Histogram of data following positively skewed distribution

Bowley's Quartile Coefficient of skewness $= \text{Sk}_1 = \dfrac{\{(Q_3 - M) - (M - Q_1)\}}{(Q_3 - Q_1)}$, where M is the Median.

If this value is equal to zero, it is symmetric distribution and there is no skewness. If this value is positive, the distribution is positively skewed and if it is negative, it is negatively skewed. The extent of skewness will be high or low depending upon the magnitude of this value.

Another simple measure of skewness is given in terms of mean and mode:

Pearson's Coefficient of skewness $= \text{Sk}_2 = \dfrac{(\text{Mean} - \text{Mode})}{\text{SD}}$ or $= \dfrac{3\,(\text{Mean-Median})}{\text{SD}}$

A third measure of skewness is given in terms of the percentiles:

Kelly's Percentile Coefficient of skewness $= \text{Sk}_3 = \dfrac{(P_{90} + P_{10} - 2\,P_{50})}{(P_{90} - P_{10})}$ where P_{50} is the Median.

4.4.1.2. Kurtosis

Another kind of deviation from normality is called kurtosis. It gives the extent of peakedness of the curve. In this type of departure, the curve may be symmetric, but the peakedness may be either high or low compared to that of normal curve. If the peakedness is high as shown in Fig. 4.6a, it is called leptokurtic and if it is low, as shown in Fig. 4.6c, it is called platykurtic. If the peakedness is moderate as shown in Fig. 4.6b, it is normokurtic or mesokurtic, which is in case of normal curve.

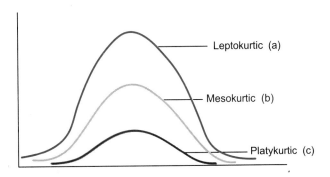

Fig. 4.6: Different types of kurtosis [a. leptokurtic; b. mesokurtic; c. platykurtic]

A simple measure of kurtosis is given in terms of the relative measures Q_1, Q_3, P_{90} and P_{10}.

$$K = \left\{ \frac{Q_3 - Q_1}{2(P_{90} - P_{10})} \right\}$$. It has been shown that if K is equal to 0.263, the curve is normokurtic; if it is greater than 0.263, it is platykurtic; and if it is less than 0.263, it is leptokurtic. The extent of kurtosis is decided based on the magnitude of this statistic.

Examples

Example 1. The following table gives the distribution of 100 women admitted in a maternal hospital. Computation of various statistical parameters (mean, median, mode, standard deviation (SD) and measures of skewness and kurtosis) and the properties of normal distribution are given below:

1. Mean and SD

Age group (years)	Mid age (X)	No. of women (f)	fx	fx²
15-19	17	10	170	2890
20-24	22	25	550	12100
25-29	27	40	1080	29160
30-34	32	20	640	20480
35-39	37	5	185	6845
Total		100	2625	71475

$$\text{Mean} = \frac{\sum fx}{\sum f} = \frac{2625}{100} = 26.25$$

$$SD = \sqrt{\frac{\sum fx^2 - \frac{\left(\sum fx\right)^2}{\sum f}}{\sum f}} = \sqrt{\frac{71475 - 68906.25}{100}} = 5.068$$

2. Median, Q_1, Q_3, P_{10} and P_{90}

Since there is discontinuity in the limits of the groups, 0.5 is subtracted from the lower class limits and 0.5 is added to the upper class limits to make the class limits continuous.

Age group (yrs.)	No. of women	Less than cumulative frequency
14.5-19.5	10	10
19.5-24.5	25	35
24.5-29.5	40	75
29.5-34.5	20	95
34.5-39.5	5	100

$$\text{Median} = \text{Lower class limit of the Median class} + \frac{\left(\dfrac{n}{2} - CF\right)w}{f}$$

Median class: 24.5-29.5, $\dfrac{n}{2} = 50$, w = 5, CF = 35, f = 40

$$\text{Median} = 24.5 + \frac{(50-35)\times 5}{40}$$

$$= 24.5 + \frac{75}{40} = 24.5 + 1.9675 = 26.375$$

$$Q_1 = LQ_1 + \frac{\left(\dfrac{n}{4} - CF\right)w}{f}$$

Where LQ_1 = Lower class limit of the Lower Quartile = 19.5, $\dfrac{n}{4} = 25$, CF = 10 f = 25

$$\therefore Q_1 = 19.5 + \left(\frac{25-10}{25}\right)5 = 19.5 + \frac{75}{25} = 22.5$$

$$Q_3 = LQ_3 + \frac{\left(\dfrac{3n}{4} - CF\right)w}{f}$$

LQ_3 = Lower class limit of the Upper Quartile group = 24.5, $\dfrac{3n}{4} = 75$, CF=35, f = 40

$$Q_3 = 24.5 + \frac{(75-35)}{40} * 5 = 29.5$$

$$P_{10} = LP_{10} + \frac{\left(\dfrac{10n}{100} - CF\right)w}{f}$$

Where LP_{10} = Lower class limit of the 10th Percentile group 14.5, $\dfrac{10n}{100} = 10$, CF = 0, f = 10

$$\therefore P_{10} = 14.5 + \frac{(10-0)5}{10} = 19.5$$

$$P_{90} = LP_{90} + \frac{\left(\frac{90n}{100} - CF\right)w}{f}$$

Where LP_{90} = Lower class limit of the 90th Percentile group = 29.5, $\frac{90n}{100}$ = 90, CF = 75, f = 20

$$\therefore P_{90} = 29.5 + \left(\frac{90-75}{20}\right) * 5$$

$$= 29.5 + \frac{75}{20} = 29.5 + 3.75 = 33.25$$

3. Mode

Modal frequency (maximum frequency) = 40

Lower class limit of the group containing the maximum frequency = 24.5 = LM

$$\text{Mode} = LM + \frac{d_1 w}{d_1 + d_2}$$

Where d_1 is the difference between the modal class frequency and the frequency preceding the modal class frequency; d_2 is the difference between the modal class frequency and the frequency succeeding the modal class frequency; w is the width of the class interval.

$$\text{Mode} = 24.5 + \left(\frac{15}{35} * 5\right)$$

$$= 24.5 + 2.14 = 26.64$$

Mean = **26.25**, median = **26.375**, mode = **26.64**

The three types of averages are almost equal and, hence, the distribution of age of 100 women admitted in the maternity hospital can be considered as normal.

$$\text{Pearson's coefficient skewness} = \frac{26.25 - 26.64}{5.068}$$
$$= -0.077$$

$$\text{Skewness in terms of the Quartiles} = \frac{(29.5 - 26.375) - (26.375 - 22.5)}{29.5 - 22.5}$$

$$= \frac{3.125 - 3.875}{7} = \frac{-0.75}{7} = -0.107$$

$$\text{Percentile coefficient of skewness} = \left\{ \frac{(33.25 + 19.5 - 52.75)}{13.75} \right\} = 0$$

$$\text{Kurtosis} = \frac{29.5 - 22.5}{2(33.25 - 19.5)} = \frac{7}{27} = 0.2593 \quad < 0.263$$

Kurtosis value is only 0.004 units less than 0.263. Hence, the distribution is normal with respect to both skewness and kurtosis

Example 2. The following table gives the distribution of ages of 100 cancer cases admitted in a cancer hospital. Computation of various statistical parameters (mean, median, mode, standard deviation (SD) and measures of skewness and kurtosis) and the properties of Normal distribution are given below:

Ag(Yrs.)	Mid Point (x)	Freq (f)	fx	f(x²)
20-29	24.5	5	122.5	3001.25
30-39	34.5	8	276.0	9522.00
40-49	44.5	15	667.5	29703.75
50-59	54.5	20	1090.0	59405.00
60-69	64.5	45	2902.5	187211.25
70-79	74.5	7	521.5	38851.75
		100	5580.0	327695.00

$$\text{Mean} = \frac{5580}{100} = 55.80$$

$$\text{SD} = \sqrt{\frac{327695 - 311364}{100}} = 12.78$$

Median

Age(Yrs.)	No. of cases	Less than cumulative frequency
19.5-29.5	5	5
29.5-39.5	8	13
39.5-49.5	15	28
49.5-59.5	20	48
59.5-69.5	45	93
69.5-79.5	7	100

Lower class of the Median class = 59.5, CF = 48, f = 45, w=10

$$\text{Mean} = 59.5 + \frac{(50 - 48) * 10}{45} = 59.94$$

Q_1 = Lower class of the Q_1 class = 39.5, CF = 13, f = 15, w=10

$$Q_1 = 39.5 + \frac{(25 - 13) * 10}{15} = 47.5$$

Q_3 = Lower class of the Q_3 class = 59.5, CF = 48, f = 45, w = 10

$$Q_3 = 59.5 + \frac{(75 - 48) * 10}{45} = 65.5$$

P_{10} = Lower class of the P_{10} class = 29.5, CF = 5, f = 8, w = 10

$$P_{10} = 29.5 + \frac{(10 - 5) * 10}{8} = 35.75$$

P_{90} = Lower class of the P_{90} class = 59.5, CF = 48, f = 45, w = 10

$$P_{90} = 59.5 + \frac{(90-48)*10}{45} = 68.83$$

Mode

Modal class frequency = 45, Lower class limit of the Modal class = 59.5

$$\textbf{Mode} = 59.5 + \frac{(45-20)*10}{(45-7)+(45-20)} = 59.5 + 3.97 = 63.47$$

Mean= 55.8; Median = 59 94; Mode = 63 .47

Values of mean, median and mode are very different. Mode is greater than mean and median. Hence, the distribution is negatively skewed.

$$\text{Pearson's Coefficient of Skewness} = \frac{55.80 - 63.47}{12.78} = -0.6$$

$$\text{Quartile Coefficient of Skewness} = \frac{(65.5-59.94)-(59.94-47.5)}{(65.5-47.5)}$$

$$= \frac{(5.56)-(12.44)}{18} = -0.382$$

Percentile coefficient of skewness = { (68.83 + 35.75 – 119.88)/33.08 = –0.4625

$$\text{Kurtosis} = \frac{(65.5-47.5)}{2(68.83-35.75)} = \frac{18}{66.17} = 0.272 > 0.263$$

Kurtosis value is only 0.009 units more than 0.263.

The distribution is negatively skewed and normokurtic.

Example 3. The distribution of systolic BP values of 60 men studied in a health survey is given below:

Sys. BP	Mid Point(x)	Freq(f)	fx	f(x²)
115-120	117.5	6	705	82837.5
120-125	122.5	14	1715	210087.5
125-130	127.5	12	1530	195075.0
130-135	132.5	10	1325	175562.5
135-140	137.5	8	1100	151250.0
140-145	142.5	6	855	121837.5
145-150	147.5	4	590	87025.0
Total		60	7820	1023675

$$\text{Mean} = \frac{7820}{60} = 130.33$$

$$\text{SD} = \sqrt{\frac{1023675 - 1019206.67}{60}} = 8.63$$

Median

SYS. BP	No. of men	Less than cumulative frequency
115-120	6	6
120-125	14	20
125-130	12	32
130-135	10	42
135-140	8	50
140-145	6	56
145-150	4	60

$n/2 = 30$, lower class limit of the median class 125, CF=20, f = 12, w = 5

$$125 + \frac{(30-20)*5}{12} = 125 + 4.16 = 129.16$$

$Q_1 = n/4 = 15$, lower class limit of the Q_1 class =120, CF = 6, f = 14, w = 5

$$Q_1 = 120 + \frac{(15-6)*5}{14} = 120 + 3.21 = 123.21$$

$Q_3 = 3n/4 = 45$, lower class limit of the Q_3 class = 135, CF = 42, f = 8, w = 5

$$Q_3 = 135 + \frac{(45-42)*5}{8} = 135 + 1.875 = 136.875$$

$P_{10} = 10n/100 = 6$, lower class limit of the P_{10} class = 115, CF = 0, f = 6, w = 5

$$P_{10} = 115 + \frac{(6-0)*5}{6} = 115 + 5 = 120$$

$P_{90} = 90n/100 = 54$, lower class limit of the P_{90} class = 140, CF = 50, f = 6, w = 5

$$Q_{90} = 140 + \frac{(54-50)*5}{6} = 140 + 3.33 = 143.33$$

Mode

Modal frequency = 14, lower class limit of the modal class = 120, d1 = (14-6), d2 = (14-12)

$$120 + \frac{(14-6)*5}{28-12-6} = 120 + 4.0 = 124$$

Pearson's Coefficient of Skewness = $\dfrac{130.33 - 124}{8.63} = 0.733$

Quartile Coefficient of Skewness = $\dfrac{(136.875 - 129.16) - (129.16 - 123.21)}{(136.875 - 123.21)}$

$$= \frac{(7.715) - (5.95)}{(13.665)}$$

$$= \frac{1.765}{13.665} = 0.129$$

Percentile Coefficient of Skewness = {143.333+120 − 258.32} / (143.333-120)
= 0.215

Since each formula uses different parameters, some of them being absolute and some others relative, it is difficult to explain the reasons for the difference in the skewness values obtained applying different formulae. Interpretation of skewness may be done based on the higher value.

$$\text{Kurtosis} = \frac{(136.875-123.21)}{2(143.33-120)} = \frac{13.665}{46.66} = 0.293$$

The distribution is positively skewed and slightly leptokurtic.

4.4.2. Other Types of Curves

Other forms of curves which are of importance in medical data are J-shaped curves and bi-modal curves.

4.4.2.1. J-shaped curves

Example of J-shaped curve (Figs 4.7-4.9): Distribution of children according to the order of birth, distribution of families in slum areas according to their income and distribution of deaths according to age.

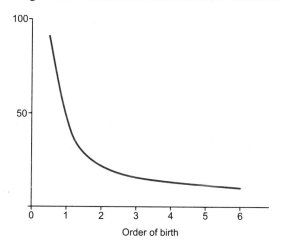

Fig. 4.7: J-shaped curve - distribution of birth order of children

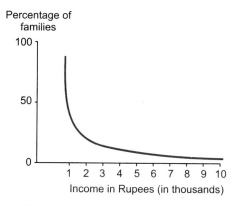

Fig. 4.8: J-shaped curve - distribution of income of families

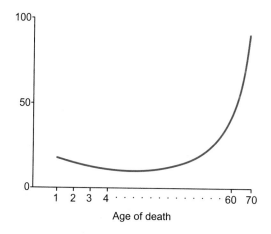

Fig. 4.9: J-shaped curve - distribution of age at deaths

4.4.2.2. Bimodal curves

Example of bi-modal curve (Figs 4.10-4.11): Distribution of weight of adults and children and distribution of age at marriage of males and females

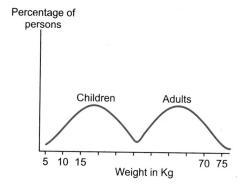

Fig. 4.10: Bi-modal curve - distribution of weights of the subjects

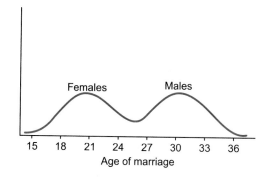

Fig. 4.11: Bi-modal curve - distribution of age at marriage of the subjects

4.4.3. Examples of the Application of Normal Distribution in Medical Problems

Example 1. The mean cholesterol of a sample of normal subjects was found to be 210 mg% and the corresponding S.D. was 20 mg%. The cholesterol value in this sample was found to be normally distributed. In a sample of 1000 individuals find the expected number of persons having cholesterol value:

    (a) >210 mg%
    (b) >260 mg%
    (c) < 250 mg%
    (d) between 210 and 230 mg%

Mean cholesterol = 210 mg%, SD= 20 mg%

For doing problems based on normal distribution, first of all a typical normal curve has to be drawn. Along the X-axis of the curve, mark the mean value of the variable (X) at the centre, which is also equal to Z =0. Also mark the other values of the variable along the X-axis at the appropriate places. The next step is to transform the X value to the corresponding Z-values by using the standard normal deviate formula. Then find out the probability of X exceeding a certain value or lying between certain values in terms of Z. Refer the normal deviate Table (Appendix 2) to find out this probability, reading the value of Z vertically and horizontally.

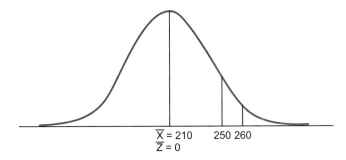

Fig. 4.12: Normal curve of the distribution of cholesterol values

  (a) $Z_1 = (210-210)/20 = 0$
     P (X>210) = P (Z>0) = 0.5
     From the normal deviate table it can be seen that probability corresponding to Z = 0 is 0.5. Expected number of persons having cholesterol value > 210 = 1000 * 0.5 = 500.

  (b) $Z_2 = \dfrac{260-210}{20} = 2.5$
     P (X>260) = P (Z>2.5) = 0.5 –P (Z value between 0 and 2.5) = 0.5 – 0.4938
                         = 0.0062
     Expected number of persons having cholesterol value > 260 = 1000 * 0.0062 = 6.2

  (c) $Z_3 = \dfrac{250-210}{20} = 2$
     P(X<250) = P (Z<2) = 0.5 + P (Z value between 0 and 2) = 0.5 + 0.4772
                        = 0.9772
     Expected number of persons having cholesterol value <250 = 1000 * 0.9772 = 977.2

(d) $Z_4 = \dfrac{230 - 210}{20} = 1$

P (X lies between 210 and 230) = P (Z lies between 0 and 1)

= 0.3413

Expected number of persons having cholesterol value between 210 and 230 = 1000 * 0.3413 = 341.3

Example 2. The mean birth weight of a sample of babies born in a hospital was found to be 2.8 kg with a SD of 0.4 kg. The birth weights in the sample were found to be normally distributed. In a sample of 500 babies, find the expected number of babies having the birth weight as:

(a) >3.5 kg

(b) < 2.5 kg

(c) between 2.5 and 3.5 kg

n = 500, mean birth weight = $\bar{x}$ = 2.8 kg, SD = 0.4 kg

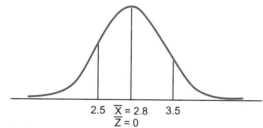

2.5 $\overline{X}$ = 2.8   3.5
$\overline{Z}$ = 0

Fig. 4.13: Normal curve of the distribution of birth weights of babies

(a) $Z_1 = \dfrac{X - \bar{X}}{SD} = \dfrac{(3.5 - 2.8)}{0.4} = 1.75$

P (X>3.5) = P (Z>1.75) = 0.5 – P (Z value between 0 and 1.75) = 0.5 – 0.4599 = 0.0401

(Refer to the normal deviate Table – Appendix 2)

Expected number of babies with birth weight > 3.5 kg = 500 * 0.0401 = 20

(b) $Z_2 = \dfrac{(2.5 - 2.8)}{0.4} = 0.75$

P(X<2.5) = P (Z<-0.75) = 0.5 –P (Z value between 0 and 0.75) = 0.5 – 0.2734 = 0.2266

(Refer to the normal deviate Table – Appendix 2)

Expected number of babies with birth weight < 2.5 kg = 500 * 0.2266 = 113

(c) P (2.5<X<3.5) = P (Z value between 0 and –0.75 + Z value between 0 and 1.75)

= P (-0.75<Z<1.75) = 0.2734 + 0.4599 = 0.7333

(Refer to the normal deviate Table – Appendix 2)

Expected number of babies with birth weight between 2.5 and 3.5 kg = 500 * 0.7333 = 367

Example 3. Assume that normotensive people have systolic blood pressures that are normally distributed with a mean of 120 mm Hg and an S.D. of 10 mm Hg. What is the probability that:

(a) A person selected at random from this group will have a systolic pressure between 120 and 130?

(b) A person selected at random will have a blood pressure less that 95?

(c) A person selected at random from this group will have a systolic blood pressure between 105 and 125?

(d) What is the blood pressure value above which 1% of the population lies?

What is the expected number of persons with these probabilities in a sample of 400 persons?

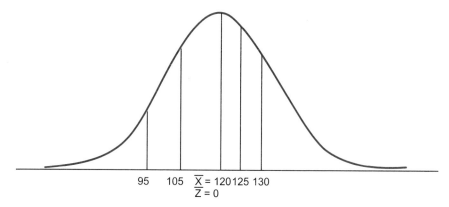

95   105 $\overline{X}$ = 120 125 130
$\overline{Z}$ = 0

Fig. 4.14: Normal curve of the distribution of systolic blood pressure values of normotensive subjects

(a) $Z_1 = \dfrac{130\text{-}120}{10} = 1$

P (120<X<130) = P (0<Z<1) = 0.3413(Refer to the normal deviate Table – Appendix 2)
Expected number of persons with sys. BP lying between 120 and 130 = 400 × 0.3413 = 136.5

(b) $Z_3 = \dfrac{95\text{-}120}{10} = -2.5$

P(X<95) = P (Z < -2.5) = 0.5 – P (Z value between 0 and 2.5)
= 0.5 – 0.4938 = 0.0062
(Refer to the normal deviate Table – Appendix 2)
Expected number of persons with sys. BP < 95 = 400 * 0.0062= 2.48

(c) $Z_4 = \dfrac{105\text{-}120}{10} = -1.5$ $Z_5 = \dfrac{125\text{-}120}{10} = -0.5$

P (105 < X <125) = P (-1.5 <Z <0.5)
= P (Z value between 0 and –1.5 + Z value between 0 and 0.5)
= 0.4332 + 0.1915(Refer to the normal deviate Table – Appendix 2)
= 0.6247
Expected number of persons with sys. BP between 105 and 125 = 400 * 0.6247 = 250

(a) Since we have to find out the X value corresponding to probability >1 % (0.01), $\dfrac{X-120}{10}$ = Z value

corresponding to probability = 0.49
= 2.33 (Refer to the normal deviate Table – Appendix 2)
X = 120 + (10 × 2.33) = 120 + 23.3 = 143.3
1 % of the sample will have their sys. BP above 143.3.

Example 4. In an intelligence test administered to 1,000 children, the average score is 90 and standard deviation 10. Assume that scores are distributed normally. Find the number of children (a) exceeding the score 100, and (b) with score less than 75.

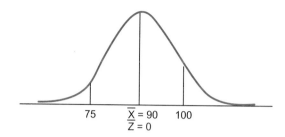

Fig. **4.15**: Normal curve of the distribution of intelligence scores of children

(a) $Z_1 = \dfrac{100-90}{10} = 1$

P (X > 100) = P (Z >1)
= 0.5 – P (0 <Z< 1) = 0.5 – P (Z value between 0 and 1)
= 0.5 - 0.3413 = 0.1587(Refer to the normal deviate Table – Appendix 2)
Expected number of children whose score is more than 100 = 0.1587 × 1000 = 158.7

(b) $Z_3 = \dfrac{75-90}{10} = 1.5$

P (X < 75) = P (0< Z < -1.5) = 0.5 – P (Z value between 0 and 1.5)
= 0.5 – 0.4332 = 0.0668 (Refer to the normal deviate Table – Appendix 2)
Expected number of children whose score is less than 75 = 0.0668 × 1000 = 66.8.

Example 5. Of a large group of men, 5% are under 60 inches in height, and 40% are between 60 and 65 inches. Assuming a normal distribution, find mean and standard deviation.

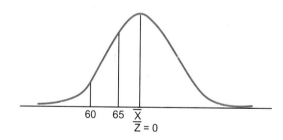

Fig. **4.16**: Normal curve of the distribution of heights of men

Since 5% are below 60, proportion of those between 60 and the mean height will be 0.45 (0.5-0.05). Similarly, since 40% are between 60 and 65, proportion of those between 65 and the mean height will be 0.05 (0.5-0.05-0.40). We have to find the Z values corresponding to the probabilities 0.45 and 0.05. Z value corresponding to P = 0.45 = 1.65 and Z value corresponding to P = 0.05 = 0.13. Since both 60 and 65 are less than the mean, these Z values will be negative.

$Z1 = \dfrac{60 - \bar{X}}{SD} = -1.65; \quad Z2 = \dfrac{65 - \bar{X}}{SD} = -0.13$

$\bar{X}$ - 0.13 SD = 65
$\bar{X}$ -1.65 SD = 60
1.52 SD = 5

$\therefore$ SD = 3.29

$\bar{X}$ = 65 + 0.13 SD

$\quad$ = 65 + (0.13 × 3.29) = 65.4277

4.5. Concept of Standard Error (SE)

The concept of standard error (SE) is very important in making inferences, i.e., making generalizations of the results obtained from a sample for the population from where the sample was randomly selected. Many times the two terms SE and SD are confused. These two terms, which are important for measuring the variability among the observations of a variable in a sample (SD) and the variability among the 'statistic' values from different samples (SE), are explained below.

Standard deviation (SD) is a measure of variability of different observations of the variable in a given sample. It represents the average amount of deviation of different sample values from the mean value. It is a measure of the extent of spread of the different sample values around the mean value.

$$SD = \sqrt{\frac{\sum(X-\bar{X})^2}{n}}$$ where, X = sample value; $\bar{X}$ = mean value; n = sample size

Standard error (SE) of a statistic is the standard deviation of the sampling distribution of that statistic. The concept of standard error is important when several samples of a population are being considered. It is the average amount of deviation of different sample mean values from the population (true) mean value. It is the standard deviation of the mean values of different samples of the same size selected from the population.

$$i.e., SE = \sqrt{\frac{\sum(\bar{X}-m)2}{r}}$$

(m = grand (combined) mean = estimate of population mean, $\bar{X}$ = individual sample means, r - no of samples)

Computation of SE empirically with repeated sampling and using the above formula is difficult and may not be feasible. Hence, SE is usually computed using statistical theoretical principles, from one randomly selected sample of adequate size, as follows:

$SE = SD/\sqrt{n}$

If the SD of the cholesterol values of 100 heart patients is equal to 20 mg%,

$SE = 20/\sqrt{100}$ = 2 mg%

The mean values obtained from different samples, of the same size, from the population of heart patients, deviate from the population (true) mean by 2 units on the average.

4.6. Statistical Hypothesis

Statistical hypothesis is a declarative statement about the parameters (of population), or the distribution form of the variable in the population. In any research study, there has to be a research question. For the purpose of statistical analysis, this research question has to be stated in terms of a statistical hypothesis, which will be confirmed or rejected based on the collected data.

Examples of hypotheses:
1. Mean systolic blood pressure ($\bar{X}_1$) in normal subjects of 30 years of age in the population is equal to 120 mm, i.e., $\bar{X}_1$ = 120.

2. Mean cholesterol value in hypertension patients $(\bar{X}_1)$ > mean cholesterol value in normals $(\bar{X}_2)$, i.e., $\bar{X}_1 > \bar{X}_2$.
3. Percent of babies born with low birth weight to anaemic women (p_1) is greater than that in normal women (p_2), i.e., $p_1 > p_2$.
4. Occurrence of lung cancer is associated with smoking.
5. Birth weights of children are normally distributed.

4.6.1. Null Hypothesis (H_o) and Alternative Hypothesis (H_1)

4.6.1.1. Null hypothesis

In any analytical research study, a hypothesis cannot be proved directly. The research question has to be framed in a specific way. It is set in terms of no difference in average values or percentages between two or several populations or no association between two or more categorical variables or factors. This type of hypothesis is called Null hypothesis. On applying an appropriate statistical test the null hypothesis is accepted or rejected.

While a null hypothesis is stated, it has to be tested against a contrasting possibility, namely, *there is a difference or there is an association*. This contrasting possibility, as a declarative statement, is called Alternative hypothesis. On applying the appropriate statistical test if the null hypothesis is rejected, the alternative hypothesis is accepted with a certain amount of error (explained later). If the null hypothesis is accepted, the corresponding power (explained later) of the test has to be stated.

Examples of Null Hypothesis (H_o):
1. Mean cholesterol value in normals $(\bar{X}_1)$ = mean cholesterol value in hypertension patients $(\bar{X}_2)$
2. Percentage of babies born with low birth weight in anaemic women (p_1) = percentage of babies born with low birth weight in normal women (p_2)
3. There is no association between lung cancer and smoking.

4.6.1.2. Alternative hypothesis

There are two types of Alternative Hypotheses: one-sided and two-sided. If the direction of the alternative hypothesis is clearly defined, then it is called one-sided and if the direction is not clearly defined it is called two-sided. In other words, if one population has its mean /proportion value of the variable clearly greater than that of the other population with which the test of comparison is done, then it is one-sided; and if one is not sure which population has its mean or proportion value greater than that of the other population and the only statement that can be made is that they are not equal, then the hypothesis is two-sided.

Examples of One-sided Alternative Hypothesis (H_1):

$$\bar{X}_1 > \bar{X}_2 \quad \text{or} \quad \bar{X}_2 > \bar{X}_1$$
$$p_1 > p_2 \quad \text{or} \quad p_2 > p_1$$

1. Mean cholesterol value in hypertension patients $(\bar{X}_1)$ > mean cholesterol value in normals $(\bar{X}_2)$.
2. Percentage of babies born with low birth weight in anaemic women $(p1)$ > percentage of babies born with low birth weight in normal women (p_2).
3. There is a positive association between lung cancer and smoking — Prevalence of lung cancer is higher in smokers than in non-smokers.

Examples of Two-sided Alternative Hypothesis:

$$\bar{X}_1 \neq \bar{X}_2$$
$$p_1 \neq p_2$$

1. Mean cholesterol value in normals $(\bar{X}_1) \neq$ mean cholesterol value in hypertension patients $(\bar{X}_2)$.

2. Percentage of babies born with low birth weight in anaemic women (p1) ≠ percentage of babies born with low birth weight in normal women (p_2).
3. There is an association between lung cancer and smoking.

4.6.2. Type-I & Type-II Errors

The concept of Type-I and Type-II errors is very important in inference statistics. While making inferences based on results from the sample, we cannot do so with a 100% certainty (confidence). Acceptance or rejection of the null hypothesis can be stated only with a certain amount of error or with a certain amount of confidence (100-error).The error can be of two types, termed Type-I and Type-II errors. The concept of these two types of errors is explained below.

Consider the following 2*2 Table:

Decision		True situation	
		Ho is True	Ho is False
Accept	Ho	(no error)	β-(type-II)
Reject	Ho	α-(type-I)	(no error)

4.6.2.1. Type-I error

Type I error involves Rejection of Ho when it is actually True or finding an effect when actually there is no effect. It measures the strength of evidence by indicating the probability that a result at least as extreme as that observed would occur by chance, when the null hypothesis is true.

It is represented as α (alpha) or p-value or level of significance.

(1-α) is called Confidence coefficient = probability of accepting Ho when it is true

= probability of not finding an effect when actually there is no effect.

4.6.2.2. Type-II error

Type II error involves acceptance of Ho when it is actually false or not finding an effect when actually there is an effect.

It is represented as β (beta).

(1-β) is called the power of the test = probability of rejecting Ho when it is false = probability of finding an effect when actually there is an effect.

Power of a statistical test is analogous to the sensitivity of a diagnostic test; α being the false positivity and β being the false negativity (refer Chapter 10).

When the null hypothesis is rejected, Type-I error is to be stated. Maximum error usually allowed —5%, i.e., minimum confidence required—95%.

When the null hypothesis is accepted, Type- II error is to be stated. Maximum error usually allowed —20 %, i.e., minimum power required — 80%.

When the null hypothesis is rejected, whatever may be the sample size, it may be adequate. But, when the null hypothesis is accepted, the adequacy of the sample size has to be checked before accepting Ho by computing the Power of the test.

In principle, the probability of making type-I error may be fixed at whatever level we want. By convention the levels – 0.05, 0.01 and 0.001 are fixed. The two types of errors must be weighed against each other in each problem, depending upon the problem. In scientific work, the consequences of erroneous claims of verification of new hypotheses are serious and the risk of type-I error is usually set very low as 0.01 or even lower as 0.001. For practical action a higher risk of Type-I error may be acceptable. But, generalization is hazardous for it is necessary to consider carefully in advance how serious are the consequences of each kind of error in each specific problem. In a legal trial an innocent person should not be punished and hence the null

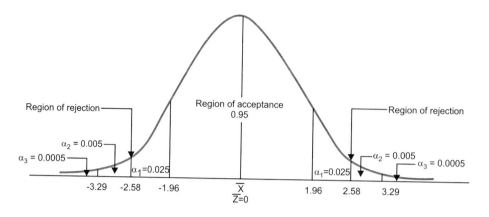

Fig. 4.17: Normal curve showing the regions of rejection and acceptance of the Null hypothesis

hypothesis that he has not committed the crime should be rejected at a very low type-I error. Similarly, a new drug, however effective it may be, but if it is expensive and having more side effects should be accepted only at a low Type-I error. In contrast to this, if no treatment is available, the new drug even if does not give a remarkable positive effect, should be accepted at a comparatively higher error, may be even at 20% Type -I error. While fixing the Type-I and Type-II errors, it should be noted that when Type-I error is lower and lower, Type-II error will be higher and higher and vice versa. Hence, these two types or errors should be well balanced depending upon the situation, experience and overall implications.

Multiple Choice Questions

Choose the correct answers in the following multiple choice questions. The correct answers are listed on p. 342.

Q.1. Probability varies between:
a. 1 and 2
b. −1 and +1
c. 0 and ∞
d. 0 and 1

Q.2. In a breast cancer-screening program, 2000 women underwent mammography and 200 were found to be positive. Out of these 200 positives, only 150 were confirmed to have breast cancer. In addition, 70 women were found to have breast cancer with their mammography showing normal. What is the probability of a woman having breast cancer, given that her mammography was negative?
a. 150/200
b. 270/ 2000
c. 70/1800
d. 70/1730

Q.3. If data on hemoglobin level of a group of 1000 persons follows normal distribution and its mean is calculated as 14.5 g% with standard deviation 2.5g%, then the number of patients having hemoglobin level between 12 and 17 g% will be:
a. 999
b. 990
c. 683
d. 954

Q.4. If the weight of 1000 adult females has a normal distribution, the percentage of females who have more than two standard deviations above the mean height will be:
a. 0.5
b. 2.5
c. 0.01
d. 0 .05

Q.5. The systolic blood pressure in patients attending a clinic was observed to have a mean of 160 mm/Hg with a standard deviation of 20 mm/Hg. Assuming normal distribution, what proportion of patients is expected to have a systolic BP more than 140 mm/Hg?

a. 50%   b.   84%
c. 68%   d.   16%

Q.6.   The mortality rate among patients suffering from a disease was found to be 3/1000. In studying the expected number of deaths of this disease in a population of 10,000 such patients, the distribution of the mortality is:

a.   Normal   b.   Binominal
c.   Chi-square   d.   Poisson

Q.7.   If the distribution of systolic blood pressure values in a sample of adults aged 20 to 25 years is bell shaped and symmetric, it is called:

a.   Binomial distribution   b.   Poisson distribution
c.   Chi-square distribution   d.   Normal distribution

Q.8.   From a previous experience on a series of allergy patients, it had been noted that 60% gave (+) ve reaction to a certain skin test. In a sample of 3 patients whose skin is going to be tested, the probability that all gave (+) ve reaction would be:

a.   0.120   b.   0.064
c.   0.216   d.   1.0

Q.9.   If it has been observed that the probability of getting a boy is equal to 0.6 and that of a girl is 0.4. The probability of getting 2 boys for a couple if they are going to have two children is:

a.   0.16   b.   0.24
c.   0.48   d.   0.36

Q. 10. The fasting blood glucose levels among diabetes patients are known to be normally distributed with a mean of 105 mg per 100 ml of blood and a standard deviation of 10 mg per 100 ml of blood. From this data it can be inferred that approximately 95% of diabetics will have their fasting blood glucose levels within the limits:

a.   95 to 115   b.   85 to 125
c.   75 to 135   d.   90 to 120

5 | Inference Statistical Methods

- Estimation of population parameters: Point estimation, interval estimation
- Testing the statistical significance of a hypothesis: Steps in testing the statistical significance, tests of statistical significance
- Continuous variables: Statistical significance of the difference in sample and population means, statistical significance of the difference in mean values between two populations
- Analysis of variance (ANOVA): Purpose, designs, completely randomized design (CRD), randomized complete block design (RCBD), repeated measures design, homogeneity of variances, multiple range tests, problems in ANOVA
- Analysis of covariance
- Discrete variables: Estimation, tests of significance, chi-square test (λ^2), Yate's corrected chi-square, chi-square test vs Z-test, Fisher's exact test, Chi-square test for association, McNemar's matched λ^2 test, Goodness of fit λ^2 test, chi-square test for testing statistical significance of a trend, partitioned chi-square

As mentioned earlier, statistical inference deals with the generalization of results obtained from the samples for the population from which the samples are selected. It is the process of drawing conclusions from the sample results based on the relevant probability laws. Conclusions based on samples cannot be drawn with 100% certainty. Methods of statistical inference help us to draw conclusions based on the sample results with a certain level of confidence, which is determined at the time of designing the study. Normally, the confidence probability is fixed as 0.95 or 0.99 or 0.999 depending upon the requirement. If a decision has to be taken in situations where it becomes beneficial due to its seriousness, confidence level can be set as 95% (drug trials for AIDS). But, if the decision has to be taken with utmost caution due to some possible hazards and or high cost, the confidence level required is usually set as 99% or even as high as 99.9%.

Thus, statistical inference is inference about a population, with respect to the study parameters or statistical hypotheses, from a random sample drawn from it. There are two important components of statistical inference: estimation of population parameters and testing the statistical significance of a hypothesis. The process of statistical inference broadly includes point estimation, interval estimation, hypothesis testing and prediction.

5.1. Estimation of Population Parameters

There are two types of estimation: point estimation and interval estimation.

5.1.1. Point Estimation

Values of mean, proportion, correlation coefficient, etc., computed from the sample serve as estimates of the population parameters. This estimate is a single value and is called **point estimate**. No confidence of any kind can be attached to this value and this value serves only as an estimate. Larger the sample size, closer will be this estimated value to the population parameter.

5.1.2. Interval Estimation (Estimation with a Defined Level of Confidence)

In interval estimate, a **lower limit (LL)** and an **upper limit (UL)** are computed from sample values and it can be said with a certain amount of **confidence** that the population value (true value) of the parameter will lie within these limits. These limits are called **confidence limits** or **interval estimates**. These limits are computed from the estimated value and its standard error value. For example: The **LL** and **UL** estimates for the population mean are given as: **mean - C* SE and mean + C*SE,**

Where C = Confidence coefficient, SE = SD/$\sqrt{n}$, n = sample size.

If 95% confidence is desired, then C = **1.96**; for 99% confidence, C = **2.58**; for 99.9% confidence, C = **3.29** (see Normal Distribution in Chapter 4).

Examples:

Example 1. In a study of a sample of 100 subjects it was found that the mean systolic blood pressure was 120 mm of Hg, with a standard deviation of 10 mm of Hg. Find out 95% confidence limits for the population mean of systolic blood pressure.

$$SE = SD/\sqrt{n} = 10/\sqrt{(100)} = 10/10 = 1$$

LL: mean – 1.96*1, = 120 – 1.96 = 118.04
UL: mean +1.96*1, = 120 + 1.96 = 121.96

Thus, the population mean value of systolic blood pressure will lie between 118.04 and 121.96 and we can have a confidence of 95% for making this statement. In other words, in repeated samples, 95 % of the estimates will have their confidence limits containing the true value of the parameter and in case of the remaining 5% samples the true value will be outside these limits.

Example 2. In a study of 10,000 persons in a town, it is found that 100 of them are affected by tuberculosis. Find out 99% confidence limits for the estimated prevalence of tuberculosis.

$$SE = \sqrt{\frac{pq}{n}} \text{ , where p = (100/10000) * 100 = 1\%}$$

q = 100 – p = 100 – 1 = 99%, E = $\sqrt{((1*99)/10000)}$ = 0.0995

LL = p - 2.58*0.0995 = 1- 0.2567 = 0.7433 = **0 .74 %**
UL= p +2.58*0.0995 = 1 +0.2567 = 1.2567 = **1.26 %**

Thus, the population prevalence rate of tuberculosis will lie between 0.74% and 1.26% and we can say this with 99% confidence.

5.2. Testing the Statistical Significance of a Hypothesis

In medical research, we set up a hypothesis to investigate or explain a real life issue or problem. A statistical hypothesis is a conjecture about the parameter of a population or form of the distribution of the variable in the population. There are two types of hypotheses, Null hypothesis and Alternate hypothesis. A null hypothesis is denoted by H_0 and the alternative hypothesis is denoted by H_A. It is the null hypothesis that is tested. Briefly, we set out the null **or** and alternative hypothesis, choose appropriate sample statistic and set out the variables to be studied; set the significance level; select an appropriate statistical test based on the variables, sample size and the form of the distribution; interpret the results of tests and then accept the null hypothesis or reject the null hypothesis and accept the alternate hypothesis based on the observed data.

In statistics, a result is called statistically significant if it is unlikely to have occurred by chance. The significance of a result is also called its p-value; the smaller the p-value, the more significant the result is said to be. Significance is usually represented by the Greek symbol, α (alpha). If a test of significance gives a p-value lower than the α-level, the null hypothesis is rejected.

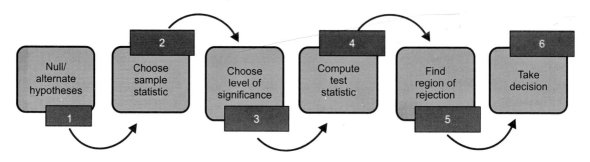

Fig. 5.1: Hypothesis testing

5.2.1. Steps in Test of Statistical Significance

Thus, testing the statistical significance of a hypothesis is the process of assessing whether the null hypothesis is true or false, using sample results (Fig. 5.1). This is one of the important aspects of statistical inference in any research study. In carrying out a test of statistical significance certain steps have to be followed in sequence. These are:

1. State the null hypothesis: Ho
2. State the alternate hypothesis: H1 (one-sided/tailed or two-sided/tailed)

   The test is called one-tailed (one-sided) if the direction of the test is clear and well defined (see Chapter 4). If the test is one-tailed, the confidence on rejecting H_0 will be more as compared to two-tailed test at the chosen level of significance. For example, if the pre-fixed p value is 0.05 (confidence = 95 %) and if the test is one-tailed, the corresponding p value in case of two-tailed test will be double this value, i.e., p will be equal to 0.1 (0.05 * 2) and the confidence will be 90%. Similarly, if p = 0.01 (confidence = 99%) and the test is one-tailed, the corresponding two-tailed p value will be equal to 0.02 and the confidence level will be equal to 98%.

   In a clinical trial, if we are certain that the improvement rate with the new drug is definitely more than that of placebo, a one-tailed test can be done. If health education is certainly going to reduce the prevalence of tobacco use, a one-tailed test can be done. However, one-tailed test should be done only if one is certain about the direction of the test. In case of one-tailed test the region of acceptance and the region of rejection will be as shown below. In the following diagram (Fig. 5.2) the region of rejection is lying on one side of the curve, the test is called one-tailed or one-sided.

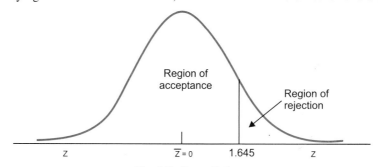

Fig. 5.2: One-tailed test

3. State the distribution of the sample statistic of the variable (normal or Student's t- or chi-square). This is based on the available information on the study variable from the literature (journals, books, etc.,) or based on the sample data.
4. State the level of significance (α or p-value or probability of type-I error) desired.
5. Compute the **Test Statistic (TS)** = (difference in parameter values)/ (SE of difference). Since the parameter values are normally unknown, these are replaced by the sample statistic values.
6. Find out the **Critical Ratio (CR)** from the statistical table at the chosen level of significance.
7. Take decision:
   a. If TS < CR: accept Ho, i.e., difference in parameter values is not statistically significant (may be due to chance).
   b. If TS > CR: reject Ho; accept H1, i.e., difference in parameter values is statistically significant (beyond chance).

If, $p < 0.05$, level of confidence (C) > 95%; if $p < 0.01$, C > 99% and if $p < 0.001$, C > 99.9%.

If the analysis is done on a computer using statistical software, the exact value of p is directly given.

5.2.2. Statistical Tests of Significance

In general, tests of hypothesis can be carried out on one, two or more than two samples. The one sample test is used to test whether the population parameter is different from a specified value, two sample test is used to test whether the difference in the parameter value between two samples is statistically significant or not and the test for more than two samples is used to test whether the differences in the parameter value among the several samples are statistically significant or not. Two sample and more than two samples tests could be unpaired (independent samples which are not related) or paired (correlated samples which are paired according to some identifiable characteristic.)

The tests can be further classified as one- tailed test and two-tailed tests. In one-tailed tests the alternate hypothesis is one-sided and we test whether the test statistic falls in the critical region on only one side of the distribution. In two-tailed test, the alternate hypothesis is formulated to test for difference in either direction (see Chapter 4 for more details).

The important statistical tests of significance have been described below in detail with examples, separately for continuous and discrete variables:

Statistical tests of significance for continuous variables:
   (a) To test the statistical significance of the difference in sample and population means (one sample test)—Z-test /normal test
   (b) To test the statistical significance of the difference in two populations means (two sample tests)

Tests used:
   (i) Large sample size—Z-test /normal test
   (ii) Small sample size with homogeneity in the populations with respect to the study variable and the two populations are independent (Student's t-test)
   (iii) Small sample size with heterogeneity in the populations with respect to the study variable and the two populations are independent (modified Student's t-test)
   (iv) Small or large sample size and the two populations are correlated (paired) (paired t-test)
   (c) To test the statistical significance of the difference among several populations means (multiple sample tests)

Tests used:
   (i) Large sample size and the multiple populations are independent (one-way ANOVA)

(ii)   Small sample size with non-normal populations with respect to the study variable and the multiple populations are independent (nonparametric Kruskal-Wally's one-way ANOVA - see Chapter 6)

(iii)   Small sample size with non-normal populations with respect to the study variable and the multiple populations are correlated (nonparametric Friedman's two-way ANOVA - see Chapter 6)

Statistical tests of significance for discrete variables:

(a)   To test the statistical significance of the difference in proportions between sample and population (Z-test/normal test)

(b)   To test the statistical significance of the difference in proportions between two independent populations/to test the statistical significance of the association between two factors (variables)

Tests used:

(i)   When the sample sizes are large and independent (proportion test/chi-square test)

(ii)   When the sample sizes are small and independent (Fisher's exact test/chi-square test with continuity correction factor)

(iii)   When the sample sizes are large and correlated (paired) (McNemar's chi-square test)

(iv)   When the sample sizes are small and correlated (paired) (McNemar's chi-square test with correction factor)

All the above mentioned statistical tests of significance have been explained below, in detail, with examples.

5.3. Continuous Variables

5.3.1. Statistical Significance of the Difference in Sample and Population Means

$H_0 : \overline{X} = \mu, H_1 : \overline{X} \neq \mu, \alpha = 0.05$

$CR = 1.96, TC = Z = (\overline{X} - m) \div S/\sqrt{n}$

Example: Mean SBP in population = 120, mean SBP in sample = 115

n = 100; SD = 20

$Z = (120 - 115) \div 20 / \sqrt{100} = 2.5$, i.e., TC > CR (1.96) . p < 0.05

Means for the population and sample are significantly different or, in other words, the sample does not represent the population with respect to SBP.

5.3.2. Statistical Significance of the Difference in Mean Values between Two Populations

(1) Large samples

Ho: Null Hypothesis: $\mu_1 = \mu_2$

μ_1 = Mean gain in weight of infants who received supplementary diet

μ_2 = Mean gain in weight of infants who did not receive supplementary diet

H_1: Alternate Hypothesis: $\mu_1 \neq \mu_2$ (two-tailed)

Since we cannot say whether the gain in weight in children who have received supplementary nutrition will be higher than those children who have not received supplementary diet, only a two-tailed test can be done.

If population distribution of gain in weight in both the groups is **normal** (either known from earlier studies or established from the random samples), or both the sample sizes are large (n_1 and $n_2 > 30$), the *test statistic* is Z and the test is called **normal (Z) Test.**

$$Z = \frac{\bar{X}_1 - \bar{X}_2}{\sqrt{\dfrac{S_1^2}{n_1} + \dfrac{S_2^2}{n_2}}}$$

Critical ratio (C.R.)

If $\alpha = 0.05$, C.R. = 1.96; if $\alpha = 0.01$, C.R. = 2.58; and if $\alpha = 0.001$, C.R. = 3.29

Taking decision	Difference in means values between the two groups
If Z < 1.96	Not significant (p > 0.05)
(Ho is acceptable)	
(a) Z > 1.96	Significant (p < 0.05)
(b) Z > 2.58	Highly significant (p < 0.01)
(c) Z > 3.29	Very highly significant (p < 0.001)

(Ho is rejected in situations 'a', 'b' and 'c')

Test of homogeneity of variances (Fisher's F-test)

One of the assumption which has to be satisfied for applying Student's t-test is homogeneity of variances in the two populations. This is tested by computing Fisher's F statistic.

$$F = \frac{\sigma_1^2}{\sigma_2^2} \text{ for } (n_1\text{-}1), (n_2\text{-}1) \text{ degrees of freedom (d.f.) } (\sigma_1 > \sigma_2)$$

Where σ_1 is the SD value of the variable in one population and σ_2 is the SD value in the second population; n_1 and n_2 are the corresponding sample sizes.

Degree of freedom (d.f.) is defined as the number of independent values in the sample. If the sample size is 10 and if 9 values and the mean of the variable in the sample are known, then the 10th value can be determined arithmetically, i.e., even though there are 10 values in the sample, the number of independent values is only 9. For example, if the birth weights (kg) of 5 babies are 3.0, 2.8, 3.2, 2.6 and 3.4 and if we know the birth weights of 4 babies and the mean birth weight, the birth weight of the fifth baby can be determined arithmetically. Mean birth weight of this sample is 5.0 and the known birth weights are only of the first 4 babies, then the birth weight of the fifth baby is

=5.0 * 5 – (3.0 + 2.8 + 3.2 + 2.6) = 3.4

In the 'F' table, the critical F value is seen for $(n_1\text{-}1)$ d.f. horizontally and $(n_2\text{-}1)$ d.f. vertically (Appendix 3).

If the computed F value is less than the critical ratio of F at $(n_1\text{-}1)$, $(n_2\text{-}1)$ d.f., then the assumption of homogeneity of variances in the two populations can be accepted. Otherwise, the variances in the two populations will be heterogeneous.

(2) Small samples (n_1 or n_2 or both n_1 & $n_2 < 30$): ($\sigma_1 = \sigma_2$)

Homogeneity of variances in the two populations is assumed and accepted.

$$t = \frac{\bar{X}_1 - \bar{X}_2}{S\sqrt{\left(\dfrac{1}{n_1} + \dfrac{1}{n_2}\right)}}; \text{ where } S = \sqrt{\frac{(n_1 - 1)S_1^2 + (n_2 - 1)S_2^2}{(n_1 + n_2 - 2)}}$$

Critical ratio values depend upon degree of freedom (n_1+n_2-2) and the CR value should be referred from the Statistical Table on Student's t-distribution (Appendix 4).

(3) Small samples (n < 30) and ($\sigma_1 \neq \sigma_2$)

Homogeneity of variances in the two populations is not accepted. In such a case, modified t-test has to be applied.

$$t = \frac{\bar{X}_1 - \bar{X}_2}{S\sqrt{\left(\frac{1}{n_1} + \frac{1}{n_2}\right)}}; \text{ compute } t = \frac{t_{(n1-1)}\dfrac{S_1^2}{n_1} + t_{(n2-1)}\dfrac{S_2^2}{n_2}}{\dfrac{S_1^2}{n_1} + \dfrac{S_2^2}{n_2}} \text{ at } \alpha = 0.05$$

where t_{n_1-1} and t_{n_2-1} are the Student's t values to be referred from the **Student's t-table** (Appendix 4), for (n_1–1) and (n_1–2) degrees of freedom.

If $n_1 = n_{2\,=}$ n, t' will be equal to t with (n-1) degrees of freedom.

If t > t', p < 0.05 (significant); if t < t', p > 0.05 (not significant)

If $\alpha = 0.01$ or 0.001, the corresponding 't' values from the Student's t-table are substituted and decisions are taken accordingly.

Examples of application of normal test (z-test), Student's t-test and modified t-test

The following are the mean and SD of weight (kg) of 100 school going (A) and 100 non-school going (B) children of 5 years of age in slum areas:

Example 1. n_1 & n_2 > 30

Population	Sample size	Mean	S.D.
A	100	17.4	3.0
B	100	13.2	2.5

Using formula, Z = 10.77 > 3.29 (p < 0.001), i.e., $\mu_A \neq \mu_B$ i.e., mean weight of school going children is significantly higher than that of non-school going children. This statement can be made with 99.9% confidence. Or, in other words, in repeated studies, only in 0.1% studies (1 in thousand), the difference observed in the mean weights between the two groups can occur by chance.

Example 2. n_1 & n_2< 30 $\sigma_1 = \sigma_2$

A	15	17.4	3.0
B	10	13.2	2.5

F = $(3.0)^2 /(2.5)^2 = 1.44 < 3.00$ (for 14 & 9 d.f. at $\alpha = 0.05$). Hence, assumption of homogeneity of variances in the two populations can be accepted.

Using formula, $t = 3.65 > 2.81$ (for 23 d.f. at $\alpha = 0.01$ from statistical Table Appendix 4) < 3.77 (for 23 d.f. at $\alpha = 0.001$)

i.e., p < 0.01, i.e., $\mu_A \neq \mu_B - \mu_A > \mu_B$

The mean weight of school going children is significantly higher than that of non-school going children. This statement can be made with 99% confidence.

Example 3. n_1 & n_2 < 30 and $\sigma_1 \neq \sigma_2$

A	15	17.4	1.8
B	10	13.2	4.2

F = $(4.2)^2 / (1.8)^2 = 5.44 > 2.65$ (for 9 & 14 d.f. at $\alpha = 0.05$) — (Appendix 2)

The assumption of homogeneous variances $(\sigma_1 = \sigma_2)$ in the two populations cannot be accepted and, hence, modified t-test has to be applied.

Using formula, t = 2.98 > 2.25 (from statistical table – Appendix 4, for 23 degrees of freedom $t'_{at \propto = 0.05}$), but < 3.22 ($t'_{at \propto = 0.01}$)

i.e., $\mu_A \neq \mu_B \longrightarrow \mu_A > \mu_B$ (p<0.05)

The mean weight of school going children is significantly higher than that of non-school going children. This statement can be made with 95% confidence.

(4) Paired samples (before and after design)

If the observations are paired, i.e., correlated, like before and after design, the test of significance to be done is called "paired" t-test.

$$|t| = \frac{\bar{d}\sqrt{n}}{Sd}$$ where $\bar{d}$: Mean of the difference, Sd: SD of the difference, degrees of freedom = n-1

Example 4. Serum cholesterol level of 12 patients, before and after giving a drug, are given below:

Patient No.	Before (X_1)	After (X_2)	$d_i = X_1 - X_2$	d_i^2
1.	201	200	-1	1
2.	231	236	5	25
3.	221	216	-5	25
4.	260	233	-27	729
5.	228	224	-4	16
6.	237	216	-21	441
7.	326	296	-30	900
8.	235	195	-40	1600
9.	240	207	-33	1089
10.	267	247	-20	400
11.	284	210	-74	5476
12.	201	209	8	64

d (Mean difference) = –20.17

$$SD = \sqrt{\frac{\sum di^2 - \frac{\left(\sum di\right)^2}{12}}{11}} = \sqrt{\frac{10766 - 4880.3}{11}} = 23.13$$

$$|t| = \frac{-20.17 * 3.464}{23.13} = -3.02$$

t' (at $\alpha = 0.05$ at 11 d.f.) = 2.20 (statistical table - Appendix 3)

t > t', i.e., mean difference in cholesterol levels before and after giving the drug is statistically highly significant (p < 0.05).

It means the drug is effective in reducing the cholesterol value in patients. This statement can be made with 95% confidence. Since t (at $\alpha = 0.01$ at 11 d.f.) = 3.106 and 3.02 < 3.106, we cannot make this statement with 99% confidence.

Example 5. Systolic blood pressure values of 10 hypertension patients before and after giving a drug are given below:

Systolic B.P	Patient number									
	1	2	3	4	5	6	7	8	9	10
Before Drug	160	150	170	130	140	170	160	160	120	140
After Drug	140	110	165	140	145	120	130	110	120	130

	Mean	S.D.
Before drug	150	17.00
After drug	131	17.13
Change (Decrease)	19	22.46

$$t = \frac{19\sqrt{10}}{22.46} = 2.67 > 2.26 \text{ (from statistical table-Appendix 3, } t_{at \propto = 0.05} \text{ with 9 d.f.), i.e., } p < 0.05$$

Thus, the decrease of 19 units, on average, in the systolic BP after giving the drug is statistically significant at 5% level of significance.

5.4. Analysis of Variance (ANOVA)

Variation is inherent in nature and one of the principal aims of statistical models is to attempt to explain the variation in measurements. This variation may be due to a variety of factors —individual variation, variation with respect to time, variation due to environment, variation due to the method of measuring, etc.

The statistical model involving a test of significance of the difference in mean values of the variable between two groups is the most familiar Student's t-test. If there are more than two groups, the corresponding appropriate statistical model is the Analysis of Variance (ANOVA).

The advantage in ANOVA is that the factors related to the measurement , if recorded, can be held fixed at each level of the main factor under consideration and the total variance can be partitioned into different components of variation due to these fixed factors. These factors are usually called 'Blocks'.

This will make the comparison of mean values between the groups of the main factor more precise, since the error variation (standard error) will be reduced due to the elimination of variation due to the blocking factors.

5.4.1. Purpose

ANOVA is used to test the statistical significance of the differences in mean values of a variable among several groups (more than *two* groups). In case of two groups, Student's t-test is applied. The added advantage in ANOVA is that the total variance can be partitioned into different components (due to several factors), which will enhance the validity of comparison of the means among the different Groups. This is not possible in the case of Student's t-test. Also, tests of significance of various hypotheses can be done simultaneously, depending upon the design of the study.

5.4.2. Designs

Basically, ANOVA is applied in three important experimental designs. These are:
1. Completely Randomized Design (CRD) (one-way ANOVA)
2. Randomized Complete Block Design (RCBD) (two or multiple-way ANOVA)
3. Repeated Measures Design (Before & after Design) (two-way, between time analysis)

5.4.2.1. CRD

If there is only *one factor* studied affecting the study variable, Completely Randomized Design (CRD)/one-way ANOVA is used.

Example: The study population consists of only children who are severely malnourished and a clinical trial is conducted to study the efficacy of three methods: diet, drug and placebo, in increasing their weight.

5.4.2.2. RCBD

If two or more factors are studied affecting the study variable or if the study elements in the population are heterogeneous with respect to the factor(s), in addition to the main factor studied, Randomized Complete Block Design (RCBD)/two or multiple-way ANOVA is used.

Example. The population consists of children who are mildly, moderately or severely malnourished and a clinical trial is conducted to study the efficacy of three methods: diet, drug and placebo in increasing their weight. Here, the children are classified according to their malnourishment status, and in each group they are randomly allocated into three methods of treatment. This design will enhance the validity of comparison of the mean weight increase among the three Groups as compared to the Completely Randomized Design

5.4.2.3. Repeated measures design

If the values of the variable of the subjects are recorded *before* and *after* an *intervention* (more than once after the intervention), Repeated Measures Design is adopted for a valid comparison of the mean values of the variable between various timings of recording, taking into consideration the variation between the subjects.

Example. Blood pressure values of hypertension patients were recorded before and after *one* week and after *two* weeks after giving a drug. To test the statistical significance of the differences in mean BP among the three timings of recording, Repeated Measures Analysis will enable us to make a more valid comparison.

5.4.3. Homogeneity of Variances

Before applying ANOVA test, the assumptions for applying ANOVA should be checked. Normality of the distributions of the variable in the different populations has to be verified from the available literature or if no information is available in the literature, normality has to be established by drawing histograms/frequency curves, verifying the properties of normal distribution for the different samples and computing the skewness and kurtosis measures. In case of larger samples, normality can be assumed. In case of non-normal distributions, transformation of the original variable into some other form may be tried and proved that the distribution is normal in terms of the transformed variable. In case of positive skewness, log transformation $\{X = \text{Log}(X)\}$ may be done and in case of negative skewness, square root transformation $\left\{X = \sqrt{(X)}\right\}$ can be done. Other transformations for getting normal distribution are reciprocal $(1/X)$, e^X, etc.

It has also to be verified whether the samples have been selected from the respective populations randomly or not. If the population parameter values are known the randomness of the selected samples can be verified by applying the normal test mentioned above. Otherwise, it has to be assumed that the samples are selected randomly.

Homogeneity (equality) of variances of the variable in the different Groups has to be tested. The most commonly used test is Bartlett's Test. If this test shows non-significance, ANOVA can be applied on the original values of the variable. If this shows statistical significance, appropriate transformation (log, square root, inverse, etc.) has to be done for the original values before applying ANOVA.

5.4.4 Multiple Range Tests

If the analysis of variance provides statistically significant F-value for the treatment variations (i.e., if the ANOVA shows statistically significant differences in the mean values among the Groups), it implies that there is at least one treatment mean that is different from the rest of the treatment means. Appropriate Multiple Range Test has to be applied to find out significantly different pairs of groups. Various Multiple Range tests are available and can be used depending upon the purpose. If comparison among all possible groups is required, the most commonly used Multiple Range Test is Student-Newman-Keul's **(SNK) Test.** If comparison of the test groups is required only with the control group, Dunnette's test is applied. Other Multiple Range tests available are Duncan's test, Tukey's test, Scheffe's test and Bonferroni's test. Here, only SNK test will be explained. For other tests, the books listed under 'references' may be referred. In the statistical software used, relevant choice of the test can be made and the results can be got.

5.4.5. Examples in ANOVA

(1) One-way ANOVA (three groups)

Example 6. Birth weights (in kg) of babies born to women classified according to their health status are given below:

Health status of women		
Good	*Fair*	*Poor*
3.1	3.0	2.4
2.9	2.6	2.2
3.5	2.5	2.0
3.6	2.7	2.3
3.4	2.6	2.2
	2.8	2.1
	2.7	2.0
		2.4
		2.3
		2.5

n =	5	7	10
Σ = Total =	16.5	18.9	22.4
Mean =	3.3	2.7	2.24

Test whether the differences in mean birth weight of babies among the three groups of women are statistically significant or not, i.e., whether birth weight is associated or not with mother's health status.

n = 5 + 7 + 10 = 22   r = No. of groups = 3

The total degrees of freedom and variation are partitioned into various components as follows:

Degrees of freedom

Total = Total observations – 1 = 22 – 1 = 21

Group = Total number of groups – 1= 3 –1 = 2

Error = Total – Group = 21-2 = 19

Compute Correction Factor (CF), Total Sum of Squares (TSS), Group Sum of Squares (GSS) and Error Sum of Squares (ESS) as follows:

$$\text{Correction factor (C.F.)} = \frac{(3.1 + 2.9 + \ldots 2.5)^2}{22} = \frac{(57.8)^2}{22} = 151.86$$

$$\text{TSS} = \left[(3.1)^2 + (2.9)^2 + \ldots (2.5)^2 \right] - \text{C.F.}$$

$$= 156.42 - 151.86 = 4.56$$

$$\text{GSS} = \frac{(16.5)^2}{5} + \frac{(18.9)^2}{7} + \frac{(22.4)^2}{10} - \text{C.F.}$$

$$= 155.66 - 151.86 = 3.80$$

ESS = TSS – GSS = 0.76

Mean Sum of Squares for Group and Error are computed as follows:

$$\text{M.S.S. (Group)} = \frac{\text{SS (Group)}}{d.f.\,(\text{Group})} = \frac{3.80}{2} = 1.9$$

$$\text{M.S.S. (Error)} = \frac{\text{SS (Error)}}{d.f.\,(\text{Error})} = \frac{0.76}{19} = 0.04$$

Fisher's F-statistics for testing the statistical significance of the differences in mean values among groups is computed as:

$$F = \frac{\text{M.S.S. (Group)}}{\text{M.S.S. (Error)}} = \frac{1.9}{0.04} = 47.5$$

All the above given details can be conveniently presented in a tabular form called 'ANOVA table'.

ANOVA Table

Source of variation	d.f.	Sum of squares (SS)	Mean sum of squares (MSS)	F-ratio	P- value
Total (T)	(n-1) = 21	4.56			
Due to mother's health status Group					
(G)	(r-1) = 2	3.80	1.90	47.5	<0.001
Error (E)	(n-1-(r-1) = (n-r) = 19	0.76	0.04		

F is distributed as Fisher's F with (r-1), (n-r) d.f., i.e., with 2, 19 d.f.

Refer to Fisher's 'F' table at $\propto = 0.05$, 2 d.f. horizontally and 19 d.f. vertically.

F (2, 19) = 3.52 at $\alpha = 0.05$ (Statistical Table - Appendix 3)

F $\propto$ = 0.01 (2, 19) = 5.93

F = 47.5 > F at $\alpha = 0.01$, p < 0.01.

Differences in mean birth weights among the three groups are statistically highly significant, i.e., birth weight of baby is significantly associated with mother's health status. Level of Confidence = 99%, i.e., better the health status of mothers, higher was the birth weight of babies.

(2) Multiple comparisons among mean values (Student-Newman-Keul's Test (SNK Test)

If ANOVA provides statistically significant F-value for the treatment variation, then SNK test is applied to find out significant pairs of groups.

Steps:

Arrange the mean values in descending order, say A, B & C.

$$\text{Find } q_1 = \frac{\bar{X}_A - \bar{X}_C}{\sqrt{\frac{\text{MESS}}{2}\left(\frac{1}{n_A} + \frac{1}{n_C}\right)}} \qquad q_2 = \frac{\bar{X}_A - \bar{X}_B}{\sqrt{\frac{\text{MESS}}{2}\left(\frac{1}{n_A} + \frac{1}{n_B}\right)}}$$

$$q_3 = \frac{\bar{X}_B - \bar{X}_C}{\sqrt{\frac{\text{MESS}}{2}\left(\frac{1}{n_B} + \frac{1}{n_C}\right)}}$$

Refer to Standardized Student Range Table (see page 746-47, Armitage et al listed under further reading), for error d.f. at $\alpha = 0.05$ at $p = 3$ for comparing A & C and $p = 2$ for comparing A & B and B & C and call them q_1', q_2', and q_3' respectively.

If $q_1 > q_1'$, then the difference between A & C is significant ($p < 0.05$).

Refer table for $\alpha = 0.01$ at $p = 3$ and find q_1''.

If $q_1 > q_1''$ then the difference is highly significant ($p < 0.01$).

Carry out the same procedure for comparing A & B (q_2 and q_2'; q_2 and q_2'') and for comparing B & C (q_3 and q_3'; and q_3 and q_3'').

For the example, ANOVA provided a significant F value for Group variation.

$$q_1 = \frac{3.3 - 2.24}{\sqrt{\frac{0.04}{2}\left[\frac{1}{5} + \frac{1}{10}\right]}} = \frac{1.06}{0.072} = 13.77$$

$$q_2 = \frac{3.3 - 2.27}{\sqrt{\frac{0.04}{2}\left[\frac{1}{5} + \frac{1}{7}\right]}} = \frac{0.6}{0.083} = 7.23$$

$$q_3 = \frac{2.7 - 2.24}{\sqrt{\frac{0.04}{2}\left[\frac{1}{7} + \frac{1}{10}\right]}} = \frac{0.46}{0.07} = 6.57$$

$q_1' = 3.593 \qquad q_2' = 2.96 \qquad q_3' = 2.96$

$q_1'' = 4.670 \qquad q_2'' = 4.046 \qquad q_3'' = 4.046$

$q_1 > q_1'' \qquad q_2 > q_2'' \qquad q_3 > q_3''$

i.e., birth weights (BW) of babies born to women of good health status are significantly higher than those of babies born to women of fair status or poor status ($p < 0.01$). Also, birth weights of babies born to women of fair health status are significantly higher than those of babies born to women of poor health status ($p < 0.01$).

If $n_A = n_B = n_C = n$, then the denominator of q_1, q_2 & q_3 is simplified to $\sqrt{\dfrac{\text{MESS}}{n}}$

Example 7. (Completely Randomized Design)

A study was conducted to investigate the effect of supplementary nutrition, a drug and placebo in increasing the weight of severely malnourished children. Fifteen severely malnourished children were randomly divided into three Groups A, B & C. Group A was given supplementary nutrition, Group B, the drug and Group C, the placebo. Gain in weight in these children was noted after one month of treatment. Results of the study are given below.

Test whether the differences in weight gain, on an average, among the three groups are statistically significant or not at 5% level of significance. Also, test whether the difference between any two groups is statistically significant or not at 5% level of significance.

	A	B	C	Total
	Gain in weight (kg)			
	0.20	0.10	0.05	0.35
	0.15	0.10	0.10	0.35
	0.10	0.05	0.05	0.20
	0.30	0.15	0.05	0.50
	0.25	0.20	0.15	0.60
Total	1.00	0.60	0.40	2.00
Mean	0.20	0.12	0.08	

Degrees of Freedom

Total = Total observations − 1 = 15 − 1 = 14

Group = Total number of groups − 1 = 3 − 1 = 2

Error = Total − Group = 14 − 2 = 12

$$\text{Correction Factor} = C.F. = \frac{(\text{Total})^2}{\text{Sample size}} = \frac{(2.00)^2}{15} = 0.2667$$

$$\text{Total Sum of Squares} = T.S.S. = (0.2)^2 + (0.15)^2 - 0.2667$$
$$= 0.35 - 0.2667 = 0.0833$$

$$\text{Group S.S.} = \frac{(1.00)^2 + (0.60)^2 + (0.40)^2}{5} - C.F.$$
$$= 0.3040 - 0.2667 = 0.0373$$

$$\text{ERROR S.S.} = T.S.S. - \text{GROUP S.S.}$$
$$= 0.0833 - 0.0373 = 0.046$$

$$\text{M.S.S. (Group)} = \frac{SS\,(\text{Group})}{d.f.\,(\text{Group})} = \frac{0.0373}{2} = 0.01865$$

$$\text{M.S.S. (Error)} = \frac{SS\,(\text{Error})}{d.f.\,(\text{Error})} = \frac{0.0460}{12} = 0.0038$$

$$F = \frac{\text{M.S.S. (Group)}}{\text{M.S.S. (Error)}} = \frac{0.01865}{0.0038} = 4.91$$

ANOVA Table

Source of Variation	d.f.	S.S.	M.S.S.	F	p
Total	14	0.0833			
Between Groups	2	0.0373	0.01865	4.91	< 0.05
Error	12	0.0460	0.0038		

By referring the F table for 2 degrees of freedom (d.f.) horizontally and 12 d.f. vertically, it can be seen that the critical ratio is 3.89 at $\alpha = 0.05$ (Statistical Tables - Appendix 3).

Computed F-value for Between Group variation is 4.91, which is greater than the critical ratio of 3.89 and, hence, the null hypothesis of no difference among the three group means is rejected, i.e., there is significant difference in the mean gain in weight among the three groups of children who received three different nutritional supplements.

Since the ANOVA has shown statistically significant difference in the mean gain in weight among the three groups, to find out the pairs of groups which are significantly different, SNK Multiple Range test is applied.

$$\sqrt{\frac{MESS}{5}} = 0.0276$$

$$q_1 = \frac{0.2 - 0.08}{0.0276} = 4.35$$

$$q_2 = \frac{0.2 - 0.12}{0.0276} = 2.90$$

$$q_3 = \frac{0.12 - 0.08}{0.0276} = 1.45$$

$q_1' = 3.77$ (at $\alpha = 0.05$ d.f. = 3, 12) $\qquad$ $q_1'' = 5.05$ (at $\alpha = 0.01$ d.f. = 3, 12)

$q_2' = 3.08$ (at $\alpha = 0.05$ d.f. = 2, 12) $\qquad$ $q_2'' = 4.32$ (at $\alpha = 0.01$ d.f. = 2, 12)

$q_3' = 3.08$ (at $\alpha = 0.05$ d.f. = 2, 12) $\qquad$ $q_3'' = 4.32$ (at $\alpha = 0.01$ d.f. = 2, 12)

(refer to page 754-55, Armitage et al)

i.e., $q_1 > 3.77$; but < 5.05

$q_2 < q_2'$ and $q_3 < q_3'$

i.e., gain in weight in severely malnourished children who received supplementary diet was significantly larger than in those who received placebo, on an average ($p < 0.05$; confidence = 95%). However, differences observed in gain in weight between those who received supplementary diet and drug or between those who received drug and placebo were statistically not significant ($p > 0.05$).

(3) Two-way ANOVA (Randomized Complete Block Design - RCBD)

Example 8. In a clinical trial to test the efficacy of two drugs and a placebo in the sleeping hours of mental patients it was thought that age of the patient could also influence the sleeping hours. Hence, the patients were stratified according to their age group and then randomly distributed into three treatment groups (each age-treatment category one patient). The results of the trial are given below:

Age group (years)	A	B	Placebo	Total
	Improvement in sleeping hours			
24-34	2.3	1.6	0.6	4.5
35-44	2.0	1.4	0.4	3.8
45-54	1.8	1.0	0.3	3.1
55 and More	1.2	0.8	0.3	2.3
Total	7.3	4.8	1.6	13.7
Mean	1.825	1.2	0.4	

The results of the two-way ANOVA are given below:

$$n = \text{Total patients} = 12, \text{Correction factor} = \frac{(13.7)^2}{12} = 15.64$$

$r = \text{No. of age groups} = 4$, $p = \text{No. of drugs} = 3$

$$\text{TSS} = \left((2.3)^2 + (2.0)^2 + \ldots (0.3)^2 - \text{CF}\right) = 20.83 - 15.64 = 5.19$$

$$\text{Age SS} = \text{(Between groups)} = \frac{(4.5)^2 + (3.8)^2 + (3.1)^2 + (2.3)^2}{3} - \text{C.F.}$$

$$= 16.33 - 15.64 = 0.89$$

$$\text{Drug SS} = \text{(Between blocks)} = \frac{(7.3)^2 + (4.8)^2 + (1.6)^2}{4} - \text{C.F.}$$

$$= 19.7225 - 15.64 = 4.0825$$

$$\text{Error SS} = \text{TSS} - \text{Age SS} - \text{Drug SS} = 0.2175$$

ANOVA Table

Source of Variation	d.f.	S.S.	M.S.S.	F	p
Total	(n-1) = 11	5.19			
Due to age	(r-1) = 3	0.89	0.2967	8.2	< 0.05
Due to drug	(p-1) = 2	4.0825	2.0412	56.4	<0.001
Error	(n-1)-(r-1)-(p-1) = n-r-p+1 = 6	0.2175	0.0362		

$$\text{F (age)} = \frac{\left((\text{MSS}) \text{Age}\right)}{\text{MESS}} = \frac{0.2967}{0.0362} = 8.20 > 4.76 (p < 0.05)$$

(3, 6)

$$\begin{bmatrix} \text{F} & (\text{at } \alpha = 0.05) = 4.76 \\ (3, 6) \ (\text{at } \alpha = 0.01) = 9.78 \end{bmatrix} \text{(From the 'F' Table (Statistical Tables-Appendix 3)}$$

$$\text{F (Drug)} = \frac{\text{MSS (Drug)}}{\text{MESS}} = \frac{2.0412}{0.0362} = 56.39 > F_{2,6 \text{ at}} \atop \alpha = 0.001 \atop (p < 0.001)$$

(2, 6)

$$\begin{bmatrix} {}^F(2,6) \text{ at } \alpha = 0.01, = 10.92 \\ \text{at } \alpha = 0.001, = \text{ much less than } 56.39 \end{bmatrix}$$

Conclusions:

1. Influence of age on treatment effect is significant (p <0.05), i.e., accounting for variation due to age has helped in reducing the error (MESS) and in improving the precision of the estimate.
2. Differences in mean improvement in sleeping hours among the three treatment groups are statistically significant (p <0.001).

Efficiency of blocking (E):

Efficiency of the RCBD compared to CRD can be studied by computing the ratio:

Approximate $E = \dfrac{\text{MESS without considering age}}{\text{MESS considering age}}$

$$= \dfrac{0.1231}{0.0362} = 3.40$$

i.e., without accounting for variation due to age, almost 3½ times for each case (or 7 for 2 cases) are required for having the same precision in the estimate. That means, for a pre-defined confidence level, say, 95%, 3½ times more cases are required if the analysis is done assuming completely randomized design, whereas the analysis should have been done for randomized complete block design when the information is available for the blocks (in this example, age groups).

(4) Multiple comparisons among treatment groups (SNK test)

ANOVA has provided significant F-value for treatment variation.

Mean improvement in sleeping hours:

Drug A: 1.825 (A), Drug B: 1.200 (B), Placebo: 1.825 (C)

Sample size n_A (Drug A) = n_b (drug B)

$\qquad\qquad = n_c$ (placebo) = 4 (because of two-way ANOVA)

Denominator of $q = \sqrt{\dfrac{\text{MESS}}{4}} = \sqrt{\dfrac{0.0362}{4}} = 0.0951$

$q_1 \dfrac{\bar{X}_A - \bar{X}_C}{\sqrt{\dfrac{\text{MESS}}{4}}} = \dfrac{1.425}{0.0951} = 14.98 \qquad q_2 \dfrac{\bar{X}_A - \bar{X}_B}{\sqrt{\dfrac{\text{MESS}}{4}}} = \dfrac{0.625}{0.0951} = 6.57 \qquad q_3 \dfrac{\bar{X}_B - \bar{X}_C}{\sqrt{\dfrac{\text{MESS}}{4}}} = \dfrac{0.8}{0.0951} = 8.41$

$q_1{}' = 4.34$, $q_2{}' = 3.46$, $q_3{}' = 3.46$

$q_1{}'' = 6.33$, $q_2{}'' = 5.24$, $q_3{}'' = 5.24$

(Error d.f. = 6, p = 3 for q_1, p = 2 for q_2 and q_3)

(refer to page 754-55, Armitage et al)

i.e., improvement in sleeping hours with drug A was significantly higher than that with drug B and placebo (p < 0.01) and that with drug B was significantly higher than that with placebo, on an average.

(5) Two-way ANOVA (RCB design where individuals themselves serve as blocks)

Example 9. Systolic blood pressure values of 10 patients, before treatment and after treatment for 1 and 2 weeks are given below. Test whether the change (reduction) in systolic blood pressure after treatment is statistically significant or not.

Sl. No.	Before	After 1 week	After 2 weeks	Total
1.	170	160	140	470
2.	165	160	135	460
3.	180	170	140	490
4.	175	165	135	475
5.	165	160	135	460
6.	180	160	140	480
7.	175	170	145	490
8.	160	150	125	435
9.	155	140	120	415
10.	165	145	120	430
Total	1690	1580	1335	4605
Mean	196	158	133.5	

C.F. = 706867.5

T.S.S. = (286250 + 250550 +178925) – C.F.

$\quad$ = 715725 – 706867.5 = 8857.5

$Patient\ SS = PSS = \dfrac{2126675}{3} - 706867.5 = 2024.17$

$TIMES\ S. = \dfrac{7134725}{10} - 706867.5 = 6605.0$

E.S.S. = T.S.S. – P.S.S. – Time SS

$\quad$ = 8857.5 – 2024.17 – 6605 = 228.33

$M.S.S\ (time) = \dfrac{6605.0}{2} = 3302.5$

$M.S.S\ (patient) = \dfrac{2024.17}{9} = 224.91$

$M.S.S\ (Error) = \dfrac{228.33}{18} = 12.685$

Two-way ANOVA Table

Source of Variation	d.f.	S.S.	M.S.S.	F	p
Total (T)	29	8857.5			
Between Time (T)	2	6605.0	3302.5	260.2	< 0.001
Between Patients (P)	9	2024.17	224.9	17.7	< 0.001
Error (E)	18	228.33	12.69		

F (P) (9, 18) = 17.7 > 3.60 (P < 0.01) (Statistical Tables - Appendix 3)

F (Time) 2, 18 = 260.2 > 6.01 (p < 0.01)

Both F (P) 9, 18 and F (time) 2, 18 are much greater than the corresponding critical ratios at a = 0.001, i.e., p < 0.001, in both cases.

Thus, variation in BP among patients is statistically significant. After accounting for this variation, the differences in mean BP among the three time periods are statistically significant (p < 0.001).

Efficiency of RCBD compared to CRD is given by:

$Approximate\ E = \dfrac{83.426}{12.69} = 6.57$

i.e., without accounting for patient variation (without pairing patients) about 6 cases are required for each case for having the same precision in the estimate. That means, for a pre-defined confidence level, say, 95%, 6½ times more cases are required if the analysis is done assuming completely randomized design, whereas the analysis should have been done for randomized complete block design when the information is available for the blocks(in this example, individual cases which are paired-before, after 1 week and after two weeks).

(6) Multiple comparisons (S N K Test)

Mean BP	Before	After 1 Week	After 2 Weeks
	169	158	133.5
	$(\bar{X}_A)$	$(\bar{X}_B)$	$(\bar{X}_C)$

$$\text{Denominator} = \sqrt{\frac{\text{MESS}}{10}} = \sqrt{\frac{12.69}{10}} = 1.13$$

$$q_1 = \frac{35.5}{1.13} = 31.4 \quad q_2 = \frac{35.5}{1.13} = 9.73 \quad q_3 = \frac{35.5}{1.13} = 21.7$$

$$q_1'' = 4.7 \quad q_2'' = 4.07 \quad q_3'' = 4.07$$

$$q_1 > q_1'', \, q_2 > q_2'', \, q_3 > q_3''$$

(refer to page 754-55, Armitage et al)

i.e., reduction in BP, 1 week after treatment and 2 weeks after treatment is statistically significant ($p < 0.001$). Reduction from 1 week to 2 weeks after treatment is also statistically significant ($p < 0.001$).

5.5. Analysis of Covariance

In ANOVA, explained above, the main variable under study is a continuous variable and the blocking factors are discrete variables with categories. If there is another continuous variable (called co-variate or concomitant variable), which may affect the main variable, then for a valid comparison of the main variable between two or more than two groups, the effect of the co-variate should be taken into consideration. This will increase the precision of the comparison. This analysis is called Analysis of Co-variance (ANOCOVA).

In any study involving a single quantitative variable, say, systolic blood pressure, design of experiment may fall into one of the following three categories.

1. Studying the difference in average values of the dependent quantitative variable between a number of categories of one or more qualitative variables.

Example. Studying the differences in average blood pressure (BP) values between various ethnic groups (first independent qualitative variable) and between sexes (second independent qualitative variable). **Analysis of variance** is the statistical technique applied for this purpose. This analysis helps us in sorting out the variation due to ethnic group and sex and thus to reduce the error variation and increase the precision of the comparison. The conclusion (acceptance or rejection) regarding the hypothesis of no difference in blood pressure between sexes and between ethnic groups will be more valid in such analysis.

2. Studying the possible changes in the dependent variable that may accompany changes in quantitative independent variable (s).

Example. Studying the possible changes in systolic BP values which may accompany changes in the age of the subjects. **Correlation and regression analysis** will be the statistical technique to be applied for this purpose.

3. Studying the differences in average values of the dependent quantitative variable between a number of categories of a qualitative variable, which may influence the quantitative variable linearly.

Example. Studying the differences in average systolic BP values between two groups of heart patients after giving two different drugs, taking into consideration that the blood pressure values after giving the drugs are influenced by values before giving the drugs, i.e., comparatively higher values may be recorded for those with higher initial values and lower values with lower initial values, showing a good correlation between initial and final B.P. values. If this fact is not taken into consideration the conclusion arrived at only from the final values would not be valid. The most appropriate analysis to be applied for such a design is **analysis of covariance (ANOCOVA).** The quantitative independent variable in **ANOCOVA** is called a **covariate** or a **concomitant variable.**

We can see from the above explanation that **analysis of covariance** combines the advantages of both **analysis of variance** and **regression**. By doing so the precision of randomized experiment is increased by controlling the extraneous variability. Controlling the variability by applying analysis of covariance is the statistical method applied at the analysis stage. This can be done at design stage also if possible and feasible, by grouping the subjects into homogeneous groups (blocks), e.g., grouping the subjects into different treatment groups according to their weight. But in many situations this may not be feasible or may be less precise. Covariance analysis can give higher precision in such situations. This gain in precision in such analysis depends upon the degree of correlation between the covariate and dependent study variable. **Precision** will be higher when the degree of correlation is higher.

5.6. Discrete Variables

Parameters and methods of estimation and tests of statistical significance in case of discrete variables are different from those for continuous variables.

5.6.1. Estimation

Point estimate: Parameters of point estimate for discrete variables are: proportion, percentage, ratio and rate. Examples are:
1. Proportion of persons diagnosed as cases in a survey of diabetes ($p = 0.14$ or 14%)
2. Proportion of smokers with lung cancer ($p = 0.24$ or 24%)
3. Sex ratio: 970 females/1000 males
    Doctor/population ratio: 1 : 10,000
4. Birth rate, death rate, etc.

Interval estimate: Interval estimates of 95% or 99% or 99.9 %
Confidence intervals for proportion, percentage ratio and rate can be computed as follows:

(1) If $p = 0.14$ and $n = 900$, S.E = $\sqrt{(pq/n)}$ = 0.0116
     95% Confidence limits: $p - 1.96$ SE and $p + 1.96$ SE: 0.1172-3 and 0.1627
(2) If $p = 24\%$ and $n = 10,000$, SE = 0.43
     99% Confidence limits: $p - 2.58$ SE and $p + 2.58$ SE; 23.2 & 24.8

5.6.2. Tests of Significance

(a) Chi-square (λ^2) test (2*2, 2*n, r*n)
(b) Z-test (proportion)
(c) Matched λ^2 test (McNemar's test) (2*2 or p*p)

Example. 2*2:
Two rows and two columns (two subgroups for each of the two discrete variables)
Example: Patients receiving two types of treatment (two groups) —rows
Response to the treatment—improved and not improved ——columns

Example. 2*n:
Two rows and n columns (two subgroups for one discrete variable and n subgroups for the other discrete variable)
Example: Patients receiving four types of treatment (4 groups)—rows
Response to the treatment improved and not improved—columns

Example. r*n:

r rows and n columns (r subgroups for one discrete variable and n subgroups for the other discrete variable)

Example: Patients receiving four types of treatment (4 groups)—rows

Response to the treatment –complete improvement, partial improvement and not improved—columns

5.6.2.1. Chi-square test (χ^2)

Purpose (A): For testing the statistical significance of the association between two discrete (qualitative) variables (test of independence)

Examples:

(1) To test whether lung cancer is associated with smoking or not.

(2) Whether diabetes is associated with type of occupation or not.

(3) Whether the drug is more effective or not in curing a particular disease compared to placebo.

Purpose (B): For testing the statistical significance of the linear trend (increase or decrease) in the magnitude of the parameter values (proportions) in relation to an ordered factor (ordinal variable).

Example. To see whether the trend of increase in the proportion of cases with respect to the socio-economic status of the subjects studied is statistically significant or not.

Purpose (C): For testing the goodness of fit of a sample distribution of a variable with respect to a standard distribution (goodness of the fitted theoretical distribution to a sample distribution).

Example. To test whether the sample distribution of cases of a particular disease is according to standard pattern or not, say, 20% of type A, 50% of type B and 30% of type C.

Formulae for the χ^2 - statistic:

$$\chi^2 = \sum \frac{(0-E)^2}{E}$$ 0- Observed number (Observed frequency)

E - Expected Number (Expected frequency

This is distributed as χ^2 with (n-1) degrees of freedom. (Appendix 5)

Degree of freedom: Number of independent observation/cells in the sample. When the marginal totals are fixed and if one of the cell frequency is known, the other three cell frequencies can be obtained by subtraction, i.e., though there are 4 cells, the number of independent cells is only one, i.e., degree of freedom (d.f.) = 1

Method for finding d.f.:

If there are r – rows and c – columns, d.f. = (r-1) (c – 1)

        If, r = 2, c = 2, d.f. = 1; If, r = 3, c = 4 d.f. = 6

Meaning of expected frequencies (2 * 2)

		Smoking		
		Yes	No	
Lung	Yes	20	10	30
Cancer	No	30	140	170
Total		50	150	200

In the above example,

Probability that a randomly selected person out of 200 persons is a cancer case, irrespective of whether he is a smoker or not	$= 30 \div 200$
	$= 0.15$
With equal probability (under Ho), expected number of cases out of 50 smokers	$= 50 \times 0.15$
	$= 7.5$
With equal probability (under Ho), expected number of cases out of 150 non-smokers	$= 150 \times 0.15$
	$= 22.5$
Probability that a randomly selected person out of 200 persons is a normal person, irrespective of whether he is smoker or not	$= 170 \div 200$
	$= 0.85$
With equal probability (under Ho), expected number of normal persons out of 50 smokers	$= 50 \times 0.85$
	$= 42.5$
With equal probability (under Ho), expected number of normal persons out of 150 smokers	$= 150 \times 0.85$
	$= 127.5$

$O_a = 20, O_b = 10, O_c = 30, O_d = 140,$
$E_a = 7.5 \; E_b = 22.5 \; E_c = 42.5 \; E_d = 127.5$

Example 10. Data on smoking habit and presence of lung cancer is given below:

		Smoking			
		Yes	No		Total
Lung	Yes	Yes	20 (a)	10 (b)	30
Cancer	No	No	30 (c)	140 (d)	170
Total		50	150	200 (n)	

$O_a = 20, O_b = 10, O_c = 30, O_d = 140$ Observed frequencies

$$E_a = \frac{50*30}{200} = 7.5 \qquad E_b = \frac{150*30}{200} = 22.5$$

Expected frequencies

$$E_c = \frac{50*170}{200} = 42.5 \qquad E_d = \frac{150*170}{200} = 127.5$$

$$\chi^2 = \frac{(20-7.5)^2}{7.5} + \frac{(10-22.5)^2}{22.5} + \frac{(30-42.5)^2}{42.5} + \frac{(140-127.5)^2}{127.5}$$

$= 32.68 > 10.83 \; (p < 0.001)$

(see Statistical Tables - Appendix 5)

χ^2 - critical value at 1 d.f. at $\alpha = 0.05, \; = 3.84$

$\qquad\qquad\qquad\qquad \alpha = 0.01, \; = 6.63$ (Statistical Tables - Appendix 5)

$\qquad\qquad\qquad\qquad \alpha = 0.001, = 10.83$

i.e., lung cancer is statistically associated with smoking and the association is highly significant. We can have a level of confidence of 99.9% in making this statement.

Percentage of cases in smokers $= 20/50 \; = 40\%$

Percentage of cases in non – smokers $= 10/150 = 6.7\%$

i.e., percentage of cases in smokers is significantly higher than in non–smokers.

A simplified formula for χ^2 statistic is $= \dfrac{(ad - bc)^2 \times n}{(a+b)(c+d)(a+c)(b+d)}$

For the above given example,

$$\chi^2 = \frac{\left[(20*140)-(30*10)\right]^2 *200}{30*170*50*150}$$

$= 32.68$ (same value as in case of the first formula)

5.6.2.2. Yate's corrected (χ^2) statistic

If any of the expected frequencies is less than 5, then a correction factor for making the 2×2 chi-square into a continuous one (Yate's) is applied. A simple formula with Yate's correction is:

$$\chi^2 \frac{\left[|ad - bc| - \dfrac{n}{2}\right]^2 \times n}{(a+b)(c+d)(a+c)(b+d)}$$

or $= \sum \dfrac{\left[|\text{O-E}| - 0.5\right]^2}{\text{E}}$

Example 11. Data on smoking habit and presence of lung cancer in another study is given below:

		Smoking		
		Yes	No	
	Yes	6	1	7
Lung cancer	No	4	19	23
Total		10	20	30

Percentage of lung cancer cases among smokers = 6/10 = 60
Percentage of lung cancer cases among non-smokers = 1/20 = 5
Observed frequencies $O_a = 6$, $O_b = 1$, $O_c = 4$, $O_d = 19$
Expected frequencies : $E_a = 2.33$ $\quad E_b = 4.67$
$\qquad\qquad\qquad E_c = 7.67$ $\quad E_d = 15.33$
$E_a = (2.3)$ and $E_b = (4.7)$ values are less than 5 and, hence, Yate's correction has to be applied in the χ^2 formula.

$$\chi^2 = \frac{\left[|(6*19)-(1*4)|-15\right]^2 *30}{7*23*10*20} \text{ OR} = \frac{(|6-2.33|-0.5)^2}{2.33} + \frac{\left[|1-4.67|-0.5\right]^2}{4.67}$$

$$+ \frac{(|4-7.67|-0.5)^2}{7.67} + \frac{\left[|19-15.33|-0.5\right]^2}{15.33}$$

$= 8.41 > 6.63$ (p < 0.01)
(see Statistical Tables - Appendix 5)

Percentage of lung cancer cases among smokers is significantly higher than that among non-smokers, i.e., **lung cancer is statistically associated with smoking (confidence = 99%).**

Example 12. Results on the improvement rate in patients with drug and placebo are given below:

Result	Drug	Placebo	
Improved	14 (70%)	5 (25%)	19
Not improved	6	15	21
Total	20	20	40

$O_a = 14$, $O_b = 5$, $O_c = 6$, $O_d = 15$
$E_a = 9.5$, $E_b = 9.5$, $E_c = 10.5$, $E_d = 10.5$
All expected frequencies are greater than 5.

$$\chi^2 = \frac{\left[\left(14*15 - (6*5)^2 *40 \right) \right]*40}{20*20*19*21} = 8.12 > 6.63 (< p \ 0.01)$$

$$\text{or } = \frac{(14-9.5)^2}{9.5} + \frac{(5-9.5)^2}{9.5} + \frac{(6-10.5)^2}{10.5} + \frac{(15-10.5)^2}{10.5} = 8.12 > 6.63 (p < 0.01)$$

(see Statistical Tables - Appendix 5)

Percentage of patients improved with the drug = 14/20 = 70%

Percentage of patients improved with the placebo = 5/20 = 25%

Thus, percentage of patients showing improvement with the drug was significantly higher than that with placebo.

Response to treatment is statistically associated with the type of drug used (confidence = 99%).

In a (2 * 2) contingency table (r = 2, c = 2) test for association can be done by applying a Proportion Test (Z-Test).

5.6.2.3. Chi-square test vs Z-test

Chi-squared (uncorrected) and Z- tests will give the same 'p' value. The relationship between them is $\sqrt{\chi^2} = Z$. χ^2 test is basically a test for association, takes no account of the sign (+/–) of difference and it is a two-tailed test. If we are interested in the size of the difference in the 2 proportions, Z- test is preferable. For one-tailed alternatives also, Z-test is preferable.

$$Z = \frac{|p_1 - p_2|}{\sqrt{pq \left(\frac{1}{n_1} + \frac{1}{n_2} \right)}} \quad \text{if } n_1 \ \& \ n_2 > 30$$

$$Z = \frac{|p_1 - p_2| - \frac{1}{2} \left[\frac{1}{n_1} + \frac{1}{n_2} \right]}{\sqrt{pq \left(\frac{1}{n_1} + \frac{1}{n_2} \right)}} \quad \text{if } n_1 \ \& \ n_2 \text{ or both } n_1 \text{ and } n_2 < 30$$

where n_1 and n_2 are sample sizes

$$p_1 = \frac{r_1}{n_1} \quad p_2 = \frac{r_2}{n_2}$$

r_1 = No. of cases with the factor in sample 1 (n_1)

r_2 = No. of cases with the factor in sample 2 (n_2)

$$p = \frac{r_1 + r_2}{n_1 + n_2} \quad q = (1 - p)$$

Example 13. For the data given in example-12, $(n_1 = n_2 = 20)$

$$Z = \frac{|0.70 - 0.25| - \frac{1}{2}\left[\left(\frac{1}{20} + \frac{1}{20}\right)\right]}{\sqrt{\left(0.475 * 0.525\left[\frac{2}{20}\right]\right)}}$$

$$= \frac{0.45 - 0.05}{0.158} = \frac{0.40}{0.158} = 2.53 > 1.96 \ (P < 0.05)$$

Critical ratio of Z (Z_{CR})

$$\begin{array}{l}
\quad\quad\quad\quad\quad\quad\quad \text{Confidence} \\
\left[\begin{array}{lll}
\text{If } \alpha = 0.05 & Z_{CR} = 1.96 & 95\% \\
\text{If } \alpha = 0.01 & Z_{CR} = 2.58 & 99\% \\
\text{If } \alpha = 0.001 & Z_{CR} = 3.29 & 99.9\% \\
\end{array}\right. \\
\text{No degree of freedom is involved and hence the statistical table need not be referred.}
\end{array}$$

Percentage of cases improved with drug (70%) was significantly higher than that with the placebo (25%) $(p < 0.05;$ confidence $= 95\%)$

Example 14. For the data given in example 10,

$n_1 = 50$ & $n_2 = 150$, i.e., both n_1 & n_2 are > 30

$p_1 = 0.4$, $p_2 = 0.067$

$$p = \frac{20 + 10}{200} = 0.15 \quad q = (1-p) = 1 - 0.15 = 0.85$$

$$z = \frac{0.4 - 0.067}{\sqrt{(0.15 * 0.85)\left[\frac{1}{50} + \frac{1}{150}\right]}} = \frac{0.0333}{0.0583} = 5.71 > 3.29$$

i.e., Lung cancer is significantly associated with smoking $(p < 0.001)$ – Confidence $= 99.9\%$

Example 15. For the data given in example 11

$$n_1 = 10 \ \& \ n_2 = 20 < 30; \ p_1 = \frac{6}{10} = 0.6 \quad p_2 = \frac{1}{20} = 0.05$$

$$Z = \frac{|0.6 - 0.5| - \left[\dfrac{1}{10} + \dfrac{1}{20}\right]}{\sqrt{(0.23 * 0.77)\left[\dfrac{1}{10} + \dfrac{1}{20}\right]}} \quad p = 0.23 \; q = 0.77$$

$$= \frac{0.55 - 0.075}{0.163} = \frac{0.475}{0.163} = 2.91 > 2.58 \; (p < 0.01)$$

i.e., Lung cancer is significantly associated with smoking ($p < 0.01$) – confidence = 99%.

5.6.2.4. Fisher's exact test

An exact method for testing the hypothesis of independence in 2*2 contingency tables is available. This test is called Fisher's exact test. This test is applied:

(1) if $(n_1 + n_2) < 40$, and
(2) one or more of the expected frequencies is <5.

Suppose the data are arranged in a 2*2 contingency table as shown below:

Group	+	–	Total
A	a	b	(a + b)
B	c	d	(c + d)
Total	(a + c)	(b + d)	n

Then the probability that the null hypothesis of no association (independence) is rejected when it is true is given by the addition of the probabilities of the smallest frequency and for all the smaller frequencies than this in the contingency table where the probability for the smallest frequency is given by:

P = {(a + b)! (c + d)! (a + c)! (b + d)!}/{n!a!b!c!d!}

Where n = a+b+c+d, '!' is called the 'factorial' as explained in Chapter-3.

The method is explained below:

Example 16. The contingency table given below shows the results (pain relief-yes or no) of two treatments (A and B) in cancer patients.

Group	Yes	No	Total
A	2(a)	8(b)	10
B	6(c)	4(d)	10
Total	8	12	20

Steps in Fisher's exact test are given below:

(1) Locate the observed smallest frequency in the table. In the example, the smallest frequency is 2.
(2) Compute the probability value using the above mentioned formula for a = 2, 1 and 0 keeping the marginal totals fixed.

The 2*2 contingency table for a = 1 is:

Group	Yes	No	Total
A	1	9	10
B	7	3	10
Total	8	12	20

The 2*2 contingency table for a = 0 is:

Group	Yes	No	Total
A	0	10	10
B	8	2	10
Total	8	12	20

$$\text{For a = 2, } P_2 = \frac{8! * 12! * 10! * 10!}{20! * 2! * 8! * 6! * 4!} = 0.0750$$

$$\text{For a = 1, } P_1 = \frac{8! * 12! * 10! * 10!}{20! * 1! * 9! * 7! * 3!} = 0.0095$$

$$\text{For a = 0, } P_0 = \frac{8! * 12! * 10! * 10!}{20! * 0! * 10! * 8! * 2!} = 0.0004$$

i.e., $p = p_2 + p_1 + p_0 = 0.0849$ (not significant at 5% level of significance-one-tailed test).

For the two tailed test (pain relief with the two treatments is statistically not the same), the above given 'p', should be multiplied by 2, i.e., $p = 0.0849*2 = 0.1698$. Thus, there is no statistically significant association between the treatment type and pain relief.

If the probability values (p) are computed for all possibilities of a (both smaller and larger than the observed value), without altering the marginal totals {(a+b), (b+d), (a+c) and (c+d), the p values obtained will be as follows:

a	d	p
0	- 80	0.0004
1	- 60	0.0095
2	- 40	0.0750
3	- 20	0.2401
4	0	0.3500
5	20	0.2401
6	40	0.0750
7	60	0.0095
8	80	0.0004
Total		1.0000

(d = Difference in percentages of patients showing pain relief between the two treatment groups)

It may be noted that the total of all these probabilities is equal to 1.

5.6.2.5. χ^2 Test for association

r = 3 rows, c = 2 columns

Example 17.

Socio-economic class	Nutritional status of children		
	Malnourished	*Normal*	*Total*
High	2 a	38 b	40
Middle	10 c	50 d	60
Low	40 e	60 f	100
Total	52	148	200

Cells	:	(a)	(b)	(c)	(d)	(e)	(f)
Observed frequencies	:	2	38	10	50	40	60
Expected frequencies	:	10.4	29.6	15.6	44.4	26.0	74.0

$$E_a = \frac{52 * 40}{200} = 10.4 \qquad E_b = \frac{148 * 40}{200} = 29.6 \qquad E_c = \frac{52 * 60}{200} = 15.6$$

$$E_d = \frac{148 * 60}{200} = 44.4 \qquad E_e = \frac{52 * 100}{200} = 26 \qquad E_f = \frac{148 * 100}{200} = 74$$

$$\chi^2 = \frac{(2 - 10.4)^2}{10.4} + \frac{(38 - 29.6)^2}{29.6} + \frac{(10 - 15.6)^2}{15.6}$$
$$+ \frac{(50 - 44.4)^2}{44.4} + \frac{(40 - 26)^2}{26} + \frac{(60 - 74)^2}{74}$$
$$= 6.78 + 2.38 + 2.01 + 0.71 + 7.54 + 2.54 + 2.65 = 22.07$$

d.f. = (r − 1) (c − 1) = (3 − 1) (2 − 1) = 2 * 1 = 2

χ^2 **at ∝ = 0.001 for 2 d.f. = 13.81** (see Statistical Tables - Appendix 5)

i.e., χ^2 computed (22.07) > χ^2 critical ratio (13 .81)

Thus, the association between nutritional status and socio–economic class of children is statistically significant.

(p < 0.001) - Confidence = 99.9%

Socio-economic class	Percentage of malnourished children
High	5.0
Middle	16.7
Low	40.0

Nutritional status of children is negatively associated with their socio-economic status – lower the status, higher the percentage of malnourished children.

5.6.2.6. McNemar's matched χ^2 test

It is applied when the data are paired or correlated.

Example 18. Results on 100 blood sample applying Test A (Standard but expensive and Test B (new and less expensive) are given below. It is required to test whether disagreement in results between tests A and B is statistically significant or not.

		Test A		
		+ ve	- ve	Total
Test B	+ ve	25 (a)	15 (b)	40
	- ve	5 (c)	55 (d)	60
	Total	30	70	100

In 25 samples both tests gave positive results and in 55 samples both tests gave negative results.

i.e Agreement in results $= \dfrac{25 + 55}{100} = \dfrac{80}{100} = 80\%$

Under H_o, i.e., no difference in the result between Test A and B, the disagreement in results will be equal. However, in the example, disagreement in the result with Test A and B is not equal (15 and 5). This difference is statistically tested for its significance by applying χ^2 statistics (d.f. = 1):

$$\chi^2 = \frac{(b - c)^2}{(b + c)} \qquad \text{If n is} > 30$$

$$\chi^2 = \frac{(|b - c| - 1)^2}{(b + c)} \qquad \text{If n is} < 30 \text{ (with correction factor)}$$

For the example, n = 100 > 30

$$\chi^2 = \frac{(15 - 5)^2}{20} = \frac{100}{20} = 5 > 3.84 \quad p < 0.05 \text{ (see Statistical Tables - Appendix 5)}$$

The difference in disagreement in results between Tests A and Tests B is statistically significant.

5.6.2.7. Goodness of fit χ^2 test

Apart from testing the statistical significance of the association between discrete variables, Chi-squared test can also be used for testing the goodness of fit of a given distribution with that of the sample. It is done by comparing the observed frequencies with the corresponding expected frequencies and seeing whether the discrepancies between them could reasonably be attributed to chance at a chosen level of significance. Goodness of fit test can be done when the expected pattern of distribution is known or it is based on a theoretical basis (for example, normal, binomial or Poisson distribution). Here we will consider only the case where the expected pattern of the distribution is known. Consider the following example:

It has already been established that the percentage distribution of three types of a disease is as: A = 20%, B = 50%, C = 30% (reported from the literature). In a study it was observed that the distribution of cases in these three types of the disease is as: A = 5, B = 30, C = 15 Total 50 (n) - Sample Size.

Expected frequencies in the sample based on the established pattern : A = 20% of 50 = 10
                                                                                                                       B = 50% of 50 = 25
                                                                                                                       C = 30% of 50 = 15

$$\chi^2 = \sum \frac{(0-E)^2}{E} = \frac{(5-10)^2}{10} + \frac{(30-25)^2}{25} + \frac{(15-15)^2}{15}$$

$$= 2.5 + 1 + 0 = 3.5 < 5.99 \qquad \text{df} = (\text{No. of type - 1})$$
$$= 3 - 1 = 2$$

(see Statistical Tables - Appendix 5)

Thus, differences between observed and expected frequencies of different types of the disease are statistically not significant. The distribution of the disease in the sample fits well to the expected distribution with respect to its various types

5.6.2.8. Chi-square test for testing statistical significance of a trend

When the grouping of the factor for which the statistical significance of the differences in proportions of a dichotomous response (positive and negative) is tested is in natural increasing or decreasing order, what is of interest is not the differences in the proportions among the different groups, but to test whether there is any linear trend in the proportions with respect to the increasing or decreasing groups of the factor. For example, the ordered grouping may be for severity of disease, socio-economic status, age groups or dosage of the drug. In such problems, the chi-squared test for trend is applied. Establishing a trend is more sensitive way of finding the association between an outcome and an exposure, as sometimes we may find there is no difference between the categories of the exposure variable, but there is an increasing or decreasing trend in the effect of exposure on the outcome.

Example 19. Consider the data given below:

Group	Score	Positive	Total	Proportion positive
1	x_1	r_1	n_1	p_1
2	x_2	r_2	n_2	p_2
k	x_k	r_k	n_k	p_k
Total		R	N	

In the above table, a score (x_i) has to be assigned for each group in a specific order. It may be mid-value of each group if the variable is a continuous one or it may be 0, 1, 2, 3, etc., or may be 3, 2,1, etc., or any other specific format. In this method, first of all a general Chi-squared test is done with (k-1) d.f., where k is the number of groups. Then, a chi-squared with 1 d.f. is computed as follows:

$$\chi^2 \text{ with 1 d.f.} = \frac{N\left[N\sum r_i x_i - R\sum n_i x_i\right]^2}{R(N-R)\left[N\sum n_i x_i^2 - \left(\sum n_i x_i\right)^2\right]}$$

The difference between χ^2 with (k-1) d.f. and χ^2 with 1 d.f. will give a χ^2 with (k-2) d.f. This is the statistic used for testing departure from linear regression of p_i on x_i. Though this will give only an approximation, for all practical purposes, provided if only small proportion of expected frequencies are less than 2 and that these do not occur in adjacent rows.

Example 20. Consider the data given below. The factor is socio-economic status which is in decreasing order (high, middle and low).

Socio-economic group	Score (x_i)	Malnourished (r_i)	Normal	Total (n_i)	Percentage malnourished (p_i)
High	0	2	38	40	0.05
Middle	1	10	50	60	0.1667
Low	2	40	60	100	0.40
Total		52	148	200	
		(R)		(N)	

χ^2 (2 d.f.) = 22.07 > 13.81(critical ratio with 2 d. f.) at 0.1% level of significance

$$\chi^2 (1 \text{ d.f.}) = \frac{N\left[N\sum r_i x_i - R\sum n_i x_i\right]^2}{R(N-R)\left[N\sum n_i x_i^2 - \left(\sum n_i x_i\right)^2\right]}$$

$\sum r_i x_i = (2*0)+(10*1)+(40*2)= 0 + 10 + 80 = 90$

$\sum n_i x_i = (40*0)+(60*1)+(100*2)= 0 + 60 + 200 = 260$

$\sum n_i x_i^2 = (40*0)+(60*1)+(100*4)= 0 + 60 + 400 = 460$

$$\chi^2 = \frac{200\left[(200*90)-(52*260)\right]^2}{52\,(148)\left[(200*460) - (260)^2\right]}$$

$$= \frac{200\left[20070400\right]}{7696*(24400)} = 21.38 > 13.81 \ (p < 0.001)$$

χ^2 for departure from linear regression = 22.07 − 21.38

$$= 0.69 < 3.84$$

(see Statistical Tables - Appendix 5)

∴ Departure from linear regression is statistically not significant, i.e., the decreasing trend in the proportion of malnourished with relation to the socio-economic groups (high to low) is statistically significant (p < 0.001)

5.6.2.9. Partitioning chi-square

If the chi-square test is done for the 2×2 contingency table, the interpretation of the result is straightforward since there are only two groups and the statistical significance of the difference between these two groups with respect to the discrete variable under study can be checked straight away. However, if there are more than two groups, the overall chi-square test will enable us only to interpret the statistical significance of the differences among the three groups, in general. If the statistical significance of the differences between selected pairs of groups is required, the overall chi-square has to be partitioned according to a pre-determined pattern where the total degrees of freedom is divided into several components. If there are three groups, the total degrees of freedom of 2 can be partitioned into one each and in case of 4 groups, the total degrees of freedom of 3 can be partitioned into 1, 1 and 1 or 2 and 1. The following examples make these aspects clear.

Example 21. The following table gives the results of a treatment in 4 stages of cancer patients.

Stage	Improved	Not improved	Total	% improved
I	25	20	45	55.6
II	30	20	50	60.0
III	10	38	48	20.8
IV	15	40	55	27.3
Total	80	118	198	

χ^2 (3 d.f.) = 23.84> 16.27 (critical ratio with 3 d.f. at 0.1 % level of significance) (p < 0.001) (see Statistical Tables – Appendix 5)

There is significant association between the stage of the disease and the improvement rate. The significant chi-square indicates that the proportion of improved cases is not the same in all the stages of the disease. However, this test does not tell us where exactly the significant differences lie. To identify the significant pairs of groups partitioned chi-squared analysis will help. It should be remembered that while partitioning a chi-square, the total of the number of subjects in each partition should be equal to the total number of subjects of the un-partitioned chi-square. By looking at the % improved column, it could be seen that the improvement rates in stages I & II are not very different and, similarly, these are not very different in stages III & IV. The total of stages I & II is 95 and that of III & IV is 103; so, the total of these two partitions will be 198, equal to the total in the un-partitioned chi-square). Hence, chi-square test may be done between stages I & II and between III & IV, each with 1 d.f.

χ^2 (I & II) = 0.578 (p = 0.447) (see Statistical Tables - Appendix 5)

χ^2 (III & IV) = 0.192 (p= 0.661)

i.e., differences in improvement rates between stages I & II and between stages III & IV were statistically not significant. Hence, stages I & II (early stage) and stages III & IV (later stage) may be combined and a chi-squared test may be done to see whether the difference in improvement rates between early and later stages is statistically significant or not.

χ^2 = 23.202 > 10.83 with 1 d.f. at 0.1% (α = 0.001) level of significance (p < 0.001) (see Statistical Tables - Appendix 5)

The difference was found to be statistically significant.

In partitioned chi-square, the total χ^2 will be equal to the sum of the χ^2 at each partition. In the example χ^2 with 3 d.f. = 23.84

χ^2 (I & II)	=	0.192
χ^2 (III & IV)	=	0.578
χ^2 (I + II & III + IV)	=	23.202
Total	=	23.838 (minor difference (0.134) from the χ^2 with 3 d.f. is due to rounding off

the figures.)

Example 22. The following data give the number of lung cancer cases detected in three types of smoking groups.

Group	Cases	Normals	Total	% of cases
> 2 packets / day	26	40	66	0.3939
< 2 packets /day	40	90	130	0.3077
No smoking	3	32	35	0.0857

χ^2 (2 d.f.) = 10.49 (p = 0.0053) (Exact 'p' value from computer output)

Statistically significant association was found between smoking and lung cancer. On doing a partitioned chi-square between the two smoking groups and between the smoking groups and the non-smoking groups, the following results were obtained.

Between the two smoking groups $\chi^2 = 1.458$ (p = 0.2273) (Exact 'p' value from computer output)

No statistically significant difference in the percentage of lung cancer cases was found between the two smoking groups. Hence, these two groups were combined and compared with the non-smoking group.

$\chi^2 = 8.93$ (p = 0.0470) (Exact 'p' value from computer output)

i.e., the difference in percentage of cases between the smoking and non-smoking groups was found to be statistically significant at 5% level of significance. The overall chi-square revealed significant differences among the two, smoking and the non-smoking, groups. But, the partitioned χ^2 showed that the difference between the two smoking groups was not significant and the difference between the combined smoking group and the non-smoking group was statistically significant.

Partitioning a chi-square and multiple comparisons in ANOVA are similar – to identify groups that are different, if there is overall significance.

Multiple Choice Questions

Choose the correct answers in the following multiple choice questions. The correct answers are listed on p. 343.

Q.1. **An investigator wants to know the similarity of the peak flow expiratory rates, on an average, among the four groups – non-smokers, light smokers, moderate smokers and heavy smokers. Which statistical test of significance will you advise?**
    a. Two-way analysis of variance   b. One-way analysis of variance
    c. Pearson's correlation coefficient   d. Contingency chi-square test

Q.2. **A drug was given to 50 hypertension patients and diastolic blood pressure (DBP) was noted down before and after giving the drug. To test whether the drug was effective or not, in reducing DBP, the statistical test to be applied is:**
    a. ANOVA   b. Student's t-test for independent samples.
    c. χ^2 test   d. Paired t-test

Q.3. **Results on the responses (Yes & No) to a question by two different methods (A & B) were cross-tabulated on a set of 1000 adult males. If we wish to assess the discordance between the responses to the question by the two methods, an appropriate statistical test would be:**
    a. Student's t-test   b. ANOVA
    c. χ^2 test for independent samples   d. McNemar's chi-square test

Q.4. **For testing the statistical significance of the difference in mean cholesterol values between obese females n = 20 and non-obese females n = 15, the statistical test to be applied is**
    a. Chi-square test   b. Paired t-test
    c. t-test for independent samples   d. Fisher's F-test

Q.5. **In a clinical trial with two groups of 50 patients each, one group receiving a standard drug and the other group the new drug, an improvement rate of 40% was observed in the former group and 60% in the latter group. To test the statistical significance of this difference, the statistical test to be applied is:**
    a. Chi-square test   b. Paired t-test
    c. T-test for independent samples   d. Fisher's F-test

Q.6. **Association of lung cancer with smoking may be studied by applying the following statistical test to the data:**
    a. Paired t-test   b. Analysis of variance
    c. Chi-square test   d. t-test for independent sample

Q.7. **A cardiologist found from his study that the mean systolic blood pressure of 20 male patients was 160 mm/Hg (SD = 15) and that of female patients was 150 (SD = 10). He wanted to see whether on an average the male patients really had higher systolic blood pressure than the female patients. The statistical test of significance he has to apply is:**

a. Chi-square test   b. Paired t-test

c. Proportion test   d. Unpaired (Independent samples) t-test

Q.8. **An investigator wants to study the association between maternal intake of iron supplements (Good or Poor) and birth weights (in grams) of newborn babies. He collects relevant data from 100 pregnant women and their newborns. What statistical test of hypothesis would you advise for the investigator in this situation?**

a. Paired t-test   b. Unpaired or independent t-test

c. Analysis of variance   d. Chi-square test

Q.9. **In a study on the association of breast cancer with usage of oral contraceptives, 200 cases of breast cancer and 200 healthy controls were studied. Oral contraceptives were reportedly used by 40 cases and 15 controls. What test of hypothesis do you suggest to assess the statistical significance?**

a. Student's t-test   b. Paired t-test

c. Analysis of variance   d. Chi-square test

Q.10. **In the diagnosis of a disease, 100 suspected cases were examined by two techniques PCR and culture. Culture detected 60 cases as having disease, while PCR detected 70 as diseased. If 58 suspected cases were declared as diseased by both the methods, what test of significance should be used to assess the agreement between the two methods?**

a. Paired t-test   b. Chi-square test

c. Bartlett's test   d. McNemar's chi-square test

6 | Non-parametric Statistical Methods

- Parametric versus non-parametric methods
- Statistical measures: Representative value, variation measurement, correlation coefficient
- Intervals for statistical measures: Quartiles and percentiles
- Non-parametric linear regression
- Non-parametric confidence limits for the median
- Statistical tests of significance: Comparison between two independent populations (Wilcoxon's rank sum test), comparison between two correlated populations (Wilcoxon's signed rank test), comparison among several independent populations (Kruskal-Wallis one-way analysis of variance), comparison among paired samples (Friedman's two-way analysis of variance)

6.1. Parametric versus Non-parametric Methods

In any study or an experiment, statistical inference methods help us to find out the truth regarding the population from the samples studied. However, in many cases the truth also cannot be clearly ascertained because of variation in the observations in the study. For example, two scientists investigating the truth based on samples may not get the same result. They may arrive at two different conclusions. Statistical methods help us in finding out the truth as far as possible correctly based on some probability rules. Laws of probability are applied in order to determine what the (chance) 'probabilities' are for various possible outcomes of the experiment, under the assumption that chance alone determines the outcome of the experiment. In a clinical trial, for example, this gives the experimenter an objective basis for deciding whether the better effect of the tested new drug was really the result of the new treatment that was applied as compared to the standard drug applied or whether it could have occurred by chance alone. Statistical methods in which probability distributions are used for making inferences from the sample of experiment in order to arrive at valid conclusions are known as **'Parametric'** statistical methods.

In the earlier chapter we discussed various methods of statistical inference such as Student's t-tests and analysis of variance by F-test. These are parametric statistical tests of significance. However, we saw that certain conditions have to be satisfied before applying these statistical inference methods. The conditions of randomness of the samples selected from the populations, normal distribution of the variable in the populations, homogeneity of variances in the values of the variable in these populations are very important for the validity of the results and for their meaningful interpretation. However, in many cases these conditions may not be satisfied, even after suitable transformation of the values of the variable. In case of large samples, normality of the observations of the variable can be assumed based on the Central Limit Theorem and parametric methods can be applied without much of inaccuracy. But, if the sample size is very small, say, less than 30 and no evidence is available from the literature about the distribution in respect of normality and if it is difficult to prove the normality of distribution based on the sample, the validity of applying parametric methods in such situations is debatable. Non-parametric methods are relatively new as compared to the parametric methods. In the late 1930s, some researchers in theoretical statistics advocated certain approximate solutions applying simple statistical methods in such situations. These methods later came to be known as **non-parametric** methods. They are known as non-parametric methods mainly since no specific parameter is involved in the computations.

For applying parametric inferences model, a specific form of distribution of the variable in the population is required. Since the assumption of specific form of distribution of the variable is not required, sometimes, the non-parametric methods are also known as **'Distribution-free methods'.** There are no parameters such as mean and standard deviation in these methods and, hence, they are called non-parametric methods.

It should be noted that non-parametric methods are not alternatives to parametric methods. They should be applied only if the conditions for applying parametric methods cannot be met with even in terms of the transformed variables. Non-parametric methods should be the last resort.

Since the development of non-parametric methods has taken place only recently, no comparable methods have been developed for all the inference methods which are used in parametric methods. However, most of the commonly used parametric inference methods have got corresponding non-parametric methods.

6.2. Statistical Measures

The following table lists the equivalent parametric and non-parametric statistical measures.

		Parametric	*Non-parametric*
1.	Representative Value (average)	Mean, Median, Mode	Median, Mode
2.	Variation	Standard Deviation (SD)	Quartile Deviation, Range
3.	Correlation	Pearson's Product Moment-corr. Coefficient (γ)	Spearman's Rank Corr. Coefficient (ρ)
4.	Intervals for the measure	Mean ± SD	Quartiles (Q_1, Q_3), Percentiles (P_3, P_{97}; P_5, P_{95}; P_{10}, P_{90})

6.2.1. Representative Value

For computing a representative value, mean, median or mode could be computed for parametric measure since all these three types of averages will be almost the same in case the variable follows normal distribution. The corresponding non-parametric representative value could be either the median or the mode since these two measures are non-parametric and are determined based on either ranks or the position.

6.2.2. Variation Measurement

Standard deviation is the best measure of variation for parametric estimation. Correspondingly, quartile deviation or the simple range, which are based on positions according to ascending or descending order and not computed arithmetically, could be computed as non-parametric measures of variation.

6.2.3. Correlation Coefficient

Pearson's Product moment correlation coefficient is the parametric measure of correlation. This coefficient is computed arithmetically (see Chapter 3). The corresponding non-parametric measure is the Spearman's Rank correlation coefficient.

Spearman's Rank Correlation Coefficient: Spearman's rank correlation coefficient 'ρ' is computed using the formula:

$$\rho = 1 - \frac{6 \sum di^2}{n(n^2 - 1)}$$

where d is the difference between the ranks of the values of the two variables/of the same variable obtained by two methods. Like Pearson's correlation coefficient, Spearman's correlation coefficient also varies from −1 (negative correlation) to +1 (positive correlation).

Examples

1. Rankings of 10 children by two educationalists (A & B) on their I.Q. are given below. Calculate Spearman's rank correlation coefficient (p).

S. No. :	1	2	3	4	5	6	7	8	9	10
A:	4	10	3	1	9	2	6	7	8	5
B:	5	8	6	2	10	3	9	4	7	1
d:	-1	2	-3	-1	-1	-1	-3	3	1	4

$$\rho = 1 - \frac{6 \sum di^2}{n(n^2 - 1)} = 1 - \frac{6*52}{10*99} = 0.685$$

2. Age (years) and systolic blood pressures (SBP) of 6 men are given below. Calculate Spearman's rank correlation coefficient (p).

Age:	25	30	36	45	65	70
SBP:	120	125	136	140	135	150

$\rho = 0.886$

3. Weight (kg) and cholesterol (mg%) values of 6 men are given below. Calculate Spearman's rank correlation coefficient (Á).

Age:	50	80	65	90	60	75
Cholesterol:	180	450	350	650	400	500

$\rho = 0.829$

6.3. Intervals for the Statistical Measures

In case of parametric intervals, mean ± 1 SD, mean ± 2 SD or mean ± 3 SD could be used depending upon the requirement. For example, for cholesterol values of healthy subjects, assuming the normality of the distribution, the limits or the reference values could be constructed based on mean ± 2 SD or mean ± 3 SD. In case of non-parametric limits, quartiles or percentiles may be used. As explained in Chapter 3, quartiles divide the sorted data set into four equal parts. Quartiles or percentiles could be computed as described below:

6.3.1. Quartiles and Percentiles (Location Measures)

$Q_1 = \{(1/4)(n+1)\}^{th}$ value, $Q_3 = \{(¾)(n+1)\}^{th}$ value of all the values in the sample arranged in an ascending order.

Q_1 is called the first quartile or lower quartile. Twenty five percent of the values in the sample will lie below Q_1 and 75% above. Similarly, Q_3 is called the 3rd quartile or upper quartile. Seventy five percent values in the sample will be below Q_3 and 25% values will above Q_3. Q_2 is called the median value. Fifty percent values will be below Q_2 and 50% will be above Q_2.

Using the notation followed for quartiles, 5th percentile is represented as P_5. Five percent values will be below P_5 and 95% will be above. $P_5 = \{5(n+1)/100\}^{th}$ value. Similarly, the other percentiles like P_3, P_{10}, P_{90}, P_{95} and P_{97} can be defined and computed.

$P_{25} = Q_1$, $P_{50} = Q_2$ = Median, $P_{75} = Q_3$.

In smaller sample sizes, the location measures may not be very accurate. When the sample size goes on increasing, the values become more accurate.

The following data gives age, arranged in order, of 15 patients admitted in a Cardiac unit of a hospital:
45, 47, 52, 55, 60, 62, 62, 64, 66, 69, 70, 72, 72, 74 and 80

The various quartiles and percentiles are calculated for this data.

Q_1 = 4th value = 55; Q_3 = 12th value = 72

P_3 = $\{(3*16)/100\}^{th}$ value = 0.48th value = 1st value = 45

P_{97} = $(0.97 *16)^{th}$ value 15.52th value = 15th value and so on.

As mentioned earlier the positions of the location measures will be better defined and the values will be more accurate in larger samples.

The limits for the statistical measure could be constructed in terms of Q_1 and Q_3 or, P_3 & P_{97} or P_5 & P_{95} or P_{10} & P_{90} depending upon the requirement. For example, for defining the different grades of malnutrition of children based on birth weight, which may not be normally distributed, various limits could be constructed in terms of the quartiles or percentiles described above.

6.4. Non-parametric Linear Regression

The linear regression equation is: Y = a + b X , where, Y is the dependent variable, X is the independent variable, *b* is the regression coefficient or slope and *a* is the Y-intercept constant. Parametric estimation of *a* and *b* values has been explained in an earlier chapter. The following the method is suggested for non-parametric estimation of a and b values.

b is obtained as the value of the median of S_{ij} values, where i = j = sample size (n) and $S_{ij} = (Y_j - Y_i)/(X_j - X_i)$ and X & Y are the sample pairs of values. If n = 10, there will be $10C_2 = 45$ S_{ij} values. After arranging them in ascending order, *b* = the median of the 45 S_{ij} values. This is called **Theil's slope estimator.**[1]

The value of a is obtained as follows:

a = median of the n (n+1)/2 pair-wise averages of the terms Yi-(b*X_i). If n =10, there will be 10 terms of Y_i-(b*X_i); and there will be 55 pair-wise averages of Y_i-(b*X_i) terms. This method is due to **Dietz**[2].

Use of Theil's and Dietz methods of computing *a* & *b* values is explained by the following example. For simplicity the method is explained for a sample size of 5. The following data give the age & systolic blood pressure of 5 males:

Age (years):	45	56	60	70	55
SBP:	130	135	150	140	150

The number of values of $(Y_j-Y_i)/(X_j-X_i)$ will be $5C_2 = 10$. They are:

(45-56)/(130-135) = 2.2; (45-60)/(130-150) = 0.75; (45-70)/(130-140) = 2.5; (45-55)/(130-150)=0.5; (56-60)/(135-150) = 0.27; (56-70)/(135-140) = 2.8; (56-55)/(135-150) = -0.067; (60-70)/(150-140); (60-55)/(150-150) = infinity; (70-55)/(140-150) = -1.5

The 10 values obtained after doing this operation are: 2.2, 0.75, 2.5, 0.5, 0.27, 2.8, -0.067, -1.0, infinity, and -1.5. These values, arranged in an ascending order, are: -1.5, -1, -0.067, 0.27, 0.5, 0.75, 2.2, 2.5, 2.8 and infinity. The median of these values is = average of 5th & 6th values = (0.5 + 0.75) / 2 = **0.625** i.e., b = 0.625.

Y_1-bX_1 = T_1=130-(0.625 * 45) = 101.875. Similarly, the values of T_2, T_3, T_4 and T_5 are computed. The five T values are: 101.875, 100, 112.5, 96.25 & 115.625.

$(T_1 + T_1)/2 = R_1 = 101.875$, $R2 = (T_1 + T_2)/2 = (101.875 + 100)/2 = 100.9375$ and so on.

There will be $(5 * 6)/2 = 15$ values of R for a sample size of 5. These 15 values are:

101.875, 100.9375, 107.1875, 99.0625, 108.75, 100, 106.25, 98.125, 107.8125, 112.5, 104.375, 114.0625, 96.25, 105.9375 and 115.625.

The median of these R values is the value occupying the 8th position when these values are arranged in ascending order. Hence, the median = **105.9375 = a**

The linear regression equation is: Y = a + b X i.e., **Y = 105.9375 + 0.625 X**

The corresponding linear regression equation obtained by applying **Parametric** least squares method is: **Y = 117.546 + 0.41 X**

The interpretations of the values of a and b are the same as those given in case of parametric regression.

It may be noted that there are differences in the values of a & b obtained by parametric and non-parametric methods. Parametric linear regression should be applied only if the conditions for applying parametric method are satisfied. Otherwise, only non-parametric regression should be applied.

6.5. Non-parametric Confidence Limits for the Median

Parametric Confidence limits for the parameter –mean, is given by mean ± 1.96 SE for 95% limits, mean ± 2.58 SE for 99% limits and mean ± 3.29 SE for 99.9 % limits, depending upon the requirement. The non-parametric confidence limits for any location measure can be constructed as follows.

For example, 95% confidence limits for the median can be given by the values, in the ascending order in the sample, occupying the positions: A & B, where

A = np - 1.96 SQRT {np (1-p)}, and   Conover[3]

B = np + 1.96 SQRT {np (1-p)},

(n is the sample size and p = 0.5)

These will be approximate values of the confidence interval for the median. In case of large sample sizes, the confidence limits computed would be more accurate.

Example

The number of cases of malaria reported in a village during the last 12 months, arranged in an ascending order, are: 10, 20, 35, 40, 60, 78, 90, 120, 132, 145, 150, 160.

If certain values occur more than once, rankings are given as consecutive numbers.

Median = Average of 6th & 7th values = (78 + 90)/2 = 84 n= 12, p = 0.5

A = $(12 \times 0.5) - 1.96\{SQRT \{12 \times 0.5 \times 0.5\}\}$ = 6- 3.3948 = **2.6052**

B = 6+ 3.3948 = **9.3948**

The values occupying these positions in the ordered series of the data can be computed by interpolation, which is explained below:

Value occupying 2nd position = 20, value occupying 3rd position = 35

Therefore, value occupying $(2.6052)^{th}$ position = 20 + {(35-20) × 0.6052} = 29.078

Value occupying 9th position=132, value occupying 10th position = 145

Therefore, value occupying $(9.3948)^{th}$ position = 132 + {(145-132) × 0.3948} = 137.1324

Thus, lower limit = 29.078 or 29 and upper limit = 137.1324 or 137.

These figures can be rounded off to the nearest integers. Value of A also could be got by rounding off to the next integer,

i.e., A =3 and B = 12+1-3 =10, i.e., values occupying the 3rd and 10th positions.

i.e., LL=35 and UL = 145

Since the actual positions are obtained by rounding off to the next integer, the confidence limits will not be exactly 95%. The value will be slightly more or less than 95%.

When n is smaller than 100, the above given method may not be applicable. In such cases another method using a specially constructed statistical table is applied. Since the procedure is a bit laborious and beyond the scope of this book, this method is not discussed here

6.6. Statistical Tests of Significance

Parametric and equivalent non-parametric statistical tests of significance for various comparisons are given below:

	Variable	Parametric test	Non-parametric test
1. Comparison between two independent populations	Continuous (Quantitative)	Z-test t-test	Wilcoxon's rank sum test
	Discrete (Qualitative)	Z-test	χ^2-test
2. Comparison between correlated populations	Continuous	Paired t-test	Wilcoxon's signed rank test
	Discrete	—	McNemar's χ^2-test
3. Comparison among several independent populations	Continuous	One- way ANOVA	Kruskal-Wallis One-way ANOVA
	Discrete	—	χ^2-test
4. Comparison among several correlated populations	Continuous	Two- way ANOVA	Freidman's Two-way ANOVA
	Discrete	—	McNemar's χ^2-test

From the above table, it can be seen that chi-square tests which are applied for categorical variables and discussed in Chapter 5 are all non-parametric tests of significance. The non-parametric tests of significance applied for continuous variables, as given in the above table are explained below.

6.6.1. Comparison between Two Independent Populations: Wilcoxon's Rank Sum Test

For testing whether two independent samples with respect to a variable come from the same population or not, Wilcoxon's rank sum test is used. This test is also called Mann-Whitney U test. This would be equivalent to checking whether one population tends to yield larger values than the other population or do the two medians tend to be equal or not. This test corresponds to the Z-test or the Student's t-test for two independent samples.

Method

Null hypothesis (Ho): The median values in the two groups are the same.

Alternate hypothesis (H1): The median values in the two groups are different.

n_1 = Sample size of the smaller group, n_2 = sample size of the larger group

Rank all the values in the two groups taken together. Tied values should be given average ranks.

T_1 = Sum of the ranks of smaller group, $T_2 = n_1 (n_1 + n_2 + 1) - T_1$

T = Smaller of T_1 and T_2

Assuming that the ranks are randomly distributed in the two groups, it is expected that the average ranks for each of the groups are approximately equal. The test statistic is given as:

$Z = \{$Modulus $(m-T) - 0.5\}/SD$

where m = mean sum of the ranks = $\{n_1 (n_1 + n_2 + 1)\}/2$

SD = Standard deviation of 'm' = SQRT $\{(n_1 * n_2) (n_1 + n_2 + 1)/12\}$

If Z is less than 1.96, Ho is accepted; if $Z > 1.96$, Ho is rejected at 5% level of significance ($p < 0.05$). If $Z > 2.58$, $p < 0.01$ and if $Z > 3.29$, $p < 0.001$.

If the sample sizes in the two groups are very small, normal approximation may not be valid. Hence, 'p' value has to be found by referring to the statistical Table (Appendix 6) for the values of n_1 taken horizontally and n_2 taken vertically, at $p = 0.05$. The value thus obtained is called the Critical Ratio (CR). If the value of T is greater than the value of CR obtained, then Ho is accepted and if it is lesser or equal to CR, Ho is rejected.

The difference in the decision making between the normal approximation method and the small sample size method, referring to the statistical Table (Appendix 6), may be noted. In case of normal approximation method, Ho is rejected if $Z > 1.96$, while in case of small sample size method, referring Appendix 6, Ho is rejected if $T < 1.96$.

Example

Intelligence Quotient (IQ) of 5 normally nourished children (NN) and 4 malnourished children (MN), aged 4 years, is given below:

NN: 60, 80, 120, 130, 100; **MN:** 50, 60, 100, 45

Null hypothesis (Ho): The median IQs in the two groups are the same.

Alternate hypothesis (H1): The median IQs in the two groups are different.

n_1 = Sample size of the smaller group (MN) = 4; n_2 = sample size of the larger group (NN) = 5.

Rank all the values in the two groups taken together. Tied values should be given average ranks. For example, 60 is repeated twice. Hence, after giving rank 1 to the smallest value 45 and 2 to 50, the next highest value is 60, which is repeated twice, average of the ranks 3 and 4 is taken and a rank of 3.5 is given to each of these two values of 60. This method is repeated whenever there are tied values.

Ranks: NN — 3.5, 5, 8, 9, 6.5 and MN — 2, 3.5, 6.5, 1

T_1 = Sum of the ranks of smaller group (MN) = 13

T_2 = $n_1 (n_1 + n_2 + 1) - 13$

= $4 (4 + 5 + 1) - 13 = 27$

T = Smaller of T_1 and T_2 = 13

Assuming that the ranks are randomly distributed in the two groups, it is expected that the average ranks for each of the groups are approximately equal.

The test statistic is given as:

$Z = \{$Modulus $(m - T) - 0.5\}/SD$

m = mean sum of the ranks = $\{n_1 (n_1 + n_2 + 1)\}/2$

= $\{4 (4 + 5 + 1)\}/2 = 20$

SD = Standard deviation of m

= SQRT $\{(n_1 * n_2) (n_1 + n_2 + 1)/12\}$

= SQRT$\{(4*5)(4 + 5 + 1) /12 \}$ = SQRT (200/12) = 4.1

$Z = \{$Modulus $(20 - 13) - 0.5\}/ 4.1 = 6.5 / 4.1 = 1.6 < 1.96$ and, hence, Ho is accepted.

Or, the hypothesis of identical median IQ values in the two groups is accepted; the difference in median IQs between the two groups is statistically not significant.

Since the sample sizes in the two groups are very small, 'p' value has to be found by referring to the statistical Table (Appendix 6).

For $n_1 = 4$ and $n_2 = 5$ at p = 0.05, the Critical Ratio = 11.

i.e., T = 13 > 11 (CR)

The difference in median IQs between the two groups is statistically not significant (p > 0.05).

6.6.2. Comparison between Two Correlated Populations: Wilcoxon's Signed Rank Test

For testing whether the differences observed in the values of the variable between two correlated populations (before and after design) are statistically different or not, Wilcoxon's signed rank test is applied. This corresponds to the paired t-test in parametric methods.

Method

H_0: There is no difference in the paired values, on an average, between the two groups.

H_1: There is difference in the paired values, on an average, between the two groups.

Compute the difference between each group of paired values in the two groups. Rank the differences from smallest, without considering the sign of the difference. After giving the ranks, the corresponding sign should be attached.

T+ = Sum of the ranks of the positive signs

T- = Sum of the ranks of the negative signs

Under Ho, it is expected that the sum of the ranks of the positive differences will be equal to the sum of the ranks of the negative differences. Assuming normal distribution for the differences, the test statistic is:

$Z = \{Modulus (T- m) -0.5\}/SD$

where T = smaller of T + and T-

m = mean sum of the ranks = $\{n (n + 1)\}/4 = \{8 (8 + 1)\}/4$

$SD = SQRT \{n (n + 1) (2n + 1)/24\}$

If Z < 1.96, Ho is accepted (p > 0.05) and if Z > 1.96, Ho is rejected (p < 0.05).

For small sample sizes, Statistical Table given in Appendix 7 should be referred for n, taken vertically under the chosen level of significance to find the Critical Ratio (CR).

If T > CR, Ho is accepted and if T < CR, Ho is rejected.

Example

IQ values of 8 malnourished children of 4 years of age, before and after giving some nutritious diet for three months (a), are given below:

Before (b):	40	60	55	65	43	70	80	60
After (a):	50	80	50	70	40	60	90	85

Diff. (d):	10	20	-5	5	-3	-10	10	25
Rank:	- 5	7	-2.5	2.5	-1	-5	5	8

where d = a-b

Rank the differences from smallest, without considering the sign of the difference. After giving the ranks, the corresponding sign should be attached.

T+ = Sum of the ranks of the positive signs = 27.5

T- = Sum of the ranks of the negative signs = 8.5

Under Ho, it is expected that the sum of the ranks of the positive differences will be equal to the sum of the ranks of the negative differences. Assuming normal distribution for the differences, the test statistic is:

$Z = \{Modulus (T- m) -0.5\}/SD$

where T = smaller of T+ and T- = 8.5

m = mean sum of the ranks = {n (n + 1)}/4 = {8 (8 + 1)}/4 = 18

SD = SQRT{n (n + 1) (2n + 1)/24}

= SQRT{8 (8 + 1) (16 + 1)/24} = 7.14

Z = {Modulus (8.5 – 18)-0.5}/7.14 = 1.26 < 1.96 (p > 0.05)

i.e., the difference in the sum of the positive ranks and the sum of the negative ranks is statistically not significant, or increase in the IQ values after giving the nutritious diet for three months is statistically not significant.

Since the sample size is small, inference should be drawn referring the Statistical Table given in Appendix 7. If the value of T, for a given sample size-n, lies within the range of values under a particular value, then the null hypothesis of no difference in the ranks before and after the intervention is rejected at that level of significance.

In the example, for a rank sum of 8.5 (T) with a sample size of 8, look along the row for n = 8. We find that for n = 8, the value of T, 8.5 lies between 5 and 31 under p = 0.1. This means that the null hypothesis of no difference can be rejected only under a p-value of 0.1, which is > 0.05. Hence the null hypothesis of no difference in the ranks before and after the intervention is accepted at 5% level of significance (p>0.05).

6.6.3. Comparison among Several Independent Populations: Kruskal-Wallis One-way Analysis of Variance

For testing whether several independent samples come from the same population or not, Kruskal-Wallis one-way analysis of variance is applied. It corresponds to one-way analysis of variance in parametric methods.

Method

Ho: The median values in the different groups are the same.

H$_1$: The median values in the different groups are different (at least median in one of the groups is different from those in other groups).

Rank the values taking all the groups together.

Test statistic $T = \dfrac{12}{n(n+1)} \sum \dfrac{R_i^2}{n_i} - 3(n+1)$, where n is the total of sample sizes in all the groups, say, 'k' groups and R$_i$ is the sum of the ranks in the ith group (i= 1 to k).

T is distributed as χ^2 distribution with k-1 degrees of freedom (d.f.), where k is the number of groups.

Degrees of freedom are the number of independent groups with respect to the averages of the values of the variable.

ANOVA shows only whether the differences in median values among the different groups are statistically significant or not. To identify the pairs of groups which are significantly different, Multiple Range test should be applied. The method is explained below when there are three groups:

Compute the absolute differences: $(R_1/n_1) - (R_2/n_2)$, $(R_2/n_2) - (R_3/n_3)$ and $(R_1/n_1) - (R_3/n_3)$.

Compute $w = \sqrt{\left[S^2 \left(\dfrac{n-1-T}{n-k} \right) \right]}$, where $S^2 = \dfrac{n(n+1)}{12}$

t = Find t from the Table (Appendix 4), at p = 0.05 for (n-k) d.f.

Compute

$w_1 = t \times w \sqrt{\left(\dfrac{1}{n_1} + \dfrac{1}{n_2} \right)}$, $w_2 = t \times w \sqrt{\left(\dfrac{1}{n_2} + \dfrac{1}{n_3} \right)}$, $w_3 = t \times w \sqrt{\left(\dfrac{1}{n_1} + \dfrac{1}{n_3} \right)}$

If $\dfrac{R_1}{n_1} - \dfrac{R_2}{n_2} > w_1$, the difference in the median values between Groups I & II is statistically significant (p <0.05); otherwise, the difference is not statistically significant.

Similarly, for $\dfrac{R_2}{n_2} - \dfrac{R_3}{n_3} > w_2$ and $\dfrac{R_1}{n_1} - \dfrac{R_3}{n_3} > w_3$ and for comparison between Groups II & III and between Groups I & III, respectively.

Example

Intelligence Quotient (IQ) of 5 normally nourished children (NN), 4 moderately malnourished children (MMN) and 5 severely malnourished children (SMN), aged 4 years, are given below:

NN: 60, 80, 120, 130, 100
MMN: 50, 60, 100, 45
SMN: 50, 40, 60, 35, 65

Rank the values taking all the three groups together.

		Total of the ranks (R)	R^2
NN (A)———	60, 80, 120, 130, 100		
Ranks:	7 10 13 14 11.5	55.5	3080.25
MMN (B)———	50, 60, 100, 45		
Ranks:	4.5 7 11.5 3	26.0	676.00
SMN (C)———	50, 40, 60, 35, 65		
Ranks:	4.5 2 7 1 9	23.5	552.25
Total		105	4308.50

Test statistic $T = \dfrac{12}{n(n+1)} \sum \dfrac{R_i^2}{n_i} - 3(n+1)$ where n is the total of all sample sizes.

T is distributed as χ^2 distribution with k-1 degrees of freedom (d.f.), where k is the number of groups.

$$T = 0.0571 \left[\frac{(55.5)^2}{5} + \frac{(26.0)^2}{4} + \frac{(23.5)^2}{5} \right] - 45$$

= (0.0571*895.55)–45 = 51.17 – 45
= 6.17 > 5.99 (χ^2 Critical value for 2 d.f. at 5% level of significance (Statistical Tables — Appendix 5)
i.e., the differences in the median IQs among the three groups are statistically significant (p < 0.05).
p-value (Parametric one-way ANOVA): 0.0195
p-value (Non-parametric one-way ANOVA): 0.0438

The difference in the p values obtained applying parametric and non-parametric ANOVAs may be noted. Hence, it can be seen that parametric ANOVA should not be applied if the assumptions for applying parametric ANOVA are not satisfied.

To identify the pairs of groups (A & B, B & C and A & C) which are significantly different, multiple range test should be applied. The method is explained below:

$S^2 = 17.5$

$w = \sqrt{\dfrac{17.5*(13-6.17)}{11}} = \sqrt{10.866} = 3.3$ 't' value at (n-k) = (14-3) = 11 degrees of freedom at 5% level of

significance =2.201(Appendix 4)

$$w_1 = 2.201 * 3.3 * \sqrt{\frac{1}{5} + \frac{1}{4}} = 4.86 \quad w_2 = 2.201 * 3.3 \sqrt{\frac{1}{5} + \frac{1}{5}} = 4.59$$

$$w_3 = 2.201 * 3.3 \sqrt{\frac{1}{4} + \frac{1}{5}} = 4.86$$

$$\frac{R_1}{n_1} - \frac{R_2}{n_2} = \frac{55.5}{5} - \frac{26.0}{4} = 4.6 < 4.86 (w_1)$$

$$\frac{R_1}{n_1} - \frac{R_3}{n_3} = \frac{55.5}{5} - \frac{23.5}{5} = 6.4 > 4.59 (w_2)$$

$$\frac{R_2}{n_2} - \frac{R_3}{n_3} = \frac{26.0}{4} - \frac{23.5}{5} = 1.8 < 4.86 (w_3)$$

i.e., the difference in median ranks of IQs between NN & SMN is statistically significant ($p < 0.05$) and the differences between NN & MMN and between MMN & SMN are not statistically significant ($p > 0.05$).

6.6.4. Comparison Among Paired (Repeated) Samples (More than Two Occasions): Friedman's Two-way Analysis of Variance

For testing whether the differences observed in the values of the variable between different time periods are statistically significant or not, Friedman's two-way analysis of variance is applied. This test corresponds to the two-way analysis of variance in parametric methods.

Method

Rank the values separately for each group, taking the average of the ranks for tied values.

Define $A = \dfrac{bk(k+1)(2k+1)}{6}$ where b is the sample size and k is the number of occasions.

Define $B = \dfrac{1}{b} \sum R_i^2$ i = 1 to k where R_i is the sum of the ranks of the ith group.

Compute $T = \dfrac{(b-1)\left[B - bk(k+1)^2/4\right]}{A - B}$

T is distributed as 'F' distribution with (k-1), (b-1) (k-1) d.f.

If T < Table value (Appendix 3) for (k-1), (b-1) (k-1) d.f., H_0 is accepted, and if T > Table value for (k-1), (b-1) (k-1) d.f., H_0 is rejected.

ANOVA shows only whether the differences in the rank values among the different groups (occasions) are statistically significant or not. To identify the pairs of groups which are significantly different, multiple range test should be applied. The method is explained below when there are three groups (occasions) — for example, before, after 3 months of medication and after 6 months of medication.

Compute $|R_b - R_{a3}|$, $|R_b - R_{a6}|$ and $|R_{a3} - R_{a6}|$
(b = before, a3 = after 3 months and a6 = after 6 months).

Find $w = t_{(b-1),|(k-1)|} \sqrt{\left[\dfrac{2b(A-B)}{(b-1)(k-1)}\right]}$

Where $t = t_{(b-1),\,(k-1)}$ at $p = 0.5$ value should be obtained from Student's 't' Statistical Table (given in Appendix 4), for $(b-1) \times (k-1)$ d.f.

The differences indicated above are statistically significant at the chosen level of significance if they are greater than w.

Example

IQ values of 8 malnourished children of 4 years of age, before and after giving some nutritious diet for three months (a3) and for six months (a6) are given below:

Before (b):	40	60	55	65	43	70	80	60
After (a3):	50	80	50	70	40	60	90	85
After (a6):	70	90	100	90	75	65	70	120

Rank the values separately for each group, taking the average of the ranks for tied values.

									Total (R)	R2
Before (b):	40	60	55	65	43	70	80	60		
Ranks:	1	1	2	1	2	3	2	1	13	169 —A
After (a3):	50	80	50	70	40	60	90	85		
Ranks:	2	2	1	2	1	1	3	2	14	196—B
After (a6):	70	90	100	90	75	65	70	120		
Ranks:	3	3	3	3	3	2	1	3	21	441—C

$$A = \frac{bk(k+1)(2k+1)}{6}$$ where b is the sample size and k is the number of occasions.

$$= \frac{8*3(4)7}{6} = 112$$

$$B = \frac{1}{b}\sum R_i^2 \quad i = 1 \text{ to } k, \text{ i.e., } B = \frac{1}{8}[169 + 196 + 441] = 100.75$$

$$T = \frac{(b-1)\left[B - bk(k+1)^2/4\right]}{A - B}$$

$$= \frac{7\left[100.75 - \dfrac{24*16}{4}\right]}{112 - 100.75} = 2.96$$

T is distributed as 'F' distribution with $(k-1)$, $(b-1)$ $(k-1)$ d.f.

For 2, 14 d.f. at $p = 0.05$, Critical Ratio from Table = 3.74 (Appendix 3)

Computed T (2.96) < 3.74, i.e., the differences in ranks among before, after 3 weeks and after 6 weeks are statistically not significant ($p > 0.05$).

p-value (Parametric): 0.006 (significant)

p- value (Non-parametric): 0.093 (not significant)

The difference in the p values obtained applying parametric and non-parametric ANOVAs may be noted. Hence, it can be seen that parametric ANOVA should not be applied if the assumptions for applying parametric ANOVA are not satisfied.

To identify the pairs of groups (A & B, B & C and A & C), which are significantly different, multiple range test should be applied. The method is explained below:

Compute $|R_b - R_{a3}|$, $|R_b - R_{a6}|$ and $|R_{a3} - R_{a6}|$

(b = before, a3 = after 3 months and a6 = after 6 months)

Find $W == t_{(b-1)(k-1)} \sqrt{\left[\dfrac{2b(A-B)}{(b-1)(k-1)} \right]}$

Where $t = t_{(b-1)(k-1)}$ at p = 0.5 value should be obtained from Student's 't' Table (Appendix-4) for (b-1) (k-1) d.f.

The differences indicated above are statistically significant at the chosen level of significance, if they are greater than w.

For example,

$|R_b - R_{a3}| = 1$, $|R_b - R_{a6}| = 8$, $|R_{a3} - R_{a6}| = 7$

$w = 2.145 \sqrt{\left(\dfrac{16*11.25}{14} \right)} = 7.69$

All the differences are less than 'w'. Hence, the differences in ranks of IQ values between any pair of occasions are statistically not significant.

The above methods can be applied by ranking the observations appropriately and doing simple computations. Though, all these methods can be applied manually, computer packages are available for applying these methods. The commonly used computer packages for non-parametric methods are BMDP, SPSS, SAS and SYSTAT. In case of comparatively large sample size, sometimes the ranking of observations, especially when there are more than two groups, may be difficult and confusing. In such a situation, sorting the problem using computer packages may be easier and quicker.

It has been shown by some researchers that the power of many non-parametric methods is lesser compared to the corresponding parametric methods. Hence, it is suggested that one should try his/her best to apply the parametric inference methods if the conditions for applying such methods are met with. This can be achieved by suitable transformation of the values of the variables. If all these approaches fail, then the only method of arriving at interpretations with some validity is by applying the non-parametric methods.

Multiple Choice Questions

Choose the correct answers in the following multiple choice questions. The correct answers are listed on p. 344.

Q.1. Which one of the following is a non-parametric test?
    a. Student's t-test for independent samples   b.   F-test
    c. Wilcoxon's rank sum test   d.   Paired t-test

Q.2. For testing the statistical significance of the difference in mean body mass index (bmi) values between males (n = 10) and females (n=12), the appropriate statistical test to be used is (assuming that the form of the distribution of bmi values in the population of males and females is not known):
    a. Wilcoxon's signed rank test   b.   Fisher's exact test
    c. Wilcoxon's rank sum test   d.   Bartlett's test

Q.3. Non-parametric test that is analogous to an unpaired t-test is:
    a. Kruskal-Wallis's test   b.   Wilcoxon's sign rank test
    c. Wilcoxon's rank sum test   d.   Freidman's test

Q.4. The equivalent non-parametric test for a paired t-test is:
    a. Kruskal-Wallis test   b.   Wilcoxon's signed rank test
    c. Wilcoxon's rank-sum test   d.   Chi-square test

Q.5. The equivalent non-parametric test for one way analysis of variance is:
    a. Kruskal-Wallis test   b.   Wilcoxon's signed rank test
    c. Wilcoxon's rank sum test   d.   Chi-square test

Q.6. **The equivalent non-parametric test for unpaired t-test is:**
a. Kruskal-Wallis test
b. Wilcoxon's signed rank test
c. Wilcoxon's rank sum test
d. Friedman's test

Q.7. **The equivalent non-parametric test for two-way analysis of variance is:**
a Kruskal-Wallis test
b. Wilcoxon's signed rank test
c. Wilcoxon's rank sum test
d. Friedman's test

Q.8. **Which statistical test do you suggest to test the equality of means from more than two non-normal and independent data sets with sample size less than 20?**
a. Student's t-test
b. One-way ANOVA(parametric)
c. Kruskal-Wallis test
d. Friedman's test

Q.9. **Nonparametric correlation coefficient is called:**
a. Pearson's correlation coefficient
b. Kendall's rank correlation coefficient
c. Kruskal-Wallis correlation coefficient
d. Friedman's correlation coefficient

Q.10. **The Mann-Whitney U test is also called:**
a. Kruskal-Wallis test
b. Wilcoxon's signed rank test
c. Wilcoxon's rank-sum test
d. Friedman's test

References

1. Theil H. A rank invariant method of linear and polynomial regression analysis. III. *Koninklijke Nederlandse Akademie Van Wetenschappen, Proceedings, Series A*. (1950); 53: 1397-1412.
2. Jacquelin Dietz E. Teaching regression in a non-parametric course. *The American Statistician*. 1989; 43: 35-40.
3. Conover WJ, ed. *Practical Non-Parametric Statistics*. 2nd. ed. New York: John Wiley; 1980.

7 | Introduction to Multivariable Regression Methods

- Importance of multivariable analysis
- Important multivariable analysis approaches: Multiple linear regression analysis, multiple logistic regression analysis, discriminant analysis, factor analysis, cluster analysis
- Multivariate Linear Regression Analysis: Steps in multivariable linear regression model
- Multiple logistic regression analysis

7.1. Importance of Multivariable Analysis

Choice of an appropriate method of analysis is one of the important steps in carrying out scientific studies. No matter whatever be the technical and scientific rigor of the study, it is of little practical use unless the data collected have been subjected to appropriate analyses. Once the data collection is over and reliable data is in our hand, certain steps have to be followed for an appropriate analysis. These steps are briefly enumerated in this chapter.

To start with, we should know the objectives of the study. Some objectives may be the primary ones and some could be secondary. We carry out statistical analysis to provide answers to these. At times, analyses on unplanned aspects are also carried out. However, results of such analyses should not be taken as conclusive. At best, they can help in generating a hypothesis, which needs to be examined as a separately planned study.

A statistical analyst should know the process of data collection used and whether there were changes in the definitions and methods over time, which may happen in studies involving considerable length of time in enrolling study participants. For every analysis, a clear understanding of the outcome — how it is defined, collected and coded — is important. The course of analysis is determined by this. Similarly, the issue of study design, sample size envisaged versus the actual number of subjects recruited, the way every variable has been collected and coded, the proportion of the subjects in which information on different variables is available for analysis and their distribution in different subgroups, etc., are very important issues for consideration before undertaking the analysis. Knowledge on these would not only help in planning an appropriate analysis strategy, but also be useful in describing the conduct of the study in the final report.

Another important aspect of the data is the inter-relationships between pairs of different study variables. This can be assessed by methods described in earlier chapters, depending upon the scales of measurement and meeting the required assumptions. Inter-correlations among different characteristics of the study population are crucial in deciding the independent factors that have an association with the study outcome.

After having a good understanding of the above mentioned aspects of the data, we proceed to assess the association of each variable with the study outcome. This process is commonly called **univariate analysis** as the association between the outcome on one side and each exposure or covariate on the other side, one at a time, is assessed. Though some authors prefer a term 'bivariate analysis' for the same, as we are considering two variables at a time, essentially both terminologies mean the same. Various techniques are available for this univariate analysis, depending on the combinations of the outcome and exposure variables with respect to the type and distribution, which are discussed in Chapter 5.

Usually, in any epidemiological or clinical investigation, we have a well defined outcome and different clinical, biochemical and socio-demographic factors that are suspected to have a role in the outcome. Studying the role of one aspect at a time on the outcome (univariate analysis) no doubt helps us to have an initial idea of the role of these different factors on the outcome. But as we know, these different suspected factors among themselves may be related or correlated. When an exposure variable shows a significant association with the outcome, it might be partly or wholly due to the influence of other factors that are associated with this exposure variable. We need to disentangle this information to identify the independent factors associated with the outcome. Otherwise, there will be a lot of redundancy in what we say about the outcome and its associated factors.

For example, univariate analysis may reveal the presence of a significantly higher proportion of smokers in a group of lung cancer cases compared to a group of persons with no lung cancer. But smoking itself is associated with gender (males are more likely to be smokers than females) and age (older persons are more likely to be smokers than youngsters) and so the observed difference of the proportion of smokers might be due to the differences of gender and /or age between the two groups compared. In our example, if all lung cancer cases are males and the group without lung cancer is of females only, the apparent association between lung cancer and smoking as observed in the univariate analysis may not be a true association, but an artifact. Similarly, if all lung cancer cases are aged 50+ years, while all those in no lung cancer group are below 20 years, we can find an association between lung cancer and smoking by way of an artifact.

Unless our two groups are exactly similar with respect to age and gender, the observed association between smoking and lung cancer is most likely the result of the imbalance between the two groups with respect to age and gender. But it is extremely impractical to assemble such groups and some differences with respect to many baseline characteristics, etc., are unavoidable in any scientific investigation. So we need to separate the effects of age and gender differences between the two groups, when we want to assess the role of smoking in lung cancer. Statistical methods that help in these aspects are called **multivariate analysis** methods. Such analyses take into consideration, the inter-correlations of several study variables before arriving at a conclusion of the association between a study factor and outcome. Again, as with the terms univariate and bivariate analyses, some authors prefer to distinguish procedures involving one outcome variable from those with more than one. Analyses involving more than one outcome are called multivariate and those with one outcome are referred to as multivariable. For practical purposes, in this book we use these two terms interchangeably.

There are many multivariate analysis procedures depending on the outcome type and the objective. Some of the most commonly used techniques are briefly described here.

7.2. Important Multivariable Analysis Approaches

7.2.1. Multiple Linear Regression Analysis

When the outcome or dependent variable is of continuous nature with a normal distribution, multiple linear regression analysis is the analysis of choice. The independent variables could be a mixture of continuous as well as categorical variables. In this analysis, the regression of Y (i.e. dependent variable) on a set of independent variables (X_1, X_2 ..., X_p) is studied. This analysis will help us in finding out whether the different variables are related to Y or not and if related, which all of them are significantly related, indicating the order of their importance. Apart from identifying the variables that are associated with the outcome phenomenon, it also helps to predict the dependent variable based on the significantly contributing independent variables, indicating the error observed in the prediction.

7.2.2. Multiple Logistic Regression Analysis

When the dependent variable is a binary (Yes/No) variable like "with disease" and "without disease" and the independent variables are categorical or continuous, multivariable logistic regression analysis is applied for identifying the factors/variables that have a significant association with the outcome. Each variable's association with the outcome is quantified in terms of an index called odds ratio (OR) along with its standard error. In etiological studies to identify the risk factors for a disease, multivariate logistic regression is very useful.

7.2.3. Discriminant Analysis

This is a multivariate technique for studying the extent to which different populations overlap or diverge from one another. This analysis is used often in classification and diagnosis, especially when all the independent variables are of quantitative nature.

When two or more diseases are often confused in diagnosis, it is helpful to learn what laboratory and clinical parameters are most effective in distinguishing the different types of diseases or even between normals and diseased persons. Discriminant analysis will help us to classify future cases into one of these groups based on their values of different clinical and laboratory parameters with minimum possible misclassification. It will also help us in identifying the best combination of parameters in the classification with minimum misclassification. The analysis also identifies the significantly contributing parameters in the classification.

7.2.4. Factor Analysis

Factor analysis is a body of methods by which a relationship among a large number of variables is explained by a smaller number of variables, known as factors, which are linear combination of the original variables. The main aim of factor analysis is to reduce the larger number of variables into smaller number of factors, each factor having a group of variables. Factors can be identified and given names. Factor analysis deals with the study of inter-correlations of several variables to determine whether the variations represented can be accounted adequately by that smaller number of factors. Another similar method, which is usually known as principal component analysis, helps us in finding out new composite sample parsimoniously. The reduced number of independent variables successively account for the major variation in the sample, the first component accounting maximum variation and so on. In factor analysis, only the inter-correlations are reproduced and studied and in principal component analysis the total variance is studied. Factor analysis is basically a technique that can be used with data of quantitative nature that follows a normal distribution.

7.2.5. Cluster Analysis

Cluster analysis is one of the ways of category-sorting, while classification is systematic arrangement of objects into established groups. Cluster analysis is done to find out the groups within which the objects are similar or homogenous. In cluster analysis little or nothing is known about the category structure. The analysis will help us in identifying the category structure. In a typical example, the sample patients, each described by the values of the different variables, are grouped into clusters such that the patients within a cluster have a high degree of similarity or natural association among themselves, different clusters being relatively distinct from one-another. The historical background of cluster analysis is in numerical taxonomy done for the classification of botanical specimens. Later, the application was extended to a variety of fields including health and medicine, especially in the fields of psychology, pathology and psychiatry. The analysis is done based on similarity or distance coefficients, i.e., correlation coefficients or differences in the values.

Since it is beyond the scope of this book to discuss all these methods of multivariate analyses, as an introduction of the concepts, only two commonly used methods - multivariable linear regression analysis and multiple logistic regression analysis are discussed here with examples. Their understandings may also facilitate in easier understanding of the other methods.

7.3. Multivariate Linear Regression Analysis

Multivariate linear regression analysis is the extension of univariate linear regression (single independent variable) analysis to several independent variables based on their inter-correlations. The aims are to identify the factors or variables that have an independent association with the outcome and improve the efficiency of prediction of the dependent variable based on several independent variables rather than on a single independent variable. This analysis will also help us in identifying the statistically significant variables in the order of their contribution in prediction.

Some examples of applications for multiple linear regression analysis are:

1. Studying the influence of maternal nutritional status, age, weight, height, gestation and order of birth on the birth weight of a newborn.
2. Identifying the factors among patient's age, gender, occupational status, income and weight, etc., that are associated with blood pressure.
3. Prediction of the prognosis (whether the patient would be cured or not) based on his/her age, sex, weight, severity of the disease, duration of the disease, cholesterol value, BP, sugar level, type of treatment received, etc.

In univariate linear regression analysis, the regression model is $Y = a + bX$ and r gives the correlation coefficient value between X and Y, say height (independent variable) and weight (dependent variable) respectively. Then, r^2 gives the percentage of total variation in Y explained by X.

If $r = 0.8$, then $r^2 = 0.64$, i.e., 64% of total variation in weight is explained by height.

In the multivariable linear regression analysis, the model is:

$$Y = a + b_1 X_1 + b_2 X_2 + \ldots\ldots + b_n X_n$$

Where X_1, X_2, ... X_n are the independent variables; b_1, b_2 .... b_n are called the regression coefficients of X_1, X_2 .... X_n, respectively. X_1 .. X_n are also referred to as explanatory variables or predictor variables and Y is referred to as explained or predicted variable.

The computations and interpretation of multiple regression analysis are explained in detail for the following example of data on weight, height and age of some nutritionally-deficient children (Table 7.1).

Table 7.1: Information on the weight (Y), height (X_1) and age (X_2) of 12 nutritionally deficient children

Sl. No.	Y (kg)	X_1 (cm)	X_2 (months)
1.	6.4	57	8
2.	7.1	59	10
3.	5.3	49	6
4.	6.7	62	11
5.	5.5	51	8
6.	5.8	50	7
7.	7.7	55	10
8.	5.7	48	9
9.	5.6	42	10
10.	5.1	42	6
11.	7.6	61	12
12.	6.8	57	9

Our objective is to assess the association of height and age on the weight among nutritionally deficient children

7.3.1. Steps in Multivariable Linear Regression Model

Find out the sum of squares (SS) and cross products (CP) and adjusted SS and CP, as follows:
Then we will have,

$$\sum x_1^2 = \sum X_1^2 - \frac{\left(\sum X_1\right)^2}{n} \qquad \sum x_2^2 = \sum X_2^2 - \frac{\left(\sum X_2\right)^2}{n}$$

$$\sum y^2 = \sum Y^2 - \frac{\left(\sum Y\right)^2}{n} \qquad \sum x_1 x_2 = \sum X_1 X_2 - \frac{\left(\sum X_1\right)\left(\sum X_2\right)}{n}$$

$$\sum x_1 y = \sum X_1 Y - \frac{\left(\sum X_1\right)\left(\sum Y\right)}{n} \qquad \sum x_2 y = \sum X_2 Y - \frac{\left(\sum X_2\right)\left(\sum Y\right)}{n}$$

Computation of sum of squares and cross products (SS and CP) and adjusted SS and CP for the data:

$$\sum X_1 = 633 \qquad \sum X_1^2 = 33903 \qquad \sum X_2 = 106$$

$$\sum X_2^2 = 976 \qquad \sum Y = 75.3 \qquad \sum Y^2 = 481.39$$

$$\sum X_1 X_2 = 5679 \qquad \sum X_1 Y = 4027 \qquad \sum X_2 Y = 679.6$$

$$\sum x_1^2 = 33903 - \frac{(633)^2}{12} = 512.25 \qquad \sum x_2^2 = 976 - \frac{(106)^2}{12} = 39.67$$

$$\sum y^2 = 481.39 - \frac{(75.3)^2}{12} = 8.88 \qquad \sum x_1 x_2 = 5629 - \frac{633*106}{12} = 87.5$$

$$\sum x_1 y = 4027 - \frac{633*73.5}{12} = 54.92 \qquad \sum x_2 y = 6796 - \frac{106*75.3}{12} = 14.45$$

$$\overline{Y} = \frac{\sum Y}{n} = \frac{75.3}{12} = 6.28 \qquad \overline{X_1} = \frac{\sum X_1}{n} = \frac{633}{12} = 52.75 \qquad \overline{X_2} = \frac{\sum X_2}{n} = \frac{106}{12} = 8.83$$

1. Univariate linear regression of Y on X_1 alone:
The linear univariate regression model is $Y = a + b_1 X_1$

Where $b_1 = \dfrac{\sum x_1 y}{\sum x_1^2} = \dfrac{54.92}{512.25} = 0.1072$

As explained in Chapter 3, a regression coefficient equal to 0.1072 implies that for every one unit increase in the independent variable, there is an increase of 0.1072 units in the dependent variable, on average. In our example, it means for every one centimeter increase in the height there is an increase of 107 g (0.107 kg) in the body weight of the children on average.

$$a = \overline{Y} - b_1 \overline{X}_1 = 6.28 - 0.1072 * 52.75 = 0.6252$$

Therefore, the regression equation of weight on height is: $Y = 0.6202 + 0.1072\ X_1$

Further, correlation coefficient between Y and X_1,

$$r_1 = \frac{\sum x_1 y}{\sqrt{\left(\sum x_1^2\right)\left(\sum y^2\right)}} = \frac{54.92}{\sqrt{512.25 * 8.88}} = 0.8143$$

Coefficient of determination $= (0.8143)^2 = 0.6631 = 66.31\%$

Or, $r_1^2 = \dfrac{b_1 \sum x_1 y}{\sum y^2} = \dfrac{0.1072 * 54.92}{8.88} = 0.6629 = 66.30\%$

It implies that height alone explains about 66% of the total variation in the weights of children.

Using the regression equation, we can predict the weight of a child for a given height. For example, the height and weight of the first child in our sample are 57 cm and 6.4 kg, respectively. As against the observed weight of 6.4 kg of this child, our regression equation based on height alone predicts the weight as:

Weight $= 0.6202 + 0.1072*57 = 6.73$ kg

So, there is an error of $6.4 - 6.73 = -0.33$ kg.

2. Univariate linear regression of Y on X_2 alone:

The linear univariate regression model is $Y = a + X_2$

$$b_2 = \frac{\sum x_2 y}{\sum x_2^2} = \frac{14.45}{39.67} = 0.3643$$

As explained for the regression coefficient of height on weight (b1), b2 implies that for every one month increase in the age, there is, on average, an increase of 365 g (0.365 kg) in the weight of the children studied.

$$a = \overline{Y} - b_2 \overline{X}_2 = 6.28 - 0.3643 * 8.83 = 3.0632$$

So, the regression equation of weight on age is: $Y = 3.0632 * 0.3643\ X_2$

$$r_2 = \frac{\sum x_2 y}{\sqrt{\left(\sum x_2^2\right)\left(\sum y^2\right)}} = \frac{14.45}{\sqrt{39.67 * 8.88}} = 0.7699$$

$$r_2^2 = 0.5927 = 59.27\%$$

Or, $r_2^2 = \dfrac{b_2 \sum x_2 y}{\sum y^2} = \dfrac{0.3643 * 14.45}{8.88} = 59.27\%$

Therefore, age alone explains about 59% of the total variation in the weight of children. For the first child in our sample, the regression equation based on age predicts the weight as $3.0632 + 0.3643*8 = 5.98$ kg, as against the 6.4 kg observed. Thus, there is an error of $6.4 - 5.98 = 0.42$ kg.

3. The multiple linear regression model

$Y = a + b_1X_1 + b_2X_2$

This equation can also be written as $y = b_1x_1 + b_2x_2$

From this equation, we can have two equations by multiplying with x_1 and x_2 respectively.

Multiplying with x_1, summing up and simplifying will give the equation:

$$b_1 \sum x_1^2 + b_2 \sum x_1x_2 = \sum x_1 y \qquad (1)$$

Multiplying with x_2, summing up and simplifying will give the equation:

$$b_1 \sum x_1 x_2 + b_2 \sum x_2^2 = \sum x_2 y \qquad (2)$$

We need to solve for b_1 and b_2 from these two normal equations and using these values solve for a as:

$a = \bar{y} - b_1 \bar{x}_1 - b_2 \bar{x}_2$

i.e. $512.25 \, b_1 + 87.5 \, b_2 = 54.925 \qquad (3)$

$\quad 87.5 \, b_1 + 39.6667 \, b_2 = 14.45 \qquad (4)$

Find equation (5) = Eq. (3) ÷ 512.25

Equation (6) = Eq. (4) ÷ 87.5

$b_1 + 0.1708 \, b_2 = 0.1072 \qquad (5)$

$b_1 + 0.4533 \, b_3 = 0.1651 \qquad (6)$

Accordingly, (6) – (5) gives: $2825 \, b_2 = 0.0579 \quad \therefore b_2 = 0.2050$

$b_1 = 0.1072 – 0.1708 \, b_2$ from Eq. (5)

$\quad = 0.1072 – 0.1708 * 0.2050 = 0.0722$

$a = \bar{Y} - b_1 \bar{X}_1 - b_2 \bar{X}_2$

$\therefore a = 6.275 – (0.0722 * 52.75) – (0.2050 * 8.83) = 0.6563$

The final multivariate regression model is:

$Y = 0.6563 + 0.0722X_1 + 0.2050 \, X_2$

$$R^2 = \text{Coefficient of determination} = \frac{b_1 \sum x_1 y + b_2 \sum x_2 y}{\sum y^2}$$

$$= \frac{(0.0722 * 54.925) + (0.2050 * 14.45)}{8.8825}$$

$$= \frac{6.9278}{8.8825} = 0.7799 = 78\%$$

i.e., both height and age together explain 78% of the total variation in weight.

Now let us try to predict the weight based on the two predictors, namely height and age. For the first child, predicted weight would be $0.6563 + 0.0722*57 + 0.2050*8$, which is equal to 6.41 kg. The resulting error in the prediction now is $6.4 – 6.41 = – 0.01$ kg, which is an improvement on the predictions based on height and age alone. This is the benefit of considering more than one predictor or independent variable simultaneously by multivariate regression analysis. Using such a model, one can have fairly good predictions for other possible values of the predictors.

Table 7.2: Results summary of univariate and multiple linear regression analysis

Model	Variables included	Regression coefficient	R^2
1.	Height	0.1072	66.30%
2.	Age	0.3643	52.80%
3.	Height	0.0722	
	Age	0.2050	78.0%

Taking the model 3 as the final, the regression coefficient of 0.0722 associated with height implies that on the average, there is an increase of 72 g in the weight, adjusting for the influence of age on weight. Similarly, the coefficient value 0.2050 associated with age indicates the average increase in the weight per one month increase in the age, adjusting for the influence of height on weight. Compare these coefficients with those obtained from univariate models. Clearly, the influence of height has been over-estimated in the univariate analysis (0.1072 vs 0.0722) as some part of it is due to age. Similarly, the influence of height on weight is over-estimated in the univariate analysis (0.3643 vs 0.2050). Multivariate analysis has helped in separating these mixed influences.

Statistical significance of the contribution of each variable X_1 and X_2 in the total variation in Y in the multiple regression analysis can be tested by applying appropriate test of significance, which is beyond the scope of this book.

As done in the above example, any number of variables can be considered in multivariable regression analysis. The variation can be explained on the basis of each of the variable alone and in various combinations, and their individual contributions can be investigated for statistical significance to enable us to have better predictions of the dependent variable.

Multivariable linear regression analysis can be done using any of the statistical software such as SPSS, SYSTAT, SAS or STATA. When the analysis is done using statistical software, regression coefficient along with its standard error and p-value for each independent variable will be given. Variables with p-value less than 0.05 could be considered as statistically significant variables contributing to the prediction of the expected value of the dependent variable. This analysis will give the contribution of each variable in predicting the value of the dependent variable.

Identification of the significantly contributing predictor variables can be done using an automated procedure or manually, trying with different combinations of the predictors. When there are a number of independent or predictor variables, it is cumbersome to select the important variables manually and so often recourse is taken to the automated procedure. Automated procedures involve telling the computer system to include a variable if its significance is below a certain level and remove if it exceeds that level, etc. There are different approaches for this, such as forward entry, backward elimination, stepwise and all possible subset regressions. These approaches are available in most of the software. Each approach has its merits and limitations, but the stepwise approach is the more common one providing results on par with the all possible subset regressions. The details of these procedures are beyond the scope of this book.

7.4. Multiple Logistic Regression Analysis

Application of this method can be explained with the help of the following examples:
1. Prediction of outcome (e.g., improved or not improved) in a clinical trial to compare the effect of a new drug with that of the standard drug in patients of a particular disease, based on patient's age, weight, BP, nutritional status, duration of the disease, diet, habits like smoking, alcohol use, etc.

2. Prediction of the prognosis (whether the patient would survive or not) based on his/her age, sex, type of treatment, severity of the disease, duration of the disease, cholesterol value, BP, sugar level, etc.

Multivariable logistic regression model can be formulated as follows:

If p is the probability of an event (e.g., treatment response) for a given covariate pattern, using the logic of linear regression, the model can be written as,

$$p = a + b_1X_1 + b_2 X_2 + \ldots\ldots + b_n X_n$$

We know that the proportion p cannot be negative and it can range only between 0 and 1, while the right hand side of the equation can theoretically vary from $-\infty$ to $+\infty$. So, there is an obvious mismatch between the two sides of the equation.

If we divide the above equation by the compliment of the proportion (1-p), the right hand side of the equation would look like the same as the values of regression coefficients (b_is) might change, but the form remains the same. But the dependent variable on the left hand side would now be p/(1-p). By doing this, the left hand side can now range from 0 to ∞, because, if p = 1 then 1-p = 0 and so the dependent variable would be infinity. On the other hand, if p = 0, p/(1-p) will be zero. But the right hand side would still range from $-\infty$ to $+\infty$, indicating that there is still some incompatibility between the two sides of the equation.

Now if we take the log of (p/(1-p)), it would range from $-\infty$ to $+\infty$, which is consistent with the range of the right hand side quantity. So, the multivariable logistic regression model can be written as:

$$\log\left[\frac{p}{(1-p)}\right] = b_0 + b_1x_1 + b_2x_2 + b_3x_3 + \ldots + e_i$$

Where b_1, b_2, b_3 etc are the logistic regression coefficients and log [p/(1-p)] is called the log odds or logit of the event.

The above form of the logistic model can also be written in terms of p as follows:

$$\log\left[\frac{p}{(1-p)}\right] = b_0 + b_1x_1 + b_2x_2 + b_3x_3 + \ldots + b_kx_k$$

$$p = (1-p) * exp(b_0 + b_1x_1 + b_2x_2 + b_3x_3 + \ldots + b_kx_k)$$

$$p = exp(b_0 + \sum b_ix_i) - p * exp(b_0 + \sum b_ix_i)$$

Dividing both sides by p,

$$1 = \frac{exp(b_0 + \sum b_ix_i)}{p} - exp(b_0 + \sum b_ix_i)$$

It implies,

$$\frac{1}{p} = \frac{1 + exp(b_0 + \sum b_ix_i)}{exp(b_0 + \sum b_ix_i)} \quad or \quad p = \frac{exp(b_0 + \sum b_ix_i)}{1 + exp(b_0 + \sum b_ix_i)}$$

The logistic model is explained with help of an example data below (Table 7.3). The data in Table 7.3 give the results of a clinical trial comparing the effect of two drugs (standard drug and the new drug) on the improvement in the condition of 30 hypertension patients (15 patients in each group). Information on other variables such as age group, gender, diet and smoking habit is also available in the study. We want to assess whether the new drug is more effective than the standard drug in improving the condition of the patients.

Table 7.3: Data on treatment with a new drug and the standard drug

A	B	C	D	E	F
1	1	2	2	2	1
1	2	2	1	2	1
1	2	2	2	2	1
1	2	2	2	2	1
1	2	1	1	1	2
1	2	2	2	2	1
1	2	2	2	2	1
1	2	2	1	1	2
1	1	2	2	2	2
1	2	1	1	2	2
1	2	2	2	1	1
1	1	2	1	2	2
1	1	2	2	2	1
1	2	2	2	2	1
1	1	1	2	2	1
2	2	2	1	1	1
2	2	1	1	2	1
2	1	1	1	1	2
2	1	1	1	1	2
2	1	2	1	1	2
2	1	1	1	1	2
2	1	2	2	1	2
2	1	1	1	1	2
2	1	2	1	2	2
2	2	1	2	1	2
2	1	1	1	2	1
2	1	1	2	2	2
2	1	1	1	1	2
2	1	1	1	2	2
2	2	1	1	1	2

A = Treatment group: 1–standard drug; 2–new drug

B = Sex : 1–female; 2–male

C = Age (years): 1–≤ 40; 2–>40

D = Diet: 1–vegetarian; 2–non-vegetarian

E = Smoking: 1–no; 2–yes

F = Response: 0–not improved; 1–improved

The results of the univariate analysis are shown in Table 7.4.

Table 7.4: Results of univariate analysis of the percentage patients showing improvement with respect to various factors

Variable	Number improved (%)	p-value*
Group		
1. Standard treatment	33.3	
2. New treatment	80.0	0.025
Gender		
1. Male	75.0	
2. Female	35.7	0.063
Age group (yrs)		
1. ≤ 40	78.6	
2. > 40	37.5	0.033
Diet		
1. Vegetarian	76.5	
2. Non-vegetarian	30.8	0.025
Smoking		
1. No	84.6	
2. Yes	35.3	0.010

* Based on Fisher's exact test

Univariate analysis shows that the percentage of patients with improved condition was more in (i) the new treatment group (80.0% vs 33.3%); (ii) in those aged ≤ 40 years (78.6% vs 37.5%); (iii) in the vegetarians (76.5% vs 30.8%); and (iv) among non-smokers (84.6% vs 35.3%). All these differences are statistically significant ($p < 0.05$). Difference between males and females is of marginal significance.

However, we are interested in comparing the effect of the two treatments in improving the condition of the patients. Univariate analysis indicated that not only there is a significant proportion of improved cases in the category of patients treated with the new drug, but the same also holds with respect to the variables gender, age group, diet and smoking habit. Also, we are not sure whether these additional factors that showed significant differences in the proportion of improved cases are equally distributed between the two treatment groups. If it is so, we can be sure that the observed effect of new treatment in the univariate analysis will hold even after removing the influence of these additional factors.

To know about the role of the factors other than the treatment on the outcome, first we need to know their distribution in each of the treatment groups. Summary of this analysis can be seen in Table 7.5. As can be seen, the differences in the distribution of patients between the two treatment groups with respect to age, diet and smoking habit were statistically significant. Only the differences in gender distribution seem to be due to chance (insignificant). Therefore, it is possible that the comparison in the improvement rate in patients between the two treatment groups could be affected by these variables, which are not evenly distributed in the two treatment groups. Hence, a multivariate analysis should be done for a valid comparison of the two treatment groups, adjusting for the differences between the two groups, with respect to age, diet and smoking habit.

Table 7.5: Summary of the analysis on the distribution of patients in the two treatment groups by different variables

Variable	p-value*
Gender	0.660
Age	0.009
Diet	0.025
Smoking	0.025

* Fisher's exact test

The actual calculations of the multiple logistic regression are intensive and extremely time consuming to do manually, especially with large data sets involving many explanatory variables. Multiple logistic regression analysis is implemented in most software and can be done using any of the statistical software such as SPSS, SYSTAT, SAS or STATA. The results are summarized in Table 7.6.

Table 7.6: Results of the multiple logistic regression analysis

Variable	p-value	OR
Group		
Standard treatment	0.58	1.0
New treatment		2.1
Gender		
Male	0.043	1.0
Female		23.9
Age group (in yrs.)		
< 45	0.192	1.0
≥ 45		5.4
Diet		
Vegetarian	0.124	1.0
Non-vegetarian		6.6
Smoking		
No	0.036	1.0
Yes		30.1

OR: Odds Ratio

The results of the multivariate logistic regression analysis show that after taking into consideration the influence of all the confounding variables such as age, diet, smoking habit and gender, the difference in the percentages of patients who showed improvement between the two treatment groups was not significant ($p = 0.58$). This is contrary to the result obtained in univariate analysis. In other words, the observed significant difference in the proportion of improved cases between the two groups might be the result of the unequal distribution of other factors between the two treatment groups. If the conclusion was drawn based only on the results of univariate analysis, it would have been wrong. Valid conclusion could be drawn only after doing an appropriate analysis — in this example – multivariable logistic regression analysis.

Similar to the explanation of Odds Ratio in an univariate scenario (Chapter 8), the OR of improvement to therapy associated the new treatment is 2.1, which implies that the odds of an improvement with the new therapy is 2.1 times of that with the standard treatment, adjusting for the influence of other factors such as age, smoking, etc. However this is not important since the difference is statistically not significant ($p = 0.58$).

Thus, to summarize, appropriate analysis of data is very important in any epidemiological/ clinical investigation. Examining one aspect at a time is not enough, as we know that the same phenomenon can be influenced by more than one factor, and the many factors that have an association with the study outcome are generally related to each other. Because of the inter-relationships, the conclusions based on one aspect at a time (univariate analysis) are likely to be misleading.

Depending on the research question, study design and the type of study variables, there are a variety of multivariate analytical techniques. It should be remembered that each technique has certain assumptions that need to be fulfilled before it can be applied. If the assumptions are not justified, the results from such an analysis are as good or as bad as those obtained from any other analysis. Unfortunately, in the present era of wide computerization and availability of statistical software, more and more applications of the advanced analytical techniques are being used with limited understanding of the basic assumptions required to be made for such analytical techniques. Added to these, the differences from software to software in the implementation of the analysis technique add to the difficulties of a beginner.

It should also be remembered that whatever the multivariate models give they are not absolutely final, because these models take into consideration only the statistical significance. As mentioned in earlier chapters, statistical significance may not mean clinical significance. Biological significance has also to be understood and be reflected in any good modeling exercise. Further, same variable can be analyzed in different ways and it adds a bit of artistry to the statistical analysis. For example, a variable such as age, collected on a yearly basis, can be analyzed (i) as it is collected, (ii) in group intervals of say 5 or 10 years and treated as continuous variable, or (iii) in group intervals of 5 or 10 years and treated as a category variable. Each approach has its own interpretation as well as adds to the overall goodness of the model. Because of such possibilities, Hosmer and Lemeshow have stated that good modeling is partly statistics, partly biology and partly an art.

There are many other issues related to multivariate regressions and multivariate analysis techniques such as interactions, multi-collinearity, validity, goodness and adequacy of the model, etc. Details on these aspects can be found in books on multivariate (multivariable) analysis.

Multiple Choice Questions

Choose the correct answers in the following multiple choice questions. The correct answers are listed on p. 344.

Q.1. **In Multiple regression analysis, the term 'R²' indicates:**
a. Correlation coefficient
b. Level of significance
c. Coefficient of determination
d. Coefficient of variation.

Q.2. **In case of qualitative dependent variables (say, prognosis of improved /not-improved) and many independent variables (say, severity of disease, age group, socio-economic status, diet group etc.), the multi-variable analysis to be used for identifying the independent variables which contribute significantly for prognosis is:**
a. Logistic regression
b. Multiple linear regression
c. Cluster analysis
d. Factor analysis

Q.3. **In case of quantitative dependent variables (say, diastolic BP after treatment in hypertension patients) and many independent variables (say, height, age, bmi, cholesterol, etc.), the multi-variable analysis to be used for identifying the independent variables, which contribute significantly to the prediction of diastolic BP, is:**
a. Logistic regression
b. Multiple linear regression
c. Discriminant analysis
d. Survival analysis

Q.4. **In case of dependent variables such as time to event, the generally used multivariable analysis is:**
a. Logistic regression
b. Multiple linear regression
c. Discriminant analysis
d. Survival analysis

Q.5. **In multiple regression analysis, the number of independent variables should be:**
    a. Only two   b. Only three
    c. More than one   d. Only one

Q.6. **In multiple regression analysis, the number of dependent variables should be:**
    a. Two   b. Three
    c. No limit (any number of variables)   d. One

Q.7. **In multiple regression model: $Y = a_1X_1 + a_2X_2 + a_3X_3 + \ldots\ldots\ldots\ldots$,Y is called:**
    a. Independent variable   b. Dependent variable
    c. Random variable   d. Constant

Q.8. **In multiple regression model: $Y = a_1X_1 + a_2X_2 + a_3X_3 + \ldots\ldots\ldots\ldots$, $X_1, X_2, X_{3,\ldots}$ are called:**
    a. Independent variables   b. Dependent variables
    c. Random variables   d. Constant

Q.9. **If OR (Odds Ratio) is = 4.3 for smokers compared to non-smokers, in relation to lung cancer, it means:**
    a. Odds of getting lung cancer in non-smokers are 4.3 times more compared to smokers.
    b. Odds of getting Lung cancer in smokers are 4.3 times more compared to non-smokers.
    c. Odds of getting lung cancer in smokers are 4.3 times less compared to non-smokers.
    d. Odds of smoking in those who didn't have lung cancer are 4.3 times more compared to those who have lung cancer.

Q.10. **One of the following analyses is not a multivariable analysis:**
    a. Logistic regression   b. Multiple linear regression
    c. Discriminant analysis   d. Analysis of variance

8 Epidemiological Methods

8.1. Evolution of Epidemiology

The word epidemiology has its origins in the Greek language where *epi* means upon and *demos* means population. Both these words combined with another word *logy* (meaning the study of) imply that epidemiology is the study of population. It has been defined in many ways. The *Dictionary of Epidemiology*[1] (2001) defines it as the study of the distribution and determinants of health related states or events in specified populations, and the application of this study to control of health problems. The *Oxford English Dictionary*[2] (2000) defines it as that branch of medical science, which treats of epidemics. MacMohan[3] (1970) defined it as the study of the distribution and determinants of disease frequency.

Hippocrates[4], the father of modern medicine, commented in the 5th century AD itself that the development of human diseases might be related to the external as well as personal and environmental factors of an individual. In 1662, John Graunt[5] analyzed the weekly reports of births and deaths in London and for the first time quantified patterns of disease in populations. He noted an excess of men compared to women in births and deaths, high infant mortality rate and the seasonal variations in mortality. He also attempted to provide numerical assessment of the impact of plague on the population of the city of London. He recognized the value of routinely collected data in providing information about human illnesses, which forms the basis of modern epidemiology. William Farr[6] in 1839 was responsible for setting up a routine system for compilation of the numbers and causes of deaths as medical statistics in the office of the Registrar General of England.

The beginning of contemporary epidemiology is often dated to the mid 20th century, when many large-scale studies were initiated to assess the causes of the shifting pattern of diseases in the developed world.

Studies on rising mortality from chronic diseases like coronary heart disease and lung cancer were some of these. Some of the earlier landmark studies are the Framingham Heart study[7] initiated in 1949 and the British physicians study[8] in 1950. The association of smoking and lung cancer from case-control studies[9] was reported in the 1940s and early 1950s. The principle of evaluating research findings for cause and effect was first proved by Robert Koch[10] in the relationship of microorganisms with sepsis.

Epidemiological findings are useful to plan and evaluate strategies to prevent illness and also as a guide to the management of patients in whom the disease has already developed. Just like the clinical findings, symptoms, history, biochemical and pathological features, the epidemiology of the disease also forms an integral part of the description of any disease. Epidemiological facts about the etiology and prognosis of a disease help a clinician or a health worker to give the best advice to the patients about how to avoid or limit the effects of the disease. The term epidemiology was exclusively used for the study of epidemics of infectious diseases for many years. Patterns of mortality are changing in developing countries with chronic diseases assuming increasing importance and, as a consequence, the concept of an epidemic has become much broader and complex, necessitating more advanced methods than those first developed by Snow[11] in the study of cholera in 1853. Looking at the evolution of epidemiology, the span between Hippocrates and Graunt was 2000 years, between Graunt and Farr was 200 years and between Farr and Snow it was less than 20 years. This trend continued and over the years, epidemiology, as a discipline, has undergone an extraordinary growth in the subject content, variety of applications and popularity. In this process, different authors defined it in different ways and depending on the specific applications, new terminologies like clinical epidemiology, population epidemiology, field epidemiology, molecular epidemiology, environmental epidemiology, etc., have been coined. Whatever be the definition and wherever be the applications, central to all these has been the understanding that it is epidemiology and the core of it has been formed by the principles of Biostatistics.

In this chapter we introduce certain principles of Biostatistics, which form the mainstay of many common epidemiological investigations.

8.2. Causal Relationships

Epidemiological principles stand on two basic assumptions, *viz.,* human disease does not occur at random, and the disease and its causal as well as preventive factors can be identified by a thorough investigation of the population. So, naturally, identification of causal relationship between a disease and suspected risk factors forms part of epidemiological research. There are 3 types of causal relationships, *viz.,* sufficient cause, necessary cause and a risk factor.

A **sufficient cause** precedes the disease occurrence. If it is present, disease always occurs. Such causes are generally rare. Genetic abnormalities leading to a specific condition come under this category of causes. Another example that might be thought of a sufficient cause could be the presence of HIV. As of now at least, presence of HIV always leads to AIDS. So HIV can be a sufficient cause for AIDS. As science progresses, new drugs could be evolved and some of the HIV contracted cases could be prevented from developing AIDS.

A **necessary cause** should also precede the disease. In addition, it must be present in all the diseased subjects. However, it may also be possible that the necessary cause may be present, but the disease may not be there. For example, all cases of tuberculosis have the *Mycobacterium* (M) *tuberculosis*, but all subjects who are infected with *M. tuberculosis* do not develop tuberculosis.

A **risk factor,** unlike the sufficient and necessary causes, increases the probability or risk of a particular condition in a group of persons compared to a similar group who do not have it. Thus, it is neither a sufficient nor a necessary cause of the disease. Epidemiological factors like smoking, drinking, exercise, etc., fall in this category. So we say these factors have an association with a particular condition. For example, exposure to asbestos filaments increases the chance of lung cancer as compared to those who are not exposed. So exposure to asbestos is a risk factor for lung cancer.

In health research or clinical medicine it is not always possible to prove causal relationship beyond any doubt. We can only increase our conviction of a cause-effect relation by empirical evidence. Towards this aim, the possibility of a postulated cause-effect relationship should be examined in different ways.

A causal association could be directly causal or indirectly causal. For instance, jumping from a multi-story building can cause multiple fractures and injuries leading to death. No other cause is required for death. Therefore, jumping from a high altitude is directly causal to death. Socio-economic status, literacy, etc., on the other hand, are proxy for many conditions like poor nutrition, hygiene, health awareness & motivation, etc. So, these can be considered as indirectly causal. Further, we may find a cause and effect relation in statistical analyses, but it may be result of some other factor. For example, we may find statistically significant association between presence of gray hair and CHD. But both these could be because of the age. So, whenever we come across any association, we have to examine whether it could be a really causal or non-causal or an artifact arising out of some other factor(s).

8.2.1. Establishing a Causal Relation

The cause and effect can be directly verified or established in an experimental setting as the investigator can maneuver the subjects and the exposure as desired, and can see the resultant effect. In the absence of such maneuverability, as in the case of observational studies, one has to rely on several lines of reasoning to establish causality. Sir Austin Bradford Hill[12], a British medical statistician was the first to propose a comprehensive list of criteria for a causal association (Fig. 8.1). These criteria, called Hill's criteria of causation, are described below.

Temporality: The absolutely essential criterion for cause-effect relationship is the temporality, i.e., the time factor. The exposure under consideration should always precede the disease. For example, in a study on coir workers in southern India (unpublished), it was observed that elephantiasis was more prevalent among coir workers. Such a finding tempts one to conclude that working in coir looms might be causing the disease. When enquires were made about the time of acquiring the disease, it was realized that the disease was mostly acquired prior to joining the profession; people who developed elephantiasis found it difficult to work in other occupations and, hence, settled in coir industry, where a clubfoot was helpful in their work on coir looms. Thus, the association found is fallacious, as the cause did not precede the disease.

Strength: The size of the risk associated with the exposure should be large enough to make us believe that the association observed is causal. If it is close to the risk of the disease among the unexposed, one might not be convinced about the cause and effect between the exposure and the disease. In other words, higher risk of disease associated with the exposure makes it less likely to be spurious or a chance observation.

Dose-response relationship: If the association between the suspected cause and the disease increases as the level of the suspected cause increases and decreases as the level decreases, it adds strength to the postulated causal relationship. For example, if cigarette smoking is a cause for lung cancer, the risk of the disease should be more in those who smoke more number of cigarettes/day or have been smoking for long duration than in those who smoke fewer cigarettes/day or have been smoking for shorter duration.

Reversibility: If the removal or reduction in the level of the suspected cause leads to the disappearance or reduction of the disease occurrence, it can be taken as indication that the association is causal. For example, reduced consumption of salt results in lower blood pressure. So the association between salt consumption and hypertension could be causal.

Consistency: If the association observed is also reported from different places by different investigators in varied setups, it adds strength to the causal hypothesis between an exposure and a disease.

Biological plausibility: The association observed should be consistent with the prevailing knowledge and should make sense with the known biological or physiological reasoning.

Specificity: A cause is said to be specific to an effect if the introduction of the suspected cause is followed by the occurrence of the effect and also removal of the suspected cause leads to the absence of the effect. If it can be established that a single cause produces a specified effect, the cause-effect relations gains more credence. This logic is too simplistic as often multiple factors lead to multiple conditions. So, specificity of an association definitely supports the causal relation but absence of specificity cannot be interpreted as absence of causal relation. Specificity is a more feasible criterion in infectious diseases than in non-communicable diseases.

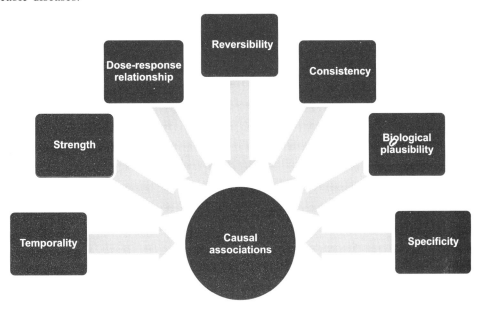

Fig. 8.1: Hill's criteria of causation

8.3. Indices of Burden of the Disease

As mentioned earlier, epidemiological methods seek to identify causes that increase or decrease the risk of a disease. Towards this objective, first we should have measures that tell us about the magnitude of the problem at hand, so that it can be compared when the exposure is present with that when the exposure is absent. The number of persons with the disease or number of events of interest is the simplest indicator of the burden of the disease. But it depends on the population size and the distribution of various characteristics in the population. Therefore, health statistics are usually expressed as 'rates' or 'ratios' with respect to different characteristics of the population. These measures can be absolute or relative. Some of the common measures are described in this section.

A **ratio** is a static quantity '*a* /*b*', where '*a*' and '*b*' are two entities such that '*a*' is not a part of '*b*'. It indicates the number of '*a*'$_s$ per one '*b*' in the population. It is more useful for comparison purposes, without regard to the sizes of populations or their characteristics. For example, sex ratio (male: female) of lung cancer cases 80:40 or 2:1in a particular place indicates that for every one female lung cancer case, there are two male cases in that place and for that particular period of time, but it does not tell anything about the total number of lung cancer cases.

A **rate** is a quantity '*a/b*', where '*a*' is a part of '*b*'. Each of the '*b*'$_s$ should have an opportunity to become '*a*'. It is usually expressed as a percentage or per 1000 or some such constant. It indicates the rapidity with which the event is occurring during a specified time-period. For example, if 400 new cases (*a*) of leukemia were observed during a 5 year period in a city with an average population of 250000 during that period (*b*), the occurrence of leukemia in that city during that particular period would be [400 ÷ (250000 * 5)]* 100000 = 32 per one lakh population per annum. For more details on rates, ratios and proportions, Chapter I may be seen.

8.3.1. Prevalence

Prevalence conveys the disease frequency in the community at a given point of time. It is the proportion of persons in a defined population who have a specific disease or condition at a point in time, usually the survey time. It is called point prevalence or just prevalence and is defined as,

$$\text{Point Prevalence} = \frac{\text{Number of subjects with the disease}}{\text{Population at risk at that time}}$$

If there were 5000 persons aged 60+ years in a town and 650 cases of coronary artery disease were found among them, the prevalence of CAD in that town at that time would be:

$$\text{Prevalence} = \frac{\text{Number of subjects with the disease}}{\text{Population at risk at that time}} = \frac{650}{5000} = 0.13 \text{ or } 13\%$$

It means that for every 100 persons aged 60+ years, we can find on average 13 persons with the CAD in that town at that particular time.

When the numerator refers to the number of persons who had the disease at any time during a specified time interval and the denominator consists of average population (or population at the mid-point of the interval) during that time period, it is called **period prevalence**.

$$\text{Period Prevalence} = \frac{\text{Number of subjects with the disease during the period}}{\text{Average population at risk during the period}}$$

In the above example on CAD, if we had 5000 population of 60+ years at the beginning of a year and 4500 at the end of the year; and if 700 cases of CAD were observed during year, the period prevalence of CAD during that year would be:

Number of CAD cases during the year = 700

To calculate the average population during the year, we assume that the change in the population size during the year is uniform and, hence, the average of the population sizes at the beginning and at the end of the period can be taken as the population at risk at the mid-point of the interval.

Average population at risk during the year = (5000 + 4500)/2 = 4750

$$\text{Prevalence of CAD for the year} = \frac{\text{Number of subjects with CAD during the year}}{\text{Average population at risk during the year}}$$

$$= \frac{700}{4750} = 0.1474 \text{ or } 14.74\%$$

It implies that on the average during the year, there were about 148 cases of CAD for every 1000 population aged 60+ years.

It can be easily noted that period prevalence is equal to the point prevalence at the beginning of the interval plus incidence during the interval. Because it is a mixture of point prevalence and incidence, it is not commonly used.

8.3.2. Incidence

While calculating prevalence, we are not concerned with the time when the disease occurred. Instead, if we ignore the old or existing cases and limit ourselves to the number of occurrences of new cases in a defined population during a certain period and adjust it to the population at risk, we get what is known as incidence rate.

$$\text{Incidence rate} = \frac{\text{Number of newly diagnosed cases during the period}}{\text{Average number of persons at risk during the period}} \ x \ \text{Constant}$$

If there were 781 new cases of uterine cervical cancer diagnosed in Delhi during 1997 (total female population at risk is 4939680), the incidence rate of cervical cancer is:

$$\frac{781}{4939680} * 100000 = 15.8$$

Or, for every 100000 females, there were 16 new cases of cervical cancer diagnosed during 1997 in Delhi.

Incidence rate can be interpreted as the average probability of developing the disease within the time interval, conditional on the absence of disease at the start of the interval.

8.3.3. Prevalence versus Incidence

Prevalence considers all the cases present at the time of data collection as compared to incidence, which considers only those cases that occurred during the study time. It is a proportion and a static quantity. The conceptual differences among point prevalence, period prevalence and incidence can be better understood with the help of Fig. 8.2. The time of occurrence of the disease and the time of recovery are indicated on the time axis during a year for ten diseased persons in a closed population, i.e., where there is no emigration and immigration. Each line represents a person with the beginning of the line indicating the time of that person acquiring the disease and the end of the line indicating recovery or death.

The line number 1 indicates that person 1 had already acquired the disease before the beginning of the year (t_1) and either recovered or was dead during the year. Same is the case with persons 2, 4 and 6 also. Person number 10 had the disease before the beginning of the year and continued to have it at the end of the year. The point prevalence at time t_1 is, therefore, 5 (Nos. 1, 2, 4, 6 and 10).

Persons numbered 3, 7 and 9 were disease-free at time t_1, acquired the disease during the year and continued to be diseased at the end of the year (t_2). In addition, person number 10 had the disease in the beginning and continued to have it at the end of the year. Therefore, the point prevalence at time t_2 is 4.

During the year, 2 persons acquired the disease and were also cured or were dead (persons 5 and 8). Adding these two cases to the 3 cases that occurred during the year, we have a total of 5 cases occurring during the year (persons 3, 5, 7, 8 and 9). So, all these 5 will be the incident cases during the year.

All the 10 cases are prevalent at some point of time during the year and so they will be accounted for in the period prevalence during the year. Note that period prevalence (10) is the sum of point prevalence at t_1 (5) and the incidence (5).

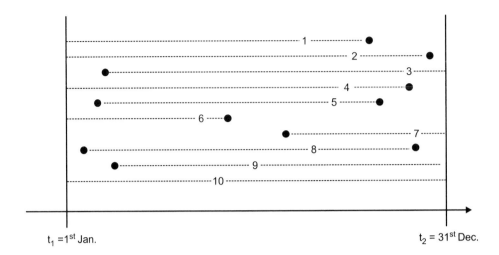

$t_1 = 1^{st}$ Jan. $t_2 = 31^{st}$ Dec.

Fig. 8.2: Diagrammatic representation of differences between prevalence and incidence

If a disease is associated with mortality immediately after onset, prevalence of such a disease will be low at any given time, though the incidence could be high. On the other hand, if the mortality associated with the disease is low, we can have a high prevalence at any time, though the incidence could be low. Thus, prevalence depends on the nature of the disease, availability and quality of treatment facilities, duration of the disease and migration. It is an appropriate measure in relatively stable conditions and is unsuitable for acute disorders. Even in chronic conditions, the manifestation of the disease could be intermittent and so a point prevalence based on a single examination tends to underestimate the load of the disease in the population. Incidence is a rate that conveys the speed with which events are occurring and it is free of the limitations associated with prevalence.

In general, if the disease under consideration is stable (no substantial changes in the incidence, management practices and case fatality, etc.), the relation between prevalence and incidence can be expressed as: Prevalence = Incidence * mean duration of disease.

8.4. Crude and Specific Rates

Incidence, prevalence, mortality or any other rate can be calculated for the population at risk as a whole or for specific subdivisions of the population at risk. The former are referred to as crude and the latter as the specific rates. The specific rates can be obtained gender-wise, age-wise, region-wise, race-wise or occupation-wise, etc., while the crude rate is only one estimate for the total population. Specific rates throw more light on the patterns or trends in the occurrence of a disease or mortality associated with it, as crude rates tend to mask the patterns. For example, incidence of gall bladder cancer in New Delhi during 1997 was 3.7 per 100000 persons per annum. If we obtain the gender specific incidence from the same data, it is 2.1 among males and 5.6 per 100000 per annum among females (Biennial Report[13]). The crude rate, though conveyed the burden of the problem in the population, masked the fact of higher incidence among females. This fact is clearly revealed by the gender specific rates. Thus, it is often helpful to examine the results for the whole population as well as to obtain specific rates with respect to different population characteristics.

8.5. Standardized or Adjusted Rates

Many times, incidence or mortality or some other rate calculated depends on the composition of population with respect to age, sex, etc. For example, consider two countries A and B such that in one country the population is relatively young (hence fewer deaths) as compared to the other country in which the population is older (hence more deaths can occur). If we compare the crude mortality rates, it will be high in the country where the population is older and may lead us to conclude that in general the health care scenario is better in the country where the crude mortality rate is lower. But it could be fallacious as the lower mortality may be due to younger population in that country rather than the availability of better health care facilities. On the other hand, if the age composition in the two countries is similar, the crude rates are comparable and lead to appropriate conclusions.

One approach to overcome the potential fallacy is to compare the age-specific mortality rates and if they also show lower mortality rates in the country with younger population, then we are right in concluding about the state of health care facilities in the two countries being compared. However, comparing many specific rates is cumbersome and also at times may be confusing with no clear indication of the direction of the differences. Because of this, a concept known as standardization or adjustment of rates with respect to age or gender, etc., is used to make the results comparable. Standardization gives us one single statistic that summarizes the comparison, allowing for the differences in the background factors such as age, gender, race or religion, etc. There are two techniques for obtaining standardized rates, viz., direct standardization and indirect standardization.

8.5.1. Direct Standardization

In this method, we compare the weighted averages of specific rates, the weights being equal to the proportion of people in each specific category. These weights are usually obtained from a convenient, known reference population. Since the rates being compared are the weighted average of specific rates with common weights, they are comparable. Alternatively, standardization can be thought of as the expected rate in the standard population if the observed specific rates of the populations being considered are applied to the standard population. We shall explain the direct method of standardization by a hypothetical example below.

Consider mortality rates in two villages A and B with a total of population of 10000 and 15000 respectively during a specified year. The age distribution of the population and the number of deaths in each age group in the two villages during the year are listed in Table 8.1.

Table 8.1: Example data for direct standardization

Age (years)	Village A			Village B		
	Population	*Deaths*	*Mortality rate*	*Population*	*Deaths*	*Mortality rate*
0 – 14	1000	2	0.0020	5000	20	0.0040
15 – 44	5000	100	0.0200	7000	245	0.0350
45 +	4000	480	0.1200	3000	390	0.1300
Total	10000	582		15000	655	

$$\text{Crude mortality rate in village A} = \frac{582}{10000} * 1000 = 58.2 \text{ per thousand}$$

$$\text{Crude mortality rate in village B} = \frac{655}{15000} * 1000 = 43.67 \text{ per thousand}$$

Looking at the crude mortality rates in the two villages, one would be tempted to conclude that mortality is higher in village A than that in village B. However, when we see the age-specific rates of mortality, they are lower in village A than those in Village B for all age groups. This is contrary to the conclusion based on crude rates.

Now let us consider a standard reference population with a known age structure and calculate the number of deaths that would have occurred in each village if the age composition in each village was the same as that of the standard population. This is same as the number of deaths expected in the standard population assuming the observed age-specific death rates in the sample population. The Table below shows the details of these calculations.

Age (years)	Standard Population S_i	Village A		Expected number of deaths in Standard Population*
		Population P_i	Observed deaths X_i	
0 – 14	9000	1000	2	(2/1000) * 9000 = 18
15 – 44	15000	5000	100	(100/5000) * 15000 = 300
45 +	6000	4000	480	(480/4000) * 6000 = 720
Total	$S = 30000$	10000	582	1038

*Expected number assuming the age-specific rates observed in the sample

Age standardized or adjusted mortality rate in village A = 1038/30000 = 34.6 per 1000.
Similarly, we can work out for village B as shown below:

Age (years)	Standard Population S_i	Village B		Expected number of deaths in Standard Population*
		Population P_i	Observed deaths X_i	
0 – 14	9000	5000	20	(20/5000) * 9000 = 36
15 – 44	15000	7000	245	(245/7000) * 15000 = 525
45 +	6000	3000	390	(390/3000) * 6000 = 780
Total	30000	15000	655	1341

Age adjusted or standardized rate of mortality in village B = 1341/30000 * 1000 = 44.7 per 1000.

In mathematical notation, the direct standardized rate = $\dfrac{\sum\limits_{i=1}^{k} \dfrac{X_i}{P_i} * S_i}{S}$

Where X_i and P_i are the number of events and the population in the ith stratum of the study population, S_i is standard population in the ith stratum and S is total of standard population with total k strata.

Comparing the age adjusted mortality rates, we see that the mortality is lower in village A than that in village B (34.4 vs. 44.7), a conclusion quite opposite to the one based on crude mortality rates.

The standard error of a direct adjusted rate is $\dfrac{\sqrt{V_1}}{S}$ where $V_i = \dfrac{E_i * S_i}{P_i * Y}$, E_i is the expected number of events in the ith stratum of the standard population and Y is the number of time-units in the reference period. For example, if the annual rates being compiled are based on 5-year data, Y will be 5 and if a monthly incidence of a disease is calculated based on 6 months data, Y will be 6 and so on.

The standard error of the direct adjusted mortality rate in village A of our example:
Since data is based on 1 year observations, Y = 1

Age (years) (years)	Standard Population S_i	Population in Village P_1	Expected deaths in Std.Pop E_i	$V_i = \dfrac{E_i * S_i}{P_i * Y}$
0 – 14	9000	1000	18	(18*9000)/ (1000*1) = 162
15 – 44	15000	5000	300	(300*15000)/((5000*1) = 900
45 +	6000	4000	720	(720*6000)/(4000*1) = 1080
Total	30000	10000	1038	2142

Standard Error = $\dfrac{\sqrt{2142}}{30000}$ = 0.0015 or 1.5427 per 1000

Therefore, the 95% CI of the direct adjusted mortality rate = Adj. Rate ± 1.96*SE
= (34.36 ± 1.96*1.5427) = (31.34 and 37.38)
Similarly, for village B, the standard error works out to be 1.7480 per 1000 and the 95% CI would then be (41.3 and 48.1).

8.5.1.1. Comparison of two direct standardized rates

For easy understanding of this procedure, we introduce some notations. Let the two adjusted or standardized rates be AR_1 and AR_2. Let the number of events, population and the event rates in the ith stratum of the two groups being compared be X_{1i}, X_{2i}; P_{1i}, P_{2i} and r_{1i} and r_{2i} respectively.
As shown earlier,

Direct standardized rate in Group 1 = $AR_1 = \dfrac{\sum\limits_{i=1}^{k} \dfrac{X_{1i}}{P_{1i}} * S_i}{S}$

Direct standardized rate in Group 2 = $AR_2 = \dfrac{\sum\limits_{i=1}^{k} \dfrac{X_{2i}}{P_{2i}} * S_i}{S}$

The variance of the difference of the two adjusted rates will be,

$$\hat{\sigma}^2 = \sum_{i=1}^{k} \left(\frac{S_i}{S}\right)^2 \left[\frac{\bar{r}_i(1-\bar{r}_i)}{P_{1i} * P_{2i}} (P_{1i} + P_{2i}) \right]$$

where $\bar{r}_i$ is the specific rate in the ith stratum for both the groups combined, i.e., $\bar{r}_i = \dfrac{(X_{1i} + X_{2i})}{(P_{1i} + P_{2i})}$

Then the equality of AR1 and AR2 can be tested by a statistic $\dfrac{(AR_1 - AR_2)^2}{\hat{\sigma}^2}$, which follows a Chi-square distribution with one degree of freedom, under the null hypothesis of equality of the two rates.
In the above example data we considered, the required quantities can be shown in a tabular form as below.

Age (years)	Standard Population S_i	Village A		Village B		$\bar{r}_i$	$\hat{\sigma}_i^2$
		Population P_{1i}	Deaths X_{1i}	Population P_{2i}	Deaths X_{2i}		
0 – 14	9000	1000	2	5000	20	0.003667	0.000000394
15 – 44	15000	5000	100	7000	245	0.028750	0.000002393
45 +	6000	4000	480	3000	390	0.124286	0.000002539
Total	$S = 30000$	10000	582	15000	655		0.000005326

We have AR1 = 34.4 per 1000 or 0.0344 and AR2 = 44.7 per 1000 or 0.0447.

Therefore, $\dfrac{\left(AR_1 - AR_2\right)^2}{\hat{\sigma}^2}$ = (0.0344 – 0.0447)² / 0.000005326 = 19.92

Comparing this with 10.83 (tabulated value of Chi-square with 1 d.f.), we conclude that the difference between the two direct adjusted rates cannot be due to chance (p < 0.001) and so both are significantly different.

8.5.2. Indirect Standardization

The direct method of standardization can be applied when we have the proportion of standard population in each specific category of age, sex, etc., and the required specific rates in our sample. If we do not have the specific rates and only the crude rate is available, the direct method cannot be applied.

In such situations, the known specific rates in a reference population are applied to the study population and the expected number of events of interest are calculated and summed up. Dividing the total expected number of events by the total study population, we obtain what is called as the index event rate. Since the expected number of events is based on the experience in the standard population, a correction factor has to be applied to get the indirect standardized rate. This correction factor is the index event rate. Crude rate in the standard population divided by the index rate in the study population is the standardization factor, and crude rate in the study population multiplied by this standardization factor yields the indirect standardized rate for the study population.

The same hypothetical data used in direct standardization will be used to illustrate the calculation of standardized rates by indirect method.

Age (years)	Village A		Standard		Expected deaths in Village A*
	Population P_i	Observed Deaths X_i	Population S_i	Deaths Y_i	
0 – 14	1000	Not known	9000	27	27/9000 * 1000 = 3
15 – 44	5000	Not known	15000	375	375/15000 * 5000 = 125
45 +	4000	Not known	6000	720	720/6000 * 4000 = 480
Total	10000	$\Sigma X_i = 582$	$\Sigma S_i = 30000$	$\Sigma Y_i = 1122$	608

*: Assuming the age-specific rates of the standard population

Crude mortality rate in Standard population = 1122/30000 = 37.4 per 1000
Index rate of mortality in village A = 608/10000 = 60.8 per 1000
Standardization factor for village A = 37.4/ 60.8 = 0.6151

Standardized mortality rate in village A = Crude mortality rate * Standardization factor
$$= 58.2 * 0.6151 = 35.8 \text{ per } 1000$$

To put it simply, the indirect adjusted rate is the ratio of total observed to the total expected events in the study population multiplied by the crude rate in the standard population.

$$\text{Indirect standardized rate} = \frac{\text{Observed number of events}}{\text{Expected number of events}} * \text{Crude rate of Standard population}$$

In mathematical notations, the Indirect standardized rate =
$$\left[\frac{\sum_{i=1}^{k} X_i}{\left(\sum_{i=1}^{k} \frac{Y_i}{S_i} * P_i \right)} \right] * \left(\frac{\sum_{i=1}^{k} Y_i}{\sum_{i=1}^{k} S_i} \right) * 1000$$

Where X_i, P_i and S_i are as defined earlier and Y_i are the known number of events in the ith stratum of the standard population.

For Village B:

Age (years)	Village B Population P_i	Village B Observed Deaths X_i	Standard Population S_i	Standard Deaths Y_i	Expected deths in Village B
0 – 14	5000	Not known	9000	27	27/9000 * 5000 = 15
15 – 44	7000	Not known	15000	375	375/15000 * 7000 = 175
45 +	3000	Not known	6000	720	720/6000 * 4000 = 360
Total	15000	$\Sigma X_i = 655$	$\Sigma S_i = 30000$	$\Sigma Y_i = 1122$	550

Standardized mortality rate in village B =

$$\frac{\text{Observed events}}{\text{Expected events}} * \text{Crude rate of Standard population} = \frac{655}{550} * 37.4 = 44.54$$

Notice that the apparent differences between the crude mortality rates of the two villages (58.20 vs. 43.67) turned opposite after adjusting for age (35.8 vs. 44.54), as we saw in direct standardization also.

Since we observed 582 deaths in village A whereas we can expect 608 (assuming the age-specific mortality rates observed in standard population), the ratio of these two numbers provides us a relative measure called standardized mortality ratio (SMR). For village A, SMR works out to be 0.957 or 95.7% and for village B it is 1.19 or 119%. Compared to the standard population, village A has about 4% less mortality and village B has 19% more mortality, after taking into account the age-wise differences in the two populations.

8.5.2.1. Comparison of two indirect standardized rates

When we have two adjusted rates, it is natural to ask whether the difference between them is statistically significant. Also we would like to know whether the SMR in each Group or population is 1 or different from 1 and also whether the two SMRs are different.

Testing whether a SMR is equal to 1 is fairly simple by using a chi-square statistic as under:

$$\chi^2 = \frac{(\text{Observed No. of Events} - \text{Expected No. of Events})^2}{\text{Expected No. of Events}},$$ which follows chi-square with one degree of freedom.

For village A, χ^2 with 1 d.f. $= = 1.11 \dfrac{(582-608)^2}{608} = 1.11$

For village B, χ^2 with 1 d.f. $= \dfrac{(655-550)^2}{550} = 20.05$

From the two chi-square statistic values we realize that the SMR in village A is not statistically different from 1, while in village B it is significantly different from 1. In other words, standardization did not change the event rate significantly in village A, but it mattered significantly in village B.

Comparing two indirect adjusted rates is equivalent to comparing the two SMRs and this is also achieved by a chi-square statistic defined as:

$$\chi^2 \text{ with 1 d.f. } = \dfrac{\left(In\ SMR_1 - In\ SMR_2\right)^2}{\left(\dfrac{1}{E_1} + \dfrac{1}{E_2}\right)},$$

where SMR_1 and E_1 are the standardized mortality ratio and expected number of events respectively in the first population and SMR_2 and E_2 in the second population. Note that logarithmic values are of natural log or with base e.

In our example, χ^2 with 1 d.f.
$$= \dfrac{\left(In\ 0.9572 - In\ 1.1909\right)^2}{\left(\dfrac{1}{608} + \dfrac{1}{550}\right)}$$
$$= \dfrac{(-0.0437 - 0.1747)}{(0.001645 + 0.001818)}$$
$$= \dfrac{0.0477}{0.003463} = 13.77$$

The obtained value of the chi-square statistic indicates a difference between the SMRs (consequently the two adjusted rates), which is statistically highly significant. Note here that taking enough number of decimals would help in the accuracy of the calculations, as we are working on logarithmic values and inverse of large numbers.

The tests for SMR being equal to 1 and for equality of two SMRs are large sample chi-square tests requiring the assumption that the ratio of the stratum specific rates of a study population to the stratum specific rates in the standard population is constant. If this does not hold, the SMRs may not be comparable.

8.5.3. Direct versus Indirect Standardization

We have discussed two methods of standardization of rates, namely, direct and indirect methods. Though both have their own advantages and disadvantages, certain points need to be noted.

- The standardized rates are imaginary and cannot be observed. They only indicate the picture as if certain conditions were present in the populations studied and in this process make the comparisons fairer than the comparison of crude rates.
- Direct method is appropriate when the studied populations are large and also when we have the specific rates in our study population. Indirect method of standardization is useful when we do not have the specific rates in our population, but we have the crude rate along with the composition with respect to

age, sex, etc., of the population being considered. Even if we have the specific rates, when the population being considered is small, the specific rates tend to fluctuate more. Indirect standardization would help to overcome this also.

- The adjusted rate depends on the standard population chosen. For example, in studying the mortality rates, if we chose a standard population that is older than the populations being compared, more weights are given for the events in the older ages. On the other hand, if we chose a younger population as standard, events at younger ages are given higher weights. In other words, two adjusted rates A and B, in which A is more than B, can be made as B more than A, by choosing another standard population.

- While interpreting the standardized rates, it should be noted that they conceal the 'interaction' between the event rate and the factor to be adjusted. Interaction is a phenomenon in which the effect of the exposure on the outcome depends on the level of a third variable. More on this phenomenon is given in Section 8.7.4. In the example we discussed above, if the effect of age on mortality is different in the two villages compared, it can be said that there is interaction. We have the age-specific mortality in village B higher than that in village A for all age groups. If the specific rates were higher in village A (say at younger ages) and some were higher in village B (say at older ages), it indicates 'interaction' between age (factor to be adjusted) and mortality (event). In particular, if the differences between the specific rates of the groups being compared are uniform, we say that there is no interaction. When interaction is present, the standardized rates may be misleading.

8.6. Types of Study Design

To assess the role of any suspected factor in the causation of a disease, we must first quantify the effect of exposure on the disease. There are different indices to measure the association between an exposure and a condition, depending upon the design of the study. There are two basic types of studies, *viz.,* observational and experimental. In observational studies, we merely observe the different characteristics of study subjects, as they exist. In contrast, experimental studies involve some manipulation by way of subjecting the study participants to specific maneuvers and observing the response to such maneuvers. Laboratory animal experiments, clinical trials, intervention studies and bio-assays, etc., fall under this category.

Observational studies can further be categorized into three broad types, namely, cross-sectional, case-control and cohort studies.

8.6.1. Cross-sectional Study

A cross sectional study, as the name itself indicates, provides a onetime snapshot of the situation that exists in the population at the specified time. The exposure under investigation and the disease status are assessed simultaneously. It provides frequency and other characteristics of a disease. Cross-sectional studies are often useful to generate, rather than test or confirm a hypothesis.

A schematic presentation of a cross-sectional study is shown in Fig. 8.3.

Generation of a hypothesis can occur in different ways. For example, if we observe a great difference in the occurrence of a disease between two groups of populations, it gives rise to a question whether one group is more prone to the disease than the other. It is called the method of difference. The observation of absence of penile cancer among Muslims by Niblock[14] (1902) is an example for generating a hypothesis by this method. Analyzing the records of a ten-year period (1892-1901) in the Madras Medical College Hospital, he observed that all the 201 patients of penile cancer were Hindus and not a single case was reported in Muslims. He ascribed this to the fact of circumcision in Muslims at a very early age and further expected that similar immunity would hold among the Jews also. This observation led to the hypothesis of a protective role of the male circumcision in the causation of penile cancer.

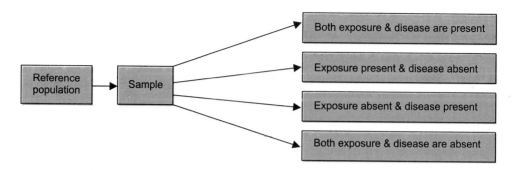

Fig. 8.3: Diagrammatic presentation of the scheme of a cross-sectional study

Another way that a hypothesis can arise is by method of agreement, that is, if the level of presence of a disease or condition agrees across some groups, it gives rise to a hypothesis that all these groups share some common factors that have a bearing on the occurrence of the disease. For example, high frequency of Acquired Immuno-Deficiency Syndrome (AIDS) is observed in intra-venous drug users, recipients of transfusions and hemophiliacs as compared to other people. This observation of agreement among these groups can lead to a hypothesis of the role of infected needles in the causation of AIDS.

Method of concomitant variation is another way in which a hypothesis can be raised. As an example, it is observed that worldwide mortality due to CHD is high where per capita cigarette consumption is high and mortality is low where cigarette consumption is low.

8.6.1.1. Measure of association in cross-sectional studies

In cross-sectional studies, the measures of association are simple proportions or averages with respect to different characteristics of the population. For instance, proportion of smokers is 50% in diseased and 30% in non-diseased individuals; average cholesterol is 200 mg/dl in white collar workers and 160 mg/dl in blue collar workers, etc. The difference between the various exposure strata could be summarized with 95% confidence intervals and also tested for statistical significance by appropriate statistical tests of significance (refer to Chapter 5).

Example:

In a school survey on smoking habits among the senior secondary boys, it was found that 15 of 150 boys from the private schools smoke as compared to 12 of the 200 from government schools. Do the proportion of boys who smoke is same in the two types of schools?

Proportion of smokers in private schools = 15 ÷ 150 = 10%

Standard Error (SE) of the proportion = $\sqrt{\dfrac{pq}{n}} = \sqrt{\dfrac{0.1 * 0.9}{150}} = 0.0245$

95% Confidence interval for the proportion = 0.1 ± (1.96*SE)
$$= (0.1 - 0.0480 \text{ and } 0.1 + 0.0480)$$
$$= (0.0520 \text{ and } 0.1480) \text{ or } (5.2\% \text{ and } 14.8\%)$$

Proportion of smokers in Government schools = 12 ÷ 200 = 6%

Standard Error of the proportion = $\sqrt{\dfrac{0.06 * 0.94}{200}} = 0.0168$

95% Confidence interval
$$= (0.06 - 0.0329 \text{ and } 0.06 + 0.0329)$$
$$= (0.0271 \text{ and } 0.0929) \text{ or } (2.71\% \text{ and } 9.29\%)$$

Since the 95% confidence intervals of the proportion of smokers in the two types of schools overlap, we can say that there is no evidence (at 5% level) to conclude that the two proportions are different.

Example:

Suppose in a survey on the elderly population (> 50 years) it was found that the average systolic blood pressure was 170 mm/Hg with a standard deviation of 15 mm/Hg in the high-income group (n = 200) and 160 mm/Hg with a standard deviation of 10 mm in the low-income group (n = 300). To test whether the differences observed are due to chance, the details of analysis are shown below.

Two-sample t test with equal variances							
Income		Obs	Mean	Std. Err.	Std. Dev.	[95% Conf.	Interval]
High		200	170	1.06066	15	167.9084	172.0916
Low		300	160	0.5773503	10	158.8638	161.1362
Combined		500	164	0.5894021	13.17943	162.842	165.158
Difference			10	1.117847		7.803723	12.19628
Degrees of freedom: 498							

The analysis indicates the number of observations, means, standard error of means, standard deviations and the 95% confidence intervals for the 2 income groups. The same details are also shown for both the groups combined.

The difference in the mean values of the two groups, its standard error and 95% CI are shown in the last row of the Table. It can be seen that there is an average difference of 10 mm/Hg (170 – 160) between the two groups and this difference would lie between 7.8 mm and 12.2 mm, 95% of times over repeated studies with the same sample size and from the same target population. Since the 95% CI does not include zero, we can conclude that the observed difference in means is beyond chance (chance probability being < 0.05).

Since computed 'k' = 8.9458 is > 3.31 for 498 d.f., chance probability will be < 0.001 (see Table in Appendix 4)

In other words, if the null hypothesis of equality of means holds true, the probability of finding a mean difference of 10 is less than one in thousand. Therefore, we conclude that the difference in the systolic blood pressure values between the high- and low-income groups is statistically significant.

When we study one variable at a time, the analysis is simple as shown above. If there are many factors or variables to be studied as to their role on the outcome, we can stratify a variable and apply the methods for one variable at a time, within each strata of the stratified variable. For example, if we wish to study the role of occupation (blue collar or white collar) in addition to the income on the blood pressure, we can assess the systolic blood pressure differences between high- and low-income groups, separately among the white-collar and blue-collar occupations.

Though stratified analysis can be intuitively extended to any number of study variables, such a method breaks down as the number of variables increases or some of the study variables are of continuous nature. Depending on the nature (quantitative or qualitative) of the outcome variable, regression analysis techniques can be applied when we have multiple study factors on a single outcome or response variable. If the response variable is of continuous nature, linear regression will be applied to quantify the influence of a study variable on the response variable (Chapter 3). If we have many study variables, the concept of simple linear regression can be extended to multiple linear regression.

When the response or outcome variable is of binary nature, such as disease present and absent, a technique called logistic regression is applied. The details of this analysis technique are presented in the section on case-control studies.

8.6.1.2. Advantages and limitations of cross-sectional studies

Cross-sectional studies are simple and easy to carry out. Since they involve one-time observation, they involve comparatively lesser costs and effort. Often, they provide a quick answer to the question at hand and are sometimes helpful to generate a hypothesis, which needs to be verified by more stringent designs.

However, in cross-sectional studies, it is not possible to determine temporal sequence, i.e., whether exposure preceded the disease. Recall the example on Elephantiasis in coir workers described earlier. Another drawback with cross-sectional studies is that the more severe cases would have already died or removed. If we wish to assess the association of cigarette smoking with CHD using a cross-sectional study, it is possible that we may not find any association. This can happen because chronic or heavy smokers, who are more likely to develop the disease, might have developed CHD and died. Those with only milder forms of the disease, who are likely to be non-smokers or light smokers, could be surviving and, hence, available at the time of the study.

A cross-sectional study is also insensitive to the change in the exposure status of study participants. For example, a person after developing cirrhosis of liver might have stopped consuming alcohol. So, now if he is asked whether he consumes alcohol, he may say no. This response at the time of the study, though a fact, may lead an investigator to a false conclusion about the association of alcohol with a specific condition being investigated. Similarly, a CHD case might have stopped smoking or a diabetic started exercise, etc.

When the suspected causal factor is stable and unlikely to change, a cross-sectional study would be a suitable design for assessing the risk of the disease associated with such risk factor. For example, blood group or religious belief of a person does not change and so association of these factors with a disease can be adequately examined by a cross-sectional study.

8.6.2. Case-Control Study

In this type of observational study, two types of subjects are enrolled - cases and controls. Cases are those in which the outcome or disease is already present and controls are those in which the disease/outcome is absent. Past exposure to a suspected cause in the case series and the control series is elicited and compared. Thus, we proceed from effect to the cause in case-control studies. Since we are taking subjects who have already developed the disease and collect information on the past exposures, it is also called a retrospective study. The scheme of the case-control study can be depicted in the Fig. 8.4 below.

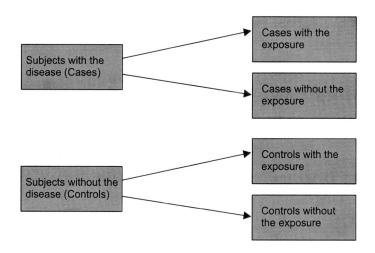

Fig. 8.4: Diagrammatic representation of the scheme of a case-control study

As an example, if one is interested in knowing the association between exposure to rubber industry and development of bladder cancer, a series of bladder cancer patients and a comparative group of normal persons without the disease can be enrolled and the past exposure to rubber industry could be ascertained. If the exposure increases (decreases) the disease risk, more (fewer) people in case series should have had the exposure as compared to the normal controls.

This straightforward logic makes the case-control study design very simple as well as popular.

8.6.2.1. *Measure of association in case-control studies*

To understand the calculation of the measure of association in a case-control study, we first arrange the available information in an R × 2 table, representing the subject status (diseased or control) on one side and the exposure status (with R possible categories) on the other. Though exposure status can have many options such as non-smoker, non-inhaling smoker, light smoker, moderate smoker and heavy smoker, etc., for easy understanding, we take the exposure status as binary only (yes/no). Now our table will have 2 rows and 2 columns with 4 cells. It is also helpful to remember that the first cell, i.e., the cell in first row and first column indicates both positive – disease as well as the exposure are present. The arrangement of the data with respect to the disease status and the exposure status can be seen in the Table 8.2 below.

Table 8.2: 2 × 2 Table showing the information on disease and exposure status

Exposure status	*Disease status*		*Total*
	Yes	*No*	
Yes	a	b	$a+b$
No	c	d	$c+d$
Total	N_1	N_2	N

Out of the N_1 cases, indicate the number with the exposure present as 'a' and those without the exposure as 'c'. Similarly, of the N_2 controls, indicate the number of controls that have the exposure as 'b' and those without the exposure as 'd'.

To test the significance of the association of the exposure with the disease, we can apply the usual chi-square test or Fisher's Exact test (Chapter 5).

To quantify the association, we use an index called Odds Ratio, which is described here. We can see that the probability of having disease among the exposed is $a/(a+b)$ and probability of not having the disease among the exposed is $b/(a+b)$. Therefore, the odds of disease among the exposed will be $a/(a+b) \div b/(a+b)$, which is equal to a/b. Similarly, the odds of disease among the unexposed can be shown to be c/d.

Now if we take the ratio of odds of disease when the exposure is present to the odds of disease when the exposure is absent, it will be $a/b \div c/d$, which is equal to ad/bc. This ratio is called the Odds Ratio (*OR*) and it measures the association between the exposure and the disease.

Note that Odds Ratio cannot be negative and it can range from zero to infinity. If the odds of disease among the exposed are more than the odds of disease among the unexposed, the *OR* will be more than one and the exposure is said to be a risk factor for the disease. On the other hand, if the odds of disease among the exposed are less than those among the unexposed, the *OR* will be less than one and the exposure is said to be a protective factor for the disease. When the odds of disease are same with or without the exposure, the *OR* will be equal to one and so the exposure has no association with the disease.

While arriving at the Odds Ratio, we took the odds of disease among the exposed and odds of disease among the unexposed. This is logical if we had really proceeded in that manner, viz., taking the exposed and unexposed and observing them to develop the disease. In a case-control study, since we already have the diseased and non-diseased persons, odds of exposure to the suspected risk factor among the cases and non-cases would be more appropriate. It can be easily verified that the odds ratio arrived at based on the odds of exposure will be same as the one obtained earlier. So, it is immaterial whether we consider odds of disease or odds of exposure as the Odds Ratio will be ad/bc in both the methods.

Example for calculation of Odds Ratio:

In a study of association of physical activity with the coronary heart disease, 20 out of 200 CHD cases were observed to be heavy exercisers compared to 40 out of 100 persons without CHD. The information is shown in a 2×2 table below:

Exposure status	Disease status		Total
	Yes	No	
Yes	20	40	60
No	180	60	240
Total	200	100	300

Odds Ratio = ad/bc = (20 * 60) / (40 * 180) = 1/6 = 0.1667
Taking the odds of exposure:
Odds of heavy exercise among diseased = 20/180
Odds of heavy exercise among non-diseased = 40/60

$$\text{Odds Ratio } = \frac{20}{180} * \frac{60}{40} = 1/6 \text{ or } 0.1667$$

Taking the odds of disease:
Odds of CHD among heavy exercisers = 20/40
Odds of CHD among non-exercisers = 180/60

$$\text{Odds Ratio } = \frac{20}{40} * \frac{60}{180} = 1/6 \text{ or } 0.1667$$

This means a person's odds of being a CHD case is about 0.17 if he is a heavy exerciser as compared to a person who is not a heavy exerciser. Therefore, heavy exercise can be said to be a protective factor for the CHD. As a measure of accuracy of the estimate, we can construct a 95% confidence interval for the *OR* obtained.

The actual distribution of the Odds Ratio is intractable, but the logarithm (natural log, with base *e*) of it has been found to be approximately Normal, especially with large samples (Woolf[15], 1955). Using this, we obtain the standard error of *ln (OR)* as:

$$\text{SE of } ln(\text{OR}) = \sqrt{\frac{1}{a} + \frac{1}{b} + \frac{1}{c} + \frac{1}{d}}$$

Therefore, an approximate 95% confidence interval for the *ln(OR)* is *ln(OR)* ± 1.96(SE).
After obtaining the confidence limits for *ln (OR)*, they are exponentiated to get back in original units. In the CHD and heavy exercise example, we have *a, b, c, d* as 20, 40, 180, 60 respectively.

$$\text{Therefore, the Standard Error} = \sqrt{\frac{1}{20} + \frac{1}{40} + \frac{1}{180} + \frac{1}{60}} = \sqrt{0.0972} = 0.3118$$

The upper 95% confidence limit of *ln (OR)* = *ln* (0.1667) + 1.96 * 0.3118 = - 1.7916 + 0.6111
   = - 1.1805
The lower 95% confidence limit of *ln (OR)* = *ln* (0.1667) - 1.96 * 0.3118 = - 1.7916 - 0.6111
   = - 2.4027
The 95% confidence interval of *ln (OR)* = [- 2.4027 and - 1.1805]
The 95% CI for the Odds Ratio = [exp(- 2.4027) and exp (- 1.1805)] = [0.09 and 0.31]

It means that over repeated studies with the same number of cases and controls, we can obtain an *OR* between 0.09 and 0.31, 95% of the times. The probability that these two limits contain the unknown *OR* in the population is 95%.

Since we deal with log values, it is important to take considerable number of decimal places (at least four) to be accurate enough.

If the exposure has more than two categories, like no smoking, light smoking and heavy smoking, calculation of odds ratio will be similar to binary exposure. One of the exposure categories is taken as a baseline (usually the one associated with least risk of disease) and the other categories are compared to the baseline category. So if we have *r* categories of the exposure, we will have *r*-1 odds ratios.

Example:

Smoking	CHD		Total	Odds Ratio
	Yes	No		
Heavy smoking	120	20	140	(120 * 40) ÷ (20 * 20) = 12.0
Light smoking	60	20	80	(60 * 40) ÷ (20 * 20) = 6.0
No	20	40	60	1.00
Total	200	100	300	

A light smoker's odds of CHD are 6.0 times and a heavy smoker's odds of CHD are 12.0 times of the odds of CHD of a non-smoker. The same data could be analyzed taking exposure as a binary variable – smoking present (light + heavy) and absent, which yields an *OR* of 9.0. By taking ordered categories of the exposure, we will be able to demonstrate a dose-response relation between the exposure and the disease, which forms a sound basis in establishing a cause-effect relation. So, wherever possible, it is better to analyze with multiple categories of exposure. The significance of the trend can also be assessed by the trend chi-square test (Chapter 5).

When more than one variable is to be studied, stratified analysis can be attempted as described in cross-sectional studies. Again, stratification may fail when there are too many strata, as the more the number of strata, the more likely it is for a strata to have zero frequency for a given sample size. An alternative is to model the risk of the event on different risk factors. Logistic regression is the technique used for this purpose. The details of this analysis technique are presented in Chapter 7.

The estimation of odds ratio and the logistic regression analysis are equally applicable in a cross-sectional study also. The only difference is in the interpretation of results, keeping the potential sources of bias in a cross-sectional study.

8.6.2.2. Matching

While selecting controls, our interest is to make the two groups of cases and controls to be similar in all respects except for the disease status. In particular, controls should be representative of all now disease-free subjects who are at risk of developing the disease. Any restrictions applied in the selection of cases should also be applied to the selection of controls. Even if we follow these requirements, it is not guaranteed that cases and controls are balanced with respect to many factors that have a bearing on the disease risk.

In view of this, we may be interested in making the two groups specifically similar to certain factor(s), so that the comparisons will be more appropriate. For example, in studying the association of heavy exercise on coronary artery disease (CAD), we can have a case series on one side and control series on another to compare the exercise habits between the two. But it is possible that the sex ratio in the two groups may not be equal. More males could be among cases and more females could be in the controls chosen. This makes the comparison inappropriate because the risk of the disease may be different among the two genders as well as the exposure under consideration (exercise) itself is likely to have different patterns in the two genders. Similarly, age differences could also make the comparisons inappropriate. Therefore, the controls can be chosen such that for every case, a control is chosen to be of similar gender and age. This concept is called matching and in the example, our controls are age-sex matched. If we do not restrict the selection of controls with respect to any such criterion, the controls are called unmatched and the study is an unmatched case-control study.

Matching forces the distribution of certain factors in the cases and controls to be identical and thus eliminates biased comparisons. Though this technique has an intuitive appeal, it is not simple to decide whether to have a matched or an unmatched design. There are several alternatives to matching. Besides, matching has a number of disadvantages also. Matching may be difficult to implement, requires more finances and is also time consuming. A matched factor can no longer be analyzed with respect to its effect on the outcome. Matching on the chosen criteria does not ensure balance of many other factors between the two groups. Analysis of a matched design is more complex than that of the unmatched design. In fact, with the availability of analytic techniques and powerful statistical software, one can adjust the effect of any imbalances between the cases and controls, obviating the need for a matching. More details on these aspects can be found in many standard books (e.g., Schlesselman[16], Hennekins[17]).

8.6.2.3. Estimation of odds ratio in a matched case-control study

Usually, one control is matched with one case. If collection of information on controls is easy and cheap, more than one matched control can be taken for each case, but same number for each case. For the sake of simplicity, we take an example of one case matched with one control and a dichotomous exposure variable.

Since in a matched case-control study each case is paired with a control, we have 4 different types of case-control pairs. Denoting the presence of exposure as + and the absence as −, we have the 4 types as + +

(exposure present in both case and its matched control); + – (exposure present in case and absent in control); – + (exposure absent in case and present in control); and – – (exposure absent in both). The arrangement of the data can be shown in the Table 8.3 below.

Table 8.3: Data lay out in a matched situation

Cases	Controls		Total
	Exposure present	*Exposure absent*	
Exposure present	*a*	*b*	*a+b*
Exposure absent	*c*	*d*	*c+d*
Total	*a+c*	*b+d*	*N*

The numbers of exposed and unexposed cases are denoted by $a+b$ and $c+d$, whereas $a+c$ and $b+d$ denote the exposed and unexposed controls, respectively. The frequency of concordant pairs in which both case and control are exposed to the risk factor or both are unexposed is denoted by a and d. The discordant pairs $(+ -)$ and $(- +)$ in which one of the paired subjects only is exposed, are indicated by b and c, respectively. N is the total number of case-control pairs studied.

The odds ratio (OR) in this set up is based only on the discordant pairs b and c and is defined as $OR = b/c$. The significance of this OR can be assessed by Mc-Nemar chi-square statistic.

$$\chi_1^2 = \frac{(|b-c|-1)^2}{(b+c)}$$

For large values of b and c, an approximate confidence interval can be constructed as:

$$\text{Variance of } In(\text{OR}) = \frac{1}{b} + \frac{1}{c}$$

95% confidence limits (if a = 0.05) are: $Z_\alpha \sqrt{\frac{1}{b} + \frac{1}{c}}$

Taking exponential of the limits of $In(OR)$, we obtain the confidence limits of OR.

Example:

In an investigation on the role of blood transfusions on cirrhosis of liver, suppose 100 cases of cirrhosis and 100 age (± 5 years) and sex matched controls were studied. 30 case-control pairs had blood transfusion history in cases but not in controls and 10 pairs indicated positive history in controls but not in cases.

OR for cirrhosis of liver associated with blood transfusion = b/c = 30/10 = 3.0

$$\text{Mc-Nemar Chi-square} = \chi_1^2 = \frac{(|b-c|-1)^2}{(b+c)} = \frac{(|30-10|-1)^2}{(30+10)} = 9.025$$

Comparing this with the tabulated value of Chi-square distribution with one degree of freedom, we conclude that the observed OR is beyond chance (Table in Appendix 5).

$$\text{The Standard error of } In(OR) = \sqrt{\frac{1}{b} + \frac{1}{c}} = \sqrt{\frac{1}{30} + \frac{1}{10}} = 0.3651$$

The 95% confidence interval for the $In(OR)$ = = (0.3830 and 1.8142)

Therefore, the 95% CI for the OR = [exp(0.3830) and exp (1.8142)] = (1.47 and 6.14)

8.6.2.4. Advantages and limitations of case-control studies

The strength or advantage of case-control studies is that they can be planned and initiated quickly. The financial requirements are also not very large. Since the available cases are utilized, this design is well suited for diseases that have a long latent period such as cancer, cardio-vascular diseases or some such degenerative diseases. Case-control design is perhaps the only optimum way to study the etiological factors of a rare disease, but may not be well suited for rare exposures. Another advantage could be that multiple factors can be studied simultaneously in a case-control design.

Though the case-control study design appears to be simple, it is prone to produce biased findings. Bias can be defined as any systematic error in a study that leads to an incorrect estimate of the association.

The first and the foremost is recall bias. Since it is a retrospective study and we elicit information about the past exposure status, there is a scope for bias in recollecting the past by the participants due to faulty memory. Further, the cases being affected by the disease, it is natural for them to think of the possible cause(s) and tend to correlate their exposure and behavior habits with disease. This in turn leads to make them remember the past exposure status and respond accordingly at the time of the study. Controls being normal (non-diseased), may not remember their exposure to the suspected risk factor and so may not be able to recall properly at the time of the study. Because of this the results may get vitiated.

Another drawback of case-control studies is their vulnerability for selection bias, i.e., the way the subjects (cases and controls) are chosen can influence the result. This can be understood by a simple analogy of drawing two lines and comparing them to decide which is bigger or smaller. Irrespective of the length of the first line drawn, we can always make it relatively smaller by drawing a bigger line adjacent to it. Alternatively, we can make the first line relatively bigger by drawing the second line smaller than the first. Similarly, depending upon the type of controls selected, the cases can be more exposed or less exposed to the suspected causal factor. This type of bias can happen if cases and controls are selected on the basis of different criteria, which in turn is related to exposure status. For example, if our objective is to study the association of smoking on lung cancer and cases of lung cancer are compared with the controls chosen from a chest clinic, the effect of smoking on lung cancer will be under-estimated. This will be because majority of patients attending a chest clinic would generally be smokers as chest problems are also associated with smoking. Thus, in this example, the selection of controls is related to the exposure under study.

Case-controls studies are also prone to observation bias or ascertainment bias. This arises due to the manner in which information is ascertained from the study participants. If the person collecting the information knew the status of the subject (case or control) and the study hypothesis, he/she may like to probe the cases more for the exposure history than the controls. This in turn produces biased exposure histories and may lead to misleading results.

These are the three main sources of bias for case control studies. As such, there are many sources of bias for epidemiological investigations. Sackett[18] (1979) compiled a list of 56 types of bias that can occur in reading-up on the data field, in specifying and selecting the study sample, in executing the experimental maneuver, in measuring exposures and outcomes, in analyzing the data and in interpreting the analysis. For fuller understanding of various types of bias, this article must be read.

8.6.3. Cohort Studies

Another popular design used in observational studies is the cohort study. A cohort can be defined as a group of similar subjects, usually free of disease. So in a cohort study we assemble a group of similar subjects and look forward for the development of an event of interest at a later date among them. We also note down the beginning time for each as well as the characteristics about the suspected causal factor and at this time all subjects must be free from disease under investigation. After follow-up over a period of time, we observe who (those with and without the exposure) and how many develop the disease, and when they develop the disease, to compare the rates of incidence in different exposure strata. Because we look for the event of interest prospectively, cohort studies can also be called as prospective studies.

The scheme of a cohort study is shown in the Fig. 8.5 below.

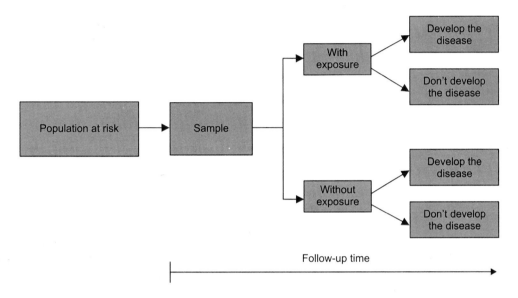

Fig. 8.5: Diagrammatic representation of the scheme of a cohort study

The cohort assembled could be of different types. If it is drawn from the community with a specified age and sex it is called a community cohort. If people exposed to specific exposures form the cohort such as radiologists or the population of Bhopal city who were exposed to Methyl Isocyanate (MIC) gas leakage during 1984, it is an exposure cohort. If school children of specific standards or all newborns in a maternity hospital during a specified period are studied it is called a birth cohort. Subjects with a similar occupation such as miners, police personnel or military personnel form an occupational cohort. Similarly, patients diagnosed with a condition will be a diagnosed cohort and patients treated for a condition forms a treated cohort.

The assembled cohort can be a fixed one, such as the Bhopal population or school children, because all the members of the cohort can be enrolled in one go. Alternatively, in a dynamic cohort, different subjects enter at different time points. Each subject's entry will be taken as beginning of observation for that subject. Diagnosed subjects or treated subjects will form such cohorts and so, generally, we come across dynamic cohorts only in a clinical set-up.

8.6.3.1. Measures of association

Like in case-control studies here also we can cross tabulate the data with respect to the exposure and the disease status. Since the exposure of each cohort member is measured initially and the outcome or development of disease is looked for prospectively, our focus is only on this aspect in a cohort study.

Table 8.4: Cross-tabulation of information in a cohort study

Exposure status	Disease status		Total
	Yes	No	
Yes	a	b	R_1
No	c	d	R_2
Total	M_1	M_2	N

We start with a cohort of N members out of whom R_1 are exposed and R_2 are unexposed to the suspected causal factor. After sufficient length of follow-up, we observed that a out of R_1 exposed individuals developed the disease or outcome of interest and so the remaining $(R_1 - a = b)$ did not develop. Similarly, out of the R_2 subjects who did not have the exposure, c developed the disease and the remaining d did not develop.

With this information we are able to assess the role of the suspected cause in the development of the disease. As presented in case-control studies, the risk of disease when the exposure is present will be a/R_1 and risk of disease when the exposure is absent will be c/R_2. Using these two estimates of risk, we can have two types of indices to convey the magnitude of association between the exposure and the disease.

Risk difference (RD). If we denote the risk of disease when the exposure is present as p_1 and the risk of disease when the exposure is absent as p_2, the risk difference is defined as $p_1 - p_2$.

$$\text{Risk Difference} = (p_1 - p_2) = \left[\frac{a}{R_1}\right] - \left[\frac{c}{R_2}\right]$$

Risk Difference (RD) indicates the amount of the disease rate that is attributable to the Exposure or Risk Factor. So, it can also be called as Attributable Risk (AR). If RD is multiplied by a constant, say 1000, we obtain the expected number of individuals (out of 1000) who would not get the disease if the risk factor is eliminated among the exposed. Risk Difference is a useful index from the public health point of view. For example, a health administrator would like to know the number of lives that would be saved if atmospheric pollution is reduced or the number of low birth weight babies that can be avoided, if folic acid supplementation is provided to the mothers.

RD can also be used as an indicator of effectiveness of different types of treatments or interventions in a trial set up. The reciprocal of RD is called the number needed to treat (NNT) and it gives the number of patients who would need to receive the specific type of treatment in order for one patient to benefit from the treatment. More the benefit of a treatment, lesser the NNT.

$$\text{Number needed to treat } (NNT) = \frac{1}{RD}$$

Example:

Suppose two treatments A and B are being compared, with 50 patients being put on each treatment. If we observe 20 in treatment A group and 35 in treatment B group have improved or cured, we show this information in a tabular form for further calculations.

Treatment	Cured	Not cured	Total
A	20	30	$n_1 = 50$
B	35	15	$n_2 = 50$
Total	55	45	100

Cure rate by treatment A: $p_1 = 20/50 = 0.40$; cure rate by B: $p_2 = 35/50 = 0.70$.

RD or cure rate difference: $p_2 - p_1 = 0.30$; number needed to treat $= 1 \div 0.3 = 3.33$.

Therefore, about 4 patients have to be treated by treatment B to have one additional case cured (or 10 cases for a benefit of 3 additional cured cases).

The 95% confidence interval for *RD* and *NNT* can be obtained as shown below.

CI for $RD = RD \pm 1.96 * SE(RD)$

Standard Error (SE) of RD is defined as $\sqrt{\left(\dfrac{p_1 * (1 - p_1)}{n_1} + \dfrac{p_2 * (1 - p_2)}{n_2} \right)}$

CI for $NNT = [1/UL \text{ and } 1/LL]$, where UL and LL are Upper and Lower confidence limits of *RD*

$$SE(RD) = \sqrt{\left(\frac{0.4 * 0.6}{50} + \frac{0.7 * 0.3}{50} \right)} = \sqrt{0.0048 + 0.0042} = 0.0949$$

Lower 95% confidence limit for $RD = 0.3 - 1.96 * 0.0949 = 0.1140$

Upper 95% confidence limit for $RD = 0.3 + 1.96 * 0.0949 = 0.4860$

95% C.I for the $RD = (0.1140 \text{ and } 0.4860)$

Therefore, 95% CI for the $NNT = [1/0.4860 \text{ and } 1/0.1140] = [2.06 \text{ and } 8.77]$ or about 2 to 9.

If we repeat the study with the same sample size in each group, we can find a *RD* between 0.1140 and 0.4860, and the *NNT* between 2 and 9, 95% of the times.

We can obtain two other useful indices from the Risk Difference or Attributable Risk, viz., attributable risk percent in the exposed group ($AR\%_{exposed}$) and population attributable risk (*PAR*) as follows.

Attributable risk percent in the exposed group ($AR\%_{exposed}$) is defined as the risk difference as a proportion of the risk in the exposed group and this conveys the proportion of risk that can be attributed to the exposure of the risk factor, among those exposed.

$$AR\%_{(exposed)} = \frac{Risk_{(Exposed)} - Risk_{(Unexposed)}}{Risk_{(Exposed)}} * 100$$

$$= \left[\frac{p_1 - p_2}{p_1} \right] * 100$$

Etiologic fraction or Population Attributable Risk is defined as the difference of the risk in total population and the risk of disease among the unexposed.

Etiologic fraction or Population Attributable Risk $(PAR) = Risk_{(total)} - Risk_{(unexposed)}$

Population attributable risk as a percentage of total risk (*PAR%*) can be calculated as,

$$PAR\% = \frac{Risk_{(total)} - Risk_{(Unexposed)}}{Risk_{(Total)}} * 100$$

Example:

To assess the association between tobacco chewing and oral cancer, suppose 5000 men with the habit of chewing tobacco and 10000 men without the habit were observed for a specified length of time. At the end of follow-up, 26 cases of oral cancers were observed among the chewing group and 14 cases among the non-chewers group. The observed data arranged in a 2 × 2 table is shown Table 8.5.

Table 8.5: Hypothetical data on tobacco chewing habit and oral cancer

Chewing tobacco	Oral cancer		Total
	Yes	No	
Yes	26 (a)	4974 (b)	5000 (R_1)
No	14 (c)	9986 (d)	10000 (R_2)
Total	40 (M_1)	14960 (M_2)	15000 (N)

Risk of oral cancer among the tobacco chewers = $\left[\dfrac{a}{R_1}\right] = p_1 = 26/5000 = 0.0052$

Risk of oral cancer among the non-chewers = $\left[\dfrac{c}{R_2}\right] = p_2 = 14/10000 = 0.0014$

Risk Difference $RD = (p_1 - p_2) = 0.0052 - 0.0014 = 0.0038$

Therefore for every 10000 men with chewing habit, 38 can be prevented from developing oral cancer if the tobacco chewing habit is removed. The 95% confidence interval for Risk Difference will be:

We have $p_1 = 0.0052, p_2 = 0.0014,$ $R_1 = 5000$ and $R_2 = 10000$

Standard Error of $RD = \sqrt{\left[(p_1 q_1 / R_1) + (p_2 q_2 / R_2)\right]}$

Where $q_1 = 1 - p_1$ and $q_2 = 1 - p_2$

$SE = \sqrt{\left[(0.0052 * 0.9948 / 5000) + (0.0014 * 0.9986 / 10000)\right]}$

$\qquad = \sqrt{0.000001174} = 0.0011$

95% CI for the $RD = [RD - 1.96*SE$ and $RD + 1.96*SE]$
$= [0.0017$ and $0.0059]$

If we repeat the study, 95% of the times we get an estimate of the risk difference between 0.0017 and 0.0059. In other words, about 17 to 59 persons per 10000 can be prevented from developing oral cancer, if tobacco-chewing habit has been eliminated in those with the habit.

Significance of the Risk Difference can be tested by the usual $\chi 2$ test or Fisher's Exact test. Z test can also be used if the sample sizes are large.

$Z = \left[\dfrac{p_1 - p_2}{SE(p_1 - p_2)}\right]$

For the example data, $RD = 0.0038$; $SE = 0.0011$
$Z = 0.0038 / 0.0011 = 3.4545$; $p < 0.01$

It implies that if the null hypothesis that the risk difference is zero is correct, the probability of finding a RD of 0.0038 with the sample sizes studied (5000 chewers and 10000 non-chewers) is less than one in 100. Since this chance is very low, we suspect our null hypothesis of $RD = 0$ and, hence, reject the null hypothesis. In other words, the observed risk difference estimate is statistically different from zero and so the association of chewing tobacco with oral cancer is significant.

The attributable risk percentage among the chewers $AR\% = \left[\dfrac{p_1 - p_2}{p_1}\right] * 100$

$$= \left[\frac{0.0052 - 0.0014}{0.0052} \right] * 100 = 73.08\%$$

Thus, nearly three quarters of the incidence of the oral cancer among the chewers can be attributed to their tobacco chewing habit.

Etiologic fraction or Population Attributable Risk (PAR) = Risk(total) – Risk(unexposed)

Risk of oral cancer among the total population (with or without the exposure) = $\text{Risk}_{(total)}$ = 40/15000 = 0.002666

$\therefore PAR = 0.002666 - 0.0014 = 0.001266$

$$PAR\% = \frac{Risk_{(total)} - Risk_{(Unexposed)}}{Risk_{(total)}} * 100 = (0.001266 / 0.002666) * 100 = 47.49\%$$

It indicates that among the men, 47.5% of the total risk of oral cancer is due to the tobacco chewing habit, and so can be avoided if chewing tobacco is eliminated in the community.

Risk ratio (RR). Another measure that quantifies the association between an exposure and a disease is the incidence risk ratio or relative risk (RR). It is the ratio of incidence risk of disease in the exposed group to the incidence risk of disease in the unexposed group. If the risk of disease in the exposed group is more than the risk in the unexposed, then the relative incidence risk is more than one and the exposure is said to be a risk factor. On the other hand, if the risk of disease in the exposed group is smaller than the risk in the unexposed, then the RR is less than one and the exposure will be a protective factor. If the risk is same when the exposure is present or absent, then the RR will be one and the factor under consideration is not associated with the disease.

Relative risk is a useful measure of association in epidemiological/etiological studies, where the aim is to identify risk factors for the disease. The Odds Ratio (OR) discussed in the Section on Case-Control or retrospective studies is an approximation of the Relative Risk (RR). This approximation holds good, if the disease incidence rate is small (< 20%). Therefore, in the retrospective studies an approximate RR can be estimated.

Using the notations introduced earlier, Risk Ratio $RR = \dfrac{p_1}{p_2} = \dfrac{a}{R_1} \div \dfrac{c}{R_2}$

$$RR = \frac{(a * R_2)}{(c * R_1)}$$

We know that,

$$AR\%_{(exposed)} = \frac{Risk_{(Exposed)} - Risk_{(Unexposed)}}{Risk_{(Exposed)}} * 100 100 = \left[\frac{p_1 - p_2}{p_1} \right] * 100$$

Using simple algebra, it can be shown that $AR\% = \left[\dfrac{RR - 1}{RR} \right] * 100$

Population Attributable Risk% $PAR\% = \dfrac{Risk_{(total)} - Risk_{(Unexposed)}}{Risk_{(total)}} * 100$

$$= \frac{p_e(RR - 1)}{1 + p_e(RR - 1)} * 100, \text{ where } p_e \text{ is the prevalence of the exposure in the community.}$$

Using the oral cancer example discussed above, we calculate the relative risk and the other measures based on it.

Risk of oral cancer among chewers = p_1 = 26 / 5000

Risk of oral cancer among non chewers = p_2 = 14 / 10000

$$\text{Relative risk } (RR) = \left[\frac{26}{5000}\right] * \left[\frac{10000}{14}\right] = 3.7143$$

This implies that a person chewing tobacco has 3.7 times the risk of developing oral cancer as compared to a person who does not chew tobacco.

To construct the 95% confidence interval for *RR*,

We have $a = 26$; $b = 4974$; $c = 14$; $d = 9986$; RR = 3.71; $ln(RR)$ = 1.3110; $R1$ = 5000 and $R2$ = 10000

$$\text{Standard Error of } In(RR) = \sqrt{\left(\frac{b}{a*R_1}\right) + \left(\frac{d}{c*R_2}\right)}$$

$$= \sqrt{\left(\frac{4974}{26*5000}\right) + \left(\frac{9986}{14*10000}\right)} = \sqrt{0.0383 + 0.0713} = 0.3310$$

95% CI of $In(RR)$ = 1.3110 ± 1.96(0.3310) = [0.6622 and 1.9598]

95% CI of RR = [exp(0.6622) and exp(1.9598)] = [1.94 and 7.10]

$$AR\% = \left[\frac{RR-1}{RR}\right] * 100 = \left[\frac{3.71-1}{3.71}\right] * 100 = 73.05\%, \text{ which is the same as that we obtained earlier with the}$$

Risk Difference.

$$\text{Population Attributable Risk Percent (PAR\%)} = \frac{p_e(RR-1)}{1 + p_e(RR-1)} * 100$$

p_e = proportion of exposed persons in the population = 5000/15000 = 0.3333

$$\therefore \text{PAR\%} = \frac{0.3333 * 2.71}{1 + (0.3333 * 2.71)} * 100 = 47.46\%, \text{ which is also same as the one obtained earlier.}$$

Since the Odds Ratio is an approximation of the *RR*, the *AR%* and *PAR%* can also be computed in a retrospective study, replacing *RR* with *OR* in the relevant expressions.

The influence of multiple factors on the event in a cohort study can also be studied by multiple logistic regression, explained in the section on case-control studies. This is possible because the Odds Ratio is same whether we consider the odds of exposure or the odds of disease. However, certain conditions have to be fulfilled to analyze cohort data by logistic regression technique as explained in the next sections.

Incidence density (ID). So far, we have analyzed the data taking each study subject or person as a unit of analysis. An implicit assumption in this process is that we followed up all subjects for the same length of time and so all the study subjects have an equal probability of developing the disease or event of interest. While this approach forms the basis for a simple first level analysis, often it may not be tenable and different subjects will have different lengths of follow-up and so different probabilities of developing the disease. In such a case, the unit of analysis cannot be a person. Similarly, if the event under consideration is of repeatable nature such as asthmatic attacks or diarrheal episodes or colds, the unit of analysis cannot be a person or subject.

Under these circumstances, we find the Person-time units of follow-up such as Person-years or Person-months and relate the number of events to the total person·time to arrive at an index called incidence density (*ID*).

$$ID = \frac{\text{Number of events}}{\text{Total person-time units followed-up}}$$

While calculating *ID*, we assume that the incidence rate is constant throughout the follow-up period. Incidence Density can vary from zero to infinity.

Suppose 5 women who were free of breast cancer initially, were planned to be followed up for 36 months and could be followed up only for 12, 24, 36, 18, 20 months respectively. Also, suppose that at the end of the study period we find that one woman developed the disease; the incidence density will be,

$$ID = \frac{1}{(12 + 24 + 36 + 18 + 20)} = \frac{1}{100} \text{ or 9 cases per 1000 woman-months of follow-up approximately.}$$

Here one might ask what happened to those women who did not develop the disease and yet were not followed up for full length as envisaged. For example, the first woman was followed-up only for 12 months and after that she was lost for follow-up as she might have shifted out of the city or died due to causes not related to the study objectives or refused to co-operate, etc. Since we have the information for 12 months, we utilize that much. Such incomplete observations are called censored observations. More details of these can be seen on the analysis of clinical trials (Chapter 9).

Comparing an observed incidence density with a known population value. Usually, in a one-sample situation, we are interested to know whether an observed incidence in a sample can be taken as a representative of the known incidence in the population. That is, we wish to test whether the observed *ID* is similar to the known *ID* in the general population.

Null hypothesis will be: $ID = ID_0$; Alternative hypothesis: $ID \neq ID_0$

Suppose, we follow-up a cohort of 100 pre-term babies with very low birth weights (< 1500 g) for the development of periventricular leukomalacia (PVL), a neuro-pathologic lesion of the brain. Since the babies are of pre-term and very low birth weight, not all babies are expected to get discharged normally as some may die. If we perform cranial ultra sound daily for detecting the development of PVL and at the end of the study suppose we have accumulated 3200 baby-days of follow-up till the last baby was either discharged or died. If we observe 30 babies developed PVLs:

ID = Incidence of PVL = 30/3200 = 0.0094 or 9.375 per 1000 baby-days of follow-up.

Now if the incidence of PVL in western countries as per the literature (ID_0) is 2 per 1000 baby-days, we would like to assess whether the incidence of PVL observed is similar to that observed in the west. Let us denote the number of babies that developed PVL in our sample as *a*, and the total person units of time of follow-up as *t*.

Assuming *a* follows a Poisson distribution, under the null hypothesis H_0, *a* has mean $m_0 = t*(ID_0)$ and variance $t*(ID_0)$.

Therefore, $m_0 = 3200 * \dfrac{2}{1000} = 6.4$

So, $\dfrac{(a - m_0)^2}{m_0} \sim \chi^2$ with 1 d.f.

$\chi_1^2 = \dfrac{(30 - 6.4)^2}{6.4} = 87.02$

This chi-square value with one degree of freedom indicates that the probability of finding 30 cases of PVL in our sample is less than one in 10000 (p < 0.0001), if the null of hypothesis of the incidence of PVL in our center is same as that in western countries.

If a is not too small (at least 10 cases), the confidence limits of the observed incidence can be easily calculated. First we calculate the confidence limits of the number of cases, i.e., c_1 and c_2 and then convert these numbers into incidence density.

$c_1 = a - Z_{(1-\alpha/2)} \sqrt{a}$; and $c_2 = a + Z_{(1-\alpha/2)} \sqrt{a}$

$(1-\alpha)\%$ confidence limits of *ID* are $(c_1/t\ c_2/t)$

In our example of PVL, $ID = 0.0094$ and $a = 30$. 5% two tailed Z value = 1.96

95% Confidence interval of a will be

$c_1 = 30 - (1.96) \sqrt{30} = 19.26$; $c_2 = 30 + (1.96) \sqrt{30} = 40.74$

Ninety five out of 100 times, we can expect about 20 to 41 PVL cases with the same sample size and follow-up, over repeated studies.

With the total person time units of 3200 days, the 95% confidence limits our incidence density would be (19.26/3200 and 40.74/3200) = (0.0060 and 0.0127) or 6 to 13 cases per 1000 days.

Comparing two estimates of incidence density. Suppose we have two groups of subjects followed up over a period of time and at the end of the follow-up, a_1 and a_2 cases were observed in the two groups with t_1 and t_2 person-units of follow-up time, respectively. We are interested in knowing whether the incidence density is similar between the two groups.

The results of such a study can be presented in tabular form as shown below (Table 8.6).

Table 8.6: Tabular presentation of results in a cohort study

Exposure	Number of events	Follow-up time (Person-units)
Yes	a_1	t_1
No	a_2	t_2
Total	$a_1 + a_2$	$t_1 + t_2$

Null hypothesis H_0: $ID_1 = ID_2$; Alternative hypothesis H_1: $ID_1 \neq ID_2$

Under the H_0, the expected events in Group1 (Exposed) will be $E_1 = (a_1 + a_2) * (t_1) / (t_1 + t_2)$

Variance of the number of events will be $V_1 = (a_1 + a_2) * (t_1) * (t_2) / (t_1 + t_2)^2$

Test statistic $Z = \dfrac{(a_1 - E_1)}{\sqrt{V_1}}$

Example:

Suppose we have the PVL data from two cities A and B as follows:

City	Number of PVLs	Follow-up time (Person-units)
A	30 (a_1)	3200 (t_1)
B	25 (a_2)	4000 (t_2)
Total	55 $(a_1 + a_2)$	7200 $(t_1 + t_2)$

Incidence Density rate in city A = 30/3200 = 0.009375

Incidence Density rate in city B = 25/4000 = 0.006250

Incidence Rate Ratio = 0.009375/0.006250 = 1.5

Testing equality of the incidence densities is equivalent to testing the rate ratio equals 1.

Under the Null hypothesis, expected number of events in City A will be,

$E_1 = 55 * 3200 / 7200 = 24.44$

Variance $= 55 * 3200 * 4000 / (7200 * 7200) = 13.58$

$$\therefore Z = \frac{(30 - 24.44)}{\sqrt{13.58}} = 1.51$$

Looking at the Tables of Normal distribution, we realize that if the null hypothesis is true, a Z with a magnitude of 1.51 or more can occur about 13% of times. Since this chance is not so small to be ignored, we conclude that the observed difference in the incidence of PVL between the 2 cities is due to chance and so we accept the null hypothesis of equality of the two incidences.

Note that the incidence rate ratio is similar to the incidence risk ratio discussed earlier. Here we use the incidence rates instead of the incidence risks. Both the ratios, namely, risk ratio and rate ratio, are referred to as relative risk (RR). However, risk ratio is used in analytical studies to compare the incidence risk of an outcome in a population exposed to a suspected risk factor with the incidence risk of the outcome in a population not exposed to the same suspected risk factor. Rate ratio is a preferred measure in analytical studies of common outcomes and in populations with a large number of people entering or leaving the different exposure groups at different times. For rare outcomes in populations in which there are few people entering or leaving the exposure groups, the risk and the rate are similar. Under such circumstances, we can use either the risk ratio or rate ratio. Because of this some people do not distinguish between a rate ratio and risk ratio, and call them both as relative risk. However, it is better to specify what one means by a relative risk – whether it is a risk ratio or a rate ratio.

8.6.3.2. Other methods of analysis

So far we have considered methods in which either the follow-up length is assumed to be equal for all subjects or it may vary, but incidence rate remains constant over time. Both these assumptions may not be valid in many practical situations. In other words, the length of the follow-up time may vary for person to person and also the risk of disease itself may not remain constant in the entire follow-up period. For example, the risk of death for a patient of CAD, who undergoes a coronary bypass surgery is maximum immediately after the surgery due to post surgery complications. Once the patient recovers from the trauma due to the surgery itself, the risk gradually comes down.

Under such conditions, we may wish to compare the number of events between two groups when the incidence varies over time. In other words, we wish to compare the incidence pattern in the two groups – exposed and unexposed to the risk factor. The collection of statistical procedures for such analysis is called survival analysis and the details of such methods are presented in Chapter 9.

8.6.3.3. Advantages and disadvantages of cohort studies

The main advantage of cohort studies is that they provide stronger case for cause-effect relationship. Generally, in cohort studies, there is less chance for bias in measuring the suspected cause, since the event has not yet happened. There will be no chance for selective recall as the data on exposure status is collected from all subjects before the occurrence of the event. Similarly, there is no scope for selective survival as all are event free initially and all are followed up prospectively. In cohort studies, it is possible to identify other diseases associated with the same suspected cause. Because of the lesser score for different biases, the results of a cohort study can be easily generalized to the population.

However, cohort studies take very long time and, hence, may not always be feasible. They are also not suitable to study rare diseases, as they require large number of subjects to be followed up. On the other hand, cohort studies are suitable for rare exposures, such as the MIC exposure to the population in the city of

Bhopal. Cohort studies are expensive, as they require a lot of money, time and personnel. The sample size required is generally large. The longer the length of follow-up, the more will be the losses in follow-up and they may introduce certain biases. Another limitation of cohort studies is that the longer the follow-up, the more the chance for change in the behavior of subjects.

8.6.4. A Comparative Summary of Study Designs

There are three main types of study designs in epidemiological investigations. Cross-sectional design is the simplest and also easy to initiate. It helps to have a quick idea of the disease burden and also to generate hypotheses about causal factors. Estimates of association obtained by this design should be viewed with caution. Case-control method is an intuitively appealing design for a quick assessment of probable etiological factors of a disease. It helps to estimate the relative risk of a disease associated with a suspected factor via the odds ratio. Careful planning is called for to avoid various types of biases in a case-control design. Cohort design enables us to have the direct estimate of the relative risk of a disease associated with a risk factor. Generally, it requires a large amount of resources.

Whatever the design of the study, to start with, the data lay out for the study of association is the same as shown below. It is the responsibility of the statistical analyst to apply the appropriate analytic techniques relevant to the design adopted, to obtain and properly interpret the obtained results to answers the research questions.

Exposure status	Disease status		Total
	Yes	*No*	
Yes	a	b	R_1
No	c	d	R_2
Total	M_1	M_2	N

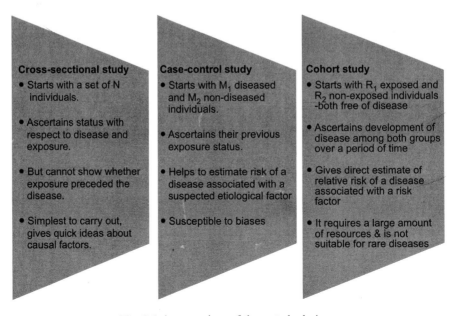

Cross-secctional study
- Starts with a set of N individuals.
- Ascertains status with respect to disease and exposure.
- But cannot show whether exposure preceded the disease.
- Simplest to carry out, gives quick ideas about causal factors.

Case-control study
- Starts with M_1 diseased and M_2 non-diseased individuals.
- Ascertains their previous exposure status.
- Helps to estimate risk of a disease associated with a suspected etiological factor
- Susceptible to biases

Cohort study
- Starts with R_1 exposed and R_2 non-exposed individuals -both free of disease
- Ascertains development of disease among both groups over a period of time
- Gives direct estimate of relative risk of a disease associated with a risk factor
- It requires a large amount of resources & is not suitable for rare diseases

Fig. 8.6: A comparison of three study designs

In the data lay-out shown above, if we start with N individuals and try to ascertain their status with respect to both the disease and the exposure (determining the frequencies of a, b, c and d), it will be a cross-sectional study. If we start with M_1 diseased and M_2 non-diseased subjects and ascertain their previous exposure status it will be case-control study. Lastly, if we start with R_1 exposed and R_2 unexposed subjects who are free of the disease now and follow them prospectively for the development of disease among them, it will be a cohort study.

8.7. Issues in Epidemiological Investigations

In any epidemiological investigation, we make inferences about the population using the information obtained from a sample. Towards this, we need to assess the validity of the findings, any alternative explanations for the findings and whether the observed associations are due to chance, systematic error(s) or due to the effect of other baseline differences. These concepts and issues are common to all designs that we have discussed. For a thorough understanding of these issues, detailed books on epidemiology (e.g., Hennekins and Buring, 1987) may be seen. A brief introduction of these is presented in this section.

8.7.1. Chance

In all investigations, inferences about the population are made based on a sample. Due to variation in the study characteristics, results vary from sample to sample. In addition, results depend on the sample size. Therefore, assessing the role of chance is an important component in any statistical investigation. This consists of 2 components - hypothesis testing and estimation of confidence interval.

In testing of a hypothesis, we make an explicit statement, called null hypothesis (H_0), asserting that there is no association (e.g., $OR = 1$). The alternative hypothesis (H_1) could then be that there is association (e.g., $OR < 1$ or $OR > 1$ or $OR \neq 1$). Then we determine the likelihood that sampling variability can be considered as an explanation for the observed results, if the null hypothesis is correct.

The likelihood is determined as a probability, usually denoted as p value. It indicates the probability of observing the association that has been found in the sample, if the null hypothesis of no association or difference is correct. The smaller the p, the less the likelihood of finding the observed result by chance alone, implying that the null hypothesis may not be true. It must be understood that the smaller the p, the higher the significance of the association, but not the magnitude of association. Conventionally, 5% ($p < 0.05$) is taken as 'statistically significant' and $p < 1\%$ is taken as 'highly significant' to conclude that chance is unlikely to explain the observed association.

It should be noted that p value only indicates whether the result is 'significant' or not. Even a small magnitude of association can be theoretically declared as 'significant' by taking a large sample and also a large effect may not achieve 'significance', if there is substantial variability. Because of these limitations, p value should be considered as a guide and not as a hard and fast rule on which to base a conclusion on the factor being studied. Even the smallest p does not rule out chance completely as a p value close to 1 also does not mean that the observed effect is due to chance only. It is also advisable to report the actual p value rather than 'significant' or 'ns' or < 0.05, etc. For example, a p value of 0.06 or 0.045 conveys more information than simply stating significant or not.

Role of chance is also assessed by a confidence interval (CI). This helps to overcome the difficulties in p value, as it is a more informative measure. It represents the range within which the true magnitude of the effect lies with a certain degree of assurance.

The CI can provide all the information of the p value (significant or not at a specified level) depending on the null value falling within the limits or not. Width of CI tells about the variability in the estimate. CI is particularly important when interpreting the results which are non-significant. A narrow CI with null value included will add support to the belief that truly there is no association. A wider interval may suggest that the sample size was not sufficient to have adequate statistical power to exclude chance as an explanation of the findings.

Therefore for evaluating the role of chance, both p value and the confidence interval together provide most information.

8.7.2. Confounding

In any investigation, the investigator ideally tries to alter one variable at a time, so that any effect he/she observes can be attributed to only that variable. But such ideal conditions may be feasible only in experimental or laboratory studies. As most epidemiological investigations are non-experimental and observational, often we have to compare people who differ in many ways – known and unknown. If such differences are associated with the risk of disease, independently of the exposure under investigation, the factors that differ among the groups being compared are said to confound the association between the exposure variable and the disease under consideration. In other words, **confounding is the mixing of effects between the exposure, the disease and a third factor**. It is a function of complex inter-relationships between various exposures and the disease under consideration. Confounding can lead to observing an apparent association when it does not truly exist (positive confounding) as well as observing no association when in fact it exists (negative confounding). It can also change in the direction of an observed effect, i.e., confounding can make a risk factor of disease appear as a protective factor and vice versa.

To be a confounder, a variable must be a risk factor for the disease, not necessarily a causal factor. It should be associated with the exposure of interest, but it is not a consequence of exposure. Alternatively, if there is no association between the exposure and the potential confounder or if the potential confounder has no relationship with the risk of disease, then there cannot be confounding due to that factor.

As an example of confounding effect, consider myocardial infarction (MI) and its association with economic status. If one estimates the association of MI with economic status without regard to other factors, the apparent association will be a mixture of the effect of economic status on MI and also the effect of other variables that are associated with economic status such as occupation, education, physical activity, etc. This is so because it is known that economic status depends on the type of occupation and which in turn determines the physical activity of an individual. Further, some factors like smoking may be more associated with certain occupations and smoking itself could be associated with MI. Therefore, the apparent association between MI and economic status could be mixed with that of physical activity with MI as well as that of occupation with MI; smoking with MI; education with MI, etc. Alternatively, if we take only one type of subjects with respect to occupation and physical activity, and relate the disease with their economic habits, the influences of the occupation and physical activity are removed and, hence, there will be no confounding with respect to these two factors.

Let us take some hypothetical data to explain these concepts further. Suppose 210 cases of MI and 179 controls were studied and it was noted that 90 cases and 99 controls were found to belong to high-income group. Rearrangement of this information in tabular form is shown below.

Income	MI	Controls	Total
High	$a = 90$	$b = 99$	189
Low	$c = 120$	$d = 80$	200
Total	210	179	389

Odds Ratio of MI with high economic status = $\dfrac{a*d}{b*c}$ = (90 * 80) ÷ (99 * 120) = 0.61

It can be verified that the Yates's corrected Chi-square associated with this Table will be 5.51 with 1 degree of freedom, implying that the odds ratio is statistically significant (p = 0.0189). Therefore, we will be tempted to conclude that higher economic status is protective against MI.

Now the same data is stratified with respect to physical activity (high and low) and analyzed separately for the association of economic status with MI among those with high and low physical activity. The results of such analysis are:

Income	MI	Controls	Total
High physical activity group			
High	a = 54	b = 81	135
Low	c = 20	d = 30	50
Total	74	111	185

Odds ratio: (54 * 30) / (81 * 20) = 1.0

Income	MI	Controls	Total
Low physical activity group			
High	a = 36	b = 18	54
Low	c = 100	d = 50	150
Total	136	68	204

(36 * 50) / (18 * 100) = 1.0

Notice that the apparent association between income status and MI observed in the crude analysis disappeared when we analyzed separately within high and low physically active persons. This is because the effect of physical activity on MI is mixed with the crude estimate of the effect of economic status on MI. Once the physical activity effect is removed, there appears no association between economic status and MI. So, physical activity has been the confounder, as it confounded the association of economic status with MI. Thus, pooling across subgroups can produce misleading results and this is referred to as **Simpson's paradox**.

To assess whether confounding is present or absent, first we find the crude estimate of association of the disease with the suspected risk factor. Then we control for the effect of the suspected confounder and estimate the association between the exposure and disease. If the adjustment results in a change in the estimate of the association, the potential confounder is actually confounding. The magnitude of confounding depends on the magnitude of associations between the confounder and the disease, and between the confounder and the exposure. The direction of confounding (positive or negative) depends on the nature of inter-relationships among the three (exposure-confounding factor-disease).

To overcome the problem of confounding and to obtain valid results, selection of potential confounders should be planned in the design stage itself. Knowledge of potential confounders can be based on the knowledge of the disease, previous studies and to some extent the judgment of the investigator.

Control of confounding can be achieved in different ways, which can be used either alone or in combination. These are randomization, restriction, matching, stratification and multivariate analysis. In all analytical studies, confounding must always be considered as an alternative explanation for the findings. Though many methods are available for controlling the confounding, no single method can be considered optimal in every situation. Each has its own strengths and limitations, which must be considered at the beginning of the study.

Most often, a combination of strategies will provide better insight into the nature of data and more efficient control of confounding than any single approach.

Coming back to the stratum specific Odds Ratios (strata can be more than 2), if they are not too different, we would like to have a common odds ratio. Mantel-Haenszel procedure, one of the most popular tools in epidemiological analyses, is used to estimate the common effect for all strata, if they are homogenous, and also to test for the significance of the common effect.

8.7.2.1. Mantel-Haenszel procedure

Recall the arrangement of information in a 2×2 table as shown in Table 8.2. If there are k strata of a variable, we can have k such 2×2 Tables and denote the frequencies as a_i, b_i, c_i and d_i for the ith strata. Let M_{1i}, M_{2i} be the column totals; R_{1i}, R_{2i} be row totals and N_i be the total of the ith 2×2 Table.

To test the heterogeneity of k Odds Ratios, Woolf[15] proposed a test, which may be referred to in standard textbooks (e.g., Schlesselman[16]).

The overall Odds Ratio adjusted for the effect of stratification variable(s) is given by,

$$OR_{MH} = \frac{\sum_{i=1}^{k} \left(\dfrac{a_i d_i}{N_1} \right)}{\sum_{i=1}^{k} \left(\dfrac{b_i c_i}{N_1} \right)}$$

The advantage of Mantel-Haenszel OR is that it can be computed even if one cell is zero in some of the strata.

To test the significance of this common OR, we have the null hypothesis H_0 that the common Odds Ratio is unity. Under this null hypothesis, the expected value of a_i will be,

$$E(a_i) = \frac{M_{1i} * R_{1i}}{N_i}$$

The variance of a_i will be given by,

$$V(a_i) = \frac{R_{1i} * R_{2i} * M_{1i} * M_{2i}}{N_i^2 (N_i - 1)}$$

Compute $E(a_i)$ and $V(a_i)$ for each 2×2 table and the Mantel-Haenszel test statistic is obtained as,

$$\frac{\left(\left| \sum_{i=1}^{k} a_i - \sum_{i=1}^{k} E(a_i) \right| \right)^2}{\sum_{i=1}^{k} V(a_i)}$$

which follows an approximate chi-square distribution with one degree of freedom under the null hypothesis.

If continuity correction is also applied, $\chi^2_{M-H} = \chi^2_{M-H} = \dfrac{\left(\left| \sum_{i=1}^{k} a_i - \sum_{i=1}^{k} E(a_i) \right| - \dfrac{1}{2} \right)^2}{\sum_{i=1}^{k} V(a_i)}$

Large values of this chi-square statistic indicate that the common OR is different from the null value of unity.

Example:

Suppose neonatal mortality from a database (n = 6652) indicates that 985 babies were of gestation less than or equal to 36 weeks; and 116 babies with gestation more than 36 weeks and 145 babies with gestation ≤ 36 weeks died before discharge from the hospital. The odds ratio of mortality associated with gestation ≤ 36 weeks would be:

Gestation (weeks)	Disease status		Total
	Dead	Alive	
≤ 36	145	840	985
> 36	116	5551	5667
Total	261	6391	6652

OR = 8.26
p = < 0.01

It is very apparent that the odds ratio is large and is also significant. Since we have not considered any other factor, this *OR* is the crude odds ratio.

Now let us consider the birth weight and stratify the data into two strata, namely, < 2000 grams and ≥ 2000 grams. The odds ratio of neonatal mortality associated with gestation within each of these two strata are:

Gestation (weeks)	Birth weight ≥ 2000 grams		Total
	Disease status		
	Dead	Alive	
≤ 36	26	463	489
> 36	99	5382	5481
Total	125	5845	5970

$OR = (26*5382) / (463*99) = 3.05$

	Birth weight < 2000 grams		
≤ 36	119	377	496
> 36	17	169	186
Total	136	546	682

$OR = (112*169) / (377*17) = 3.14$

Notice that if the effect of birth weight is ignored, the strength of association between gestation and neonatal mortality appears greater than it is for either of the two birth weight groups. This is illogical and can happen because of the relationship between gestation and mortality is mixed up with the relationship of the third factor – birth weight on the outcome. Failure to control the effect of birth weight led to the over estimation of the effect of gestation.

In both the birth weight groups, the observed odds of neonatal mortality are higher in the lower gestational groups. It is also possible that both the odds ratios are estimating the same population value and differ only because of the sampling variability or fluctations. In such a situation, we can combine the information from each stratum and make one overall estimate of the odds ratio. In our example data, both the stratum specific odds ratios are close to each other with considerable overlap in their confidence intervals. So it is not inappropriate to obtain an overall estimate using Mantel-Haenszel procedure.

We show the computations in a tabular form below.

Birth weight stratum	a_i	b_i	ci	d_i	n_i	a_i*d/n_i	b_i*c/n_i	$E(a_i)$	$V(a_i)$
< 2000 g	119	377	17	169	682	29.49	9.40	98.9091	21.6277
≥ 2000 g	26	463	99	5382	5970	23.44	7.68	10.2387	9.2048
Total	145					52.93	17.08	109.1478	30.8325

$$OR_{MH} = \frac{\sum_{i=1}^{k}\left(\frac{a_i d_i}{N_i}\right)}{\sum_{i=1}^{k}\left(\frac{b_i c_i}{N_i}\right)} = \frac{52.93}{17.08} = 3.10$$

Notice that the summary *OR*, called adjusted estimate for birth weight, is very different from the crude *OR* obtained earlier and also lies in between the two stratum specific *OR*s. It is now logical to understand that the summary estimate lies in between the two stratum specific values.

To test this overall *OR* estimate is significantly different from 1,

$$\chi^2_{M-H} = \frac{\left(\left|\sum_{i=1}^{k}a_i - \sum_{i=1}^{k}E(a_i)\right| - \frac{1}{2}\right)^2}{\sum_{i=1}^{k}V(a_i)} = \frac{\left[(145 - 109.1478) - \frac{1}{2}\right]^2}{30.8325} = 40.53$$

The Chi-square value obtained is highly significant, indicating that the overall *OR* is significantly different from the null value of one.

8.7.3. Bias

Bias can be defined as any systematic error in a study that leads to an incorrect estimate of the association. It can occur due to the manner in which subjects are selected, the way information is obtained, reported or interpreted. The details of major types of biases are discussed in the section on case-control studies.

Even the most rigorously designed study can have one or more types of bias. Evaluating the role of bias as an alternative explanation is necessary for any study. The role of bias cannot be quantified and its effects are more difficult to evaluate and even impossible to adjust in the analysis. Therefore, every possibility for bias should be foreseen and steps should be taken to minimize it.

Prevention and control of bias must be largely through a careful study design. While there are no specific measures for this, general considerations are proper care in the choice of study population, methods of data collection and construction of questionnaires. If the study population is well defined with specific inclusion and exclusion criteria, the scope for selection bias gets reduced. If the questionnaire contains highly objective, closed-ended questions, there is minimal scope for any bias. Similarly, if the questionnaire administration is standardized the interviewer is blinded to the main objectives of study and the status of the respondent (wherever feasible), it helps in reducing the chance for bias.

8.7.4. Interaction

Interaction or effect modification is a phenomenon in which the association between an exposure and disease varies by levels of a third factor. In other words, the effect of the exposure is modified by the level of a third variable or the exposure and the third variable interact. The objective is to explain or describe this phenomenon rather than control or eliminate or adjust.

Presence of an interaction can be seen by the association of exposure with disease in each strata of the suspected effect modifier. We can statistically test the uniformity of the effect across the strata and if the effect of exposure on the disease is uniform across the different strata of the suspected modifier, we say that there is no effect modification by the suspected factor. If the strata specific effects vary substantially, it indicates effect modification and pooling of results across strata may be illogical.

Example:

In a case-control study to evaluate suspected risk factor for stroke following coronary-artery bypass surgery, a total of 54 cases and 53 controls were studied. It was noted that of the 17 subjects with carotid bruit, 13 were cases (had post-surgical stroke). A total of 17 subjects had prior history of stroke (14 cases and 3 controls) of which 6 were cases. Among the 90 subjects with prior history of stroke (40 cases and 50 controls), 7 were cases.[19]

This information can be shown in a 2 × 2 Table:

Bruit	Post-surgical stroke		Total
	Yes	*No*	
Yes	13	4	17
No	41	49	90
Total	54	53	107

$OR = 3.9$

The *OR*s for post-surgical stroke associated with the presence of carotid bruit, separately for with and without prior history of stroke are:

Bruit	No prior history of stroke		Total
	Post-surgical stroke		
	Yes	*No*	
Yes	7	2	9
No	33	48	81
Total	40	50	90

$OR = 5.09$

	Prior history of stroke		
Yes	6	2	8
No	8	1	9
Total	14	3	17

$OR = 0.38$

Notice that the *OR* in the group with no prior history is close to the crude *OR* (5 and 4 respectively), but the *OR* in the group with prior history is not only far from the crude *OR*, but also the direction of the effect is opposite. Testing the homogeneity of the two stratum-specific *OR*s yields a *p* value of 0.08, which indicates there is marginally significant difference between the two. In other words, there is heterogeneity between the two stratum specific estimates and, hence, obtaining a summary *OR* is illogical. We conclude that among patients without any prior history of stroke, carotid bruits were associated with an increased risk of development of stroke; and in contrast, among patients with prior history of stroke, carotid bruits were associated with a decreased risk of post-surgical stroke. We say that presence of carotid bruits and prior history of stroke interact with each other in causing post-surgical stroke.

Just as two factors interact, more than two can also interact and modify the effect of each other. When only two factors interact, it is called the first order interaction; when three factors are involved it is second order interaction and so on. Formal estimation and testing of the interaction effect involves building up of a mathematical model, which is beyond the scope of this book.

Since the concepts of confounding and interaction both involve stratum specific estimates of association, often one may be confused about the differences between the two. Note that both are conceptually different. If the stratum specific estimates of association are different from the crude estimate, but are uniform among them, then we say there is confounding but no interaction or effect modification. The example of gestation effect on neonatal mortality (Section 8.7.2.1) conveys this, as both the birth weight stratum specific odds ratios are similar, but are different from the crude *OR*. On the other hand, if the stratum specific estimates are different among themselves, with some estimates not very different from the crude estimate, we say there is an interaction effect but no confounding (example of carotid bruits and post-surgical stroke shown above).

Both confounding and effect modification are indicated if the stratum specific estimates are different from the crude estimate as well as among themselves. This can be seen in the following example.

In a case-control study on the effect of physical activity on CHD, 260 cases and 240 controls were studied. Among the cases, 200 were of low physically activity as compared to 80 among the controls.

The Odds Ratio of CHD associated with physical activity is:

Physical activity	CHD		Total
	Yes	No	
Low	200	80	280
High	60	160	220
Total	260	240	500

OR = (200*160)/(80*60) = 6.67

The *OR*s for CHD, analyzed separately for males and females are:

Males			
Physical activity	CHD		Total
	Yes	No	
Low	102	36	138
High	24	108	132
Total	126	144	270

OR = 12.75

Physical activity	Females		Total
	CHD		
	Yes	No	
Low	98	44	142
High	36	52	88
Total	134	96	230

$OR = 3.22$

Looking at the crude OR and the stratum specific ORs, we realize that both the stratum specific ORs are not only different among themselves, but are also different from the crude OR. Hence, we can say that the gender has a confounding and interactive role in the association of CHD with physical activity. Therefore, for any association under study, a given factor can both be a confounder and an effect modifier; or a confounder but not an effect modifier; or an effect modifier and not a confounder; or neither a confounder nor an effect modifier.

To conclude, in any epidemiological investigation, we should rule out the chance; assess the role of confounding and we should remove it or adjust for it; assess the role of possible bias and evaluate it as an alternative explanation for the observed results; and describe and explain any interactions present.

8.8. Validity and Generalizability of Results

Validity refers to the correctness of the conclusions made on the basis of the results from the sample studied. Generalization of the results implies that the conclusions based on the studied sample are applicable for other populations or other situations/set-ups. Evaluation of the chance, bias and confounding as an alternative explanation to the observed findings will help us to conclude whether the observed association is valid (real) or invalid (spurious). Generalizability of the observed findings depends on the type of the disease studied and the factors associated it, selection criteria adopted for the sampled subjects, etc. We cannot generalize the results of every study to every other population. It can be done on case-to-case basis only with appropriate reasoning.

It is important to note that validity of a study's findings is more crucial than generalizability. If the results are not valid, the question of generalization does not arise. On the other hand, if the results are valid but not generalizable to other situations or set-ups, the findings are still useful, albeit for local conditions.

8.9. Role of Different Study Designs in Disease Control Activities

Though we discussed different types of study designs and as each has its own advantages and disadvantages, one should not jump to a conclusion that only a certain design is the best. We should realize that each design has its own role in the general steps in disease control activities.

To begin with, a cross-sectional study would help to assess the burden of the disease in the community and also to generate certain hypotheses about the possible causes, etc. Using these preliminary leads, one can then plan a case-control study to identify etiological factors associated with the disease. The identified etiological factors in a case-control study would then need to be established by a well-planned cohort study before an intervention can be planned and initiated.

These steps can be shown in the diagram 8.7 below.

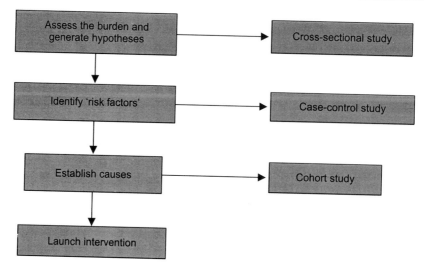

Fig. 8.7: Schematic presentation of general steps in disease control

Multiple Choice Questions

Choose the correct answers in the following multiple choice questions. The correct answers are listed on p. 344.

Q.1. **The causality between an outcome and an exposure can be more certain in which study design?**
a. Case seriesb
c. Cohort

b. Cross-sectional
d. Case report

(For questions 2 & 3)
If there are 90 nurses and 10 doctors in a small town, then:

Q.2. **The figure 10/90 or 1/9 is called a:**
a. Rate
c. Ratio

b. Proportion
d. None of the above

Q.3. **10/100 or 1/10 is called a:**
a. Rate
c. Ratio

b. Proportion
d. None of the above

Q.4. **An investigator trying to study the effect of asbestos exposure on lung cancer observed that 24 of the 120 lung cancer cases had the asbestos exposure as compared to 40 of the 1000 persons without lung cancer. What is the Odds Ratio for exposure to asbestos for getting lung cancer?**
a. 1
c. 0.17

b. 6
d. 96

Q.5. **In an attempt to study the effect of 2 drugs in reducing the blood sugar, an investigator administered Drug 1 on first half of the patients and Drug 2 on the other half of patients. After noting the response, he administered Drug 2 on the first half and Drug 1 on the second half of patients. What study design is being used on the assumption that the gap in the usage between the two drugs is sufficient enough to wash out the effect of the previous drug?**
a. Cross-over design
c. Cohort study

b. Parallel design
d. Case-control study

Q.6. **Prevalence of a disease includes:**
a. All existing cases during the defined period of time
c. Only old cases during the defined period of time

b. Only new cases during the defined period of time
d. None of the above

Q.7. **In defining incidence density, the denominator is:**
a. Number of persons exposed
c. Total population

b. Person years
d. None of the above

Q.8. **Epidemiology is the study of:**
- a. Only the distribution of diseases
- b. Only the determinants of diseases
- c. Both the distribution and determinants of diseases
- d. None of the above

Q.9. **An investigator trying to study the effect of asbestos exposure on lung cancer collects relevant data on asbestos exposure retrospectively on 200 lung cancer patients and 200 persons without lung cancer. Assume that the two groups are otherwise comparable, what is the study design he has used?**
- a. Cross sectional study
- b. Cohort study
- c. Experimental study
- d. Case-control study

Q.10. **If the association between a factor (A) and the occurrence of the disease can be explained by another factor (B) which is associated with both the disease and the factor under study, the factor B is called:**
- a. A constant
- b. A concomitant factor
- c. A confounder
- d. A chance factor

References

1. Last John M, ed. *A Dictionary of Epidemiology*. 4th ed. Oxford: Oxford University Press; 2001.
2. *Oxford English Dictionary*. 2nd ed. Oxford: Oxford University Press; 2000.
3. MacMohan B, Pugh TF. *Epidemiology: Principles and Methods*. Boston: Little Brown; 1970.
4. Hippocrates. On airs, waters and places. *Med. Classics;* 3: 19, 1938.
5. Graunt J. *Natural and Political Observations Made Upon the Bills of Mortality: London, 1662*. Baltimore: Johns Hopkins Press; 1939.
6. Humphreys NA, ed. *Vital Statistics: A Memorial Volume of Selections from the Reports and Writings of Wlliam Farr, 1807-1883*. London: Sanitary Institute of Great Britain; 1885.
7. Dawber TR. *The Framingham Study: The Epidemiology of Atherosclerotic Disease*. Cambridge, MA: Harvard University Press; 1980.
8. Doll R, Hill AB. Lung cancer and other causes of death in relation to smoking: A second report on the mortality of British doctors. *Br Med J*. 1956; 2: 1071.
9. Doll R, Peto R. Mortality in relation to smoking: Twenty years' observations on male British doctors. *Br Med J*. 1975; 2: 1525.
10. Koch Robert. Untersuchungen über die Aetiologie der Wundinfektions-krankheiten. Leipzig, 1878. (Mettler Cecilia C. As quoted in *History of Medicine*. Mettler Fred A, ed. Toronto: The Blakiston Company; 1947).
11. Snow J. *On the Mode of Communication of Cholera*. 2nd ed. London: Churchill; 1855. Reproduced in *Snow on Cholera*. New York: Hafner; 1965.
12. Hill AB. The environment and disease: association or causation. *Proc R Soc Med*. 1965; 58: 295-300.
13. *Biennial Report 1994-95*, Delhi Cancer Registry, Institute of Rotary Cancer Hospital, All India Institute of Medical Sciences, New Delhi.
14. Niblock WJ. Cancer in India. *Indian Med Gaj*. 1902; 37:161-163.
15. Woolf B. On estimating the relation between blood group and disease. *Annals of Human Genetics*. 1955; 19, 251-253.
16. Schlesselman JJ. *Case-Control Studies. Design, Conduct, Analysis*. Oxford: Oxford University Press; 1982.
17. Hennekins CH, Buring JE. *Epidemiology in Medicine*. Boston: Little, Brown and Company; 1987.
18. Sackett DL. Bias in Analytical Research. *J Chron Dis*. 1979; 32: 51-63.
19. Reed GL 3rd, Singer DE, Picard EH, DeSanctis RW. Stroke following Coronary-artery bypass surgery. A case-control estimate of the risk from carotid bruits. *N Engl J Med*. 1988; 319: 1246-50.

9 | Principles of Clinical Trials

Every experiment may be said to exist only in order to give the facts a chance of disproving the null hypothesis.

R.A. Fisher

Clinical trials are now well-accepted tools not only to evaluate medical treatments but also to evaluate educational & health intervention programmes. They may help in the development of newer drugs and procedures, testing new combinations of existing drugs or new dose schedules and routes of administration, evaluating supportive care methods and comparing various educational programmes on lifestyle changes. In general, design of a clinical trial refers to a research design, which means the procedures and methods to be adhered to in conducting a clinical trial. Although a host of literature is available on various aspects of clinical trials, attempts are made here to briefly describe randomized controlled clinical trials (RCTs) and the issues related to their designs and analysis, which are more relevant to the beginners in this area.

9.1. Definition of Trials

In a literal sense, a trial means a planned experiment designed to assess the effect of a new treatment/intervention by comparing the outcomes of interest in a group exposed to it with those observed in a comparable group receiving a control treatment/ intervention. The control treatment/ intervention may be the existing drug, dose, method, or procedure for the treatment of the disease or condition. In the absence of such treatments/ interventions, placebo or no treatment/ intervention is considered as a control treatment. In other words, one of the interventions is regarded as a standard of comparison or control, and the group of participants who receive it is called the control or standard group. This is why clinical trials are generally referred to as controlled trials. The other group who receives the new intervention/ treatment is called the experimental group.

For example, in carrying out a clinical trial on remnant ablation among thyroid cancer patients, the participants who receive the conventional higher dose of radioactive iodine will be known as control/ standard group, whereas those receiving the proposed lower dose will be the experimental group. An event is termed as outcome whose presence or absence is noted after participants receive the intervention/ treatment. This pre-determined outcome (e.g., occurrence of disease, deaths, recovery, or other appropriate outcome) is measured and compared between the study groups. In the remnant ablation example, complete ablation is the outcome. There may, however, be more than one outcome in a clinical trial. Further, in addition to considered outcomes, additional end points (e.g., blood pressure control and glycemic control) may also be used for comparison.

Clinical trials are experimental studies, because the investigators have direct control on the study conditions (e.g., the types of interventions; the number of proposed new treatments; and the dose, route, and frequency of the regimen). The investigators may consist of clinicians, epidemiologists, biologists, social scientists and biostatisticians. The persons who are being studied in clinical trials are called study participants (subjects). They do not necessarily have to be patients, because the study can be conducted in healthy volunteers, in family members of patients, or in general population, depending upon the outcome of interest. For example, to assess the impact of anti-smoking intervention programme among the adolescents, the participants will be all the selected adolescents with the smoking habit.

9.2. Types of Trials

There are many types of trials based on different criteria and objectives.

9.2.1. Therapeutic and Prophylactic Trials

A clinical trial dealing with efficacy or effectiveness of chosen treatment regimens is generally referred to as a therapeutic trial. Under such trials, the unit of allocation to receive a test or standard regimen is generally an individual human being. For example, the trials on two different doses of depin for control of blood pressure among hypertensive patients, the patients can be allocated to experimental and control groups. This trial is usually done in a hospital set up.

On the other hand, a clinical trial dealing with the preventive role of an intervention program is referred to as a prophylactic trial. In general, under such trials, the unit of allocation to receive a preventive regimen is an entire community/ specified geographical area. For example, the trials on fluoridation of drinking water for the prevention of tooth decay where the whole community may be allocated to experimental and control groups. They are sometimes referred to as "Community Trials".

9.2.2. Controlled and Uncontrolled Trials

The therapeutic/ prophylactic trials where a new treatment/intervention is studied without any direct concurrent comparison with a similar group of patients on standard treatment/ therapy or placebo may be categorized as an uncontrolled trial. On the other hand, the controlled trials refer to those where a new treatment is studied along with its direct concurrent comparison with standard treatment/ therapy or placebo on a similar group of patients.

9.2.3. Randomized and Non-randomized Controlled Trials

The controlled trials may further be categorized in two ways: non-randomized and randomized controlled trials. In the first category, patients are allocated to the experimental/control groups without adopting any random procedure. To be very specific, the studies that use even pseudo-random or quasi-random methods of allocation (e.g., division into the different study groups according to date of birth (odd or even years), the registration number of their hospital records (odd or even numbers), the date at which they are invited to participate in the study (odd or even days), or alternative inclusion or other systematic method), are also known as non-randomized controlled trials. They neither provide each of the participants the same chance to be included in each of the study groups nor make the study less prone for biases. Under the randomized controlled trials, patients are allocated using a specified random process that is reproducible.

9.2.4. Efficacy and Effectiveness Trials

A controlled trial may further be categorized as an **efficacy trial** if it measures the benefit resulting from an intervention for a given health problem under the ideal conditions of an investigation. To be more specific, such trial tends to be an explanatory trial, which tries to provide clear evaluation of the interventions. For this, the investigators adopt strict inclusion criteria that may provide highly homogeneous study groups. For example, an explanatory study of the effects of radioactive iodine doses on remnant ablation among thyroid cancer patients may decide to include only thyroid cancer patients aged between 40 and 50 years, with no coexisting diseases and exclude those receiving other interventions. These trials may also tend to use fixed regimens (i.e., first dose as 100 mci), and placebo controls. Here, focus is on hard outcome (that is, complete ablation after six months of first dose). In summary, such trials reveal the success of an intervention in an ideal setting.

An **effectiveness trial**, on the other hand, measures the benefit resulting from an intervention for a given health problem under the usual conditions of clinical care for a particular group. In addition, it also measures acceptance of the intervention by those to whom it is offered. The investigators of such a trial try to evaluate the effects of the intervention in circumstances similar to those found by clinicians in their daily practice. An effectiveness trial falls in the category of the pragmatic trials that are planned not only to determine whether the intervention works, but also to assess all the consequences of its use (beneficial or harmful). For this, in contrast to explanatory trials, stringent inclusion criteria are not used so that participants with heterogeneous characteristics, similar to those seen by clinicians in their daily practice, are included. In addition to this, pragmatic trials tend to use flexible regimens. Further, these trials also involve the use of soft outcome measures (e.g., partial ablation) and/ or additional or surrogate end points like reduction in blood pressure or in blood sugar levels. In summary, such trials refer the success of an intervention in an actual practice.

9.2.5. Superiority and Equivalence Trials

A controlled clinical trial is known as a superiority trial if its objective is to study superiority of one treatment in comparison to another. However, this is always not necessary to establish superiority, especially when the standard treatment involves invasive procedures, is expensive and/ or has toxic side effects. Also, the new treatment may have lesser side effects, may be cheaper and / or easy to adapt. Under such circumstances, one may be interested in showing that the new treatment is equivalent in efficacy to the standard treatment. In other words, under equivalence, attempt is made only to demonstrate that the new treatment is not significantly worse than the standard treatment. Accordingly, one does not try to prove that the new treatment is better than the standard treatment. Such trials are called equivalence trials.

The equivalence does not mean to find a non-significant difference in the means/ proportions. Under testing of equivalence, there is involvement of an additional parameter "d" that indicates the maximum clinical difference allowed for an experimental treatment to be considered equivalent with a standard treatment. For example, in view of the lesser side effects and lower cost of the new treatment in comparison to standard treatment, new treatment may be considered equally effective even if its cure rate is at most 10% less than that of the standard treatment. Such trials are also known as non-inferiority trials.

9.3. Phases of Clinical Trials

As a first step in the development of a new drug, the probable dose, frequency and effect of experimental treatments/ interventions (beneficial as well as harmful) are assessed through animal studies. Based on these results, taking into account the observed effects along with side effects, the expected safer doses and their frequencies are considered for an experimental study on human beings before its use in clinical practice. Such studies in general are known as **clinical trials**. There are basically four phases of clinical trials.

9.3.1. Phase I Trials

After successful completion of animal studies on a new drug, these are the initial trials in human beings to assess the toxicity concerned with safety of a new drug. In the development of a new drug for human beings, the first phase may be devoted to understanding its maximum tolerable dose in a small number of individuals. Such trials are usually performed on healthy human volunteers. Sometimes, the volunteers would be patients who might have not shown any improvement on the standard treatments/ interventions. As such, the primary objective of Phase I study is to identify tolerable dose without causing serious side effects. This also involves assessment of other clinical aspects of the drug such as its pharmacokinetics (maximum concentration, duration of action, half life, etc.). As a rule of thumb, Phase-I studies may require at least 20 patients on a pre-specified dose.

9.3.2. Phase II Trials

This phase of study involves initial clinical investigations for treatment effect. In other words, this involves fairly small-scale investigations to determine the effect and safety of a new treatment/ dose or to assess the probable benefits that may outweigh risks. An exploratory study to select drugs/ doses having genuine potential effects out of the large number of drugs/ doses, which are inactive or over-toxic, also comes under this phase. Although there need not be any randomization of the subjects in the different groups studied, Phase II studies involve comparable groups.

9.3.3. Phase III Trials

Full-scale evaluation of treatment is planned under this phase. This phase of study is carried out to compare a reasonably effective new drug/ treatment to a standard drug/ treatment or placebo under a well-defined protocol. This is a most rigorous and extensive type of scientific clinical investigation involving randomization and a substantial number of patients that may be decided in view of the objective and other theoretical/ statistical considerations (discussed in Chapter 10). The present chapter will mainly concentrate on the issues related to design and analysis of Phase-III trials.

9.3.4. Phase IV Trials

This phase of study may sometimes be called as post-marketing surveillance. This phase of clinical trial is generally referred to as a promotion exercise aimed at bringing a new drug to the attention of a large number of practicing clinicians/ physicians. As such, there is neither involvement of sample size determination nor control group under this phase of study. Once a drug is approved for marketing after phase III trial, there is need of monitoring for adverse effects on a larger scale. Long-term studies of morbidity and mortality due to the use of the drug are also included in this phase.

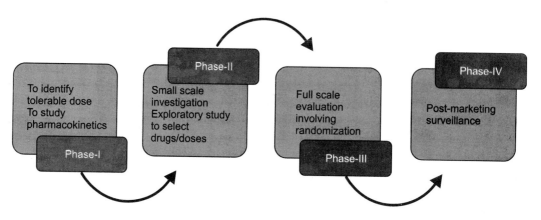

Fig. 9.1: Phases of clinical trial

To summarize, the randomized controlled clinical trial (RCT) is the most reliable method of hypothesis testing in conducting clinical research that is the main focus of the present chapter. RCTs are designed to answer questions concerning the efficacy of treatment with statistical validity. Main focus of the trials is to compare the experience of a group of patients on the new treatment with that of a control group of similar patients receiving a standard treatment or placebo. Therefore, there is need to make efforts to follow the basic principles of experimental design (such as randomization, etc.) to ensure that an experiment will give valid results. In the absence of a good design, major problems like bias and confounding may occur that are described in an earlier chapter on epidemiological methods. Further discussion in this chapter mainly focuses on issues related to RCTs.

9.4. Designs of RCTs

There are various experimental designs based on the procedures adopted regarding participants' exposure to the treatments/ interventions. They may be categorized and summarized briefly as follows.

9.4.1. Parallel Designs

Under parallel design, each of the participants receives only one of the study treatments/ interventions. These studies may sometimes be addressed as parallel trials or RCTs with parallel group design. For example, under a parallel design, to evaluate the effect of a new drug in comparison with that of a standard drug in patients with a particular disease, the new drug has to be given to one group of patients and the standard drug to another group of similar patients. Most of the RCTs have a parallel design. Following are the commonly used parallel designs.

9.4.1.1. Completely randomized design

In a completely randomized experiment, random allocation of patients to the various treatment groups may be carried out using the random number table. For example, a simple randomization list can be prepared using random number table. For this, on any page of the random number table, one can identify the starting point by putting pen/pencil after closing the eyes. From the starting point one can move row wise or column wise or even diagonally in any direction. Thus, a set of distinct one digit numbers ranging between 0 and 9 may be obtained in a listed manner. Marking the starting point as serial number "1", one has to fix serial numbers of the patients. Further procedure is described below.

(i) In case of two alternative treatments, one may consider that patients at serial numbers corresponding to digits 0-4 will receive treatment A; and those corresponding to digits 5-9 will receive treatment B so that this process provides equal probability for each patient to be included in either of the groups. This is described with the following example:

Selected row of random number table:	0	5	2	7	8	4	3	7	4	1	6	8	3	8	-	-	-
Serial numbers of the patients:		1	2	3	4	5	6	7	8	9	10	11	12	13	14	-	-	-
Sequence of treatment:		A	B	A	B	B	A	A	B	A	A	B	B	A	B	-	-	-

(ii) In case of three alternative treatments, one may consider that patients at serial numbers corresponding to digits 1-3 will receive treatment A; those corresponding to digits 4-6, treatment B; and those corresponding to digits 7-9, treatment C. Further, digit 0 is ignorable (*) so that this process provides equal probability for each patient to be included in any of the three groups. This procedure is illustrated with the following example:

Selected row of random number table:	0	5	2	7	8	4	3	7	4	1	6	8	3	8	-	-	-
Serial numbers of the patients:		1	2	3	4	5	6	7	8	9	10	11	12	13	14	-	-	-
Sequence of treatment:		*	B	A	C	C	B	A	C	B	A	B	C	A	C	-	-	-

Another method of randomization can be used when the trial size (n) is pre-fixed, other than sequential trial. In this method, after making a random start, as explained earlier, only those random numbers between 1 and n are selected from a column of random numbers (Appendix 1) that have width equal to the number of digits in the trial size. For example, if the trial size is of two digits (say, 50), select only those random numbers between 01 and 50 in the randomly chosen column of two digits. Ignore any numbers between 51 and 99 that are also two digits with similar width but larger than the trial size 50, repetitions and 00. Similarly, if the trial size is of three digits (say, 200), select only those random numbers between 001 and 200 in the randomly chosen column of three digits ignoring numbers between 201 and 999 (since the total sample size for random allocation is 200) repetitions and 000. Thus, the first 100 selected random numbers between 001 and 200 will correspond to the serial number of the subjects to whom treatment A will be given and the rest of the random numbers between 001 and 200 will correspond to the serial number of the subjects to whom treatment B will be given.

This design may provide fairly unbiased comparisons, especially if appropriate blinding is adopted. This design generally ensures equal number in various treatment groups. However, it does not make any effort to control or reduce the random variation. But, to further enhance the power of the study, the random (error) variation needs to be made as small as possible. For this, other sources of variation need to be identified. To achieve this, use of other appropriate designs is encouraged.

9.4.1.2. Randomized block design

This design involves stratified randomization. For stratification, potential prognostic factors may be considered that are basically demographic, disease-specific, or co-morbid characteristics. These characteristics generally have strong association with outcomes of a condition, for example, type of tumour and tumour size among cancer patients. They indicate prediction of the eventual development of these outcomes. In other words, prognosis means the likelihood that each one of the possible outcomes of a disease or condition will occur in presence of a factor. For example, status of disease that is often difficult to be measured may indicate probable outcome. As stated earlier, because randomization alone does not guarantee that the treatment groups will be comparable in terms of baseline characteristics, stratification before randomization (e.g., by age group, gender, disease stage, or other important prognostic factors) may be used as an additional means of ensuring balance in the treatment groups for known variables. Stratification is usually used when there are important known prognostic factors, such as age and tumor stage that can be measured before randomization. For this, the treatment group may be divided into homogeneous subgroups based on levels of prognostic factors at the start of the trial and the desired number of subjects may be included from each subgroup (strata). A stratum may be defined on the basis of single or multiple prognostic factors. For example, investigators designing an RCT to study the effects of varying doses of radioactive iodine on remnant ablation among thyroid cancer patients may decide to group thyroid cancer patients in the following manner:

Prognostic factors	Levels of factors
Thyroid cancer stage:	I+II, III+IV
Age :	30-45 years, more than 45 years

There may be four (2×2) strata as under:
1. Stage I+II and age between 30 and 45 years
2. Stage III+IV and age between 30 and 45 years
3. Stage I+II and age more than 45 years
4. Stage III+IV and age more than 45 years

Under this design, those strata of patients are considered that have generally number of patients either equal to the number of treatments or its multiples. Further, the strata are considered in such a way that the patients in each stratum are inherently similar individuals. Each stratum will have equal number of patients and patients are randomized to treatments randomly within each stratum. Restricting the stratum size to multiples of the number of treatments being compared is necessary to ensure that similar and equal subjects are allocated to each treatment. Under single blocking structure, in an experiment involving three treatment groups (e.g., T_1, T_2, T_3), the block wise randomization may be done as follows:

Disease stage and age blocks	Random allocation of treatments		
Stage I+II and age between 30 and 45 years	T_1	T_3	T_2
Stage III+IV and age between 30 and 45 years	T_2	T_1	T_3
Stage I+II and age more than 45 years	T_3	T_2	T_1
Stage III+IV and age more than 45 years	T_1	T_2	T_3

This randomization may be extended if the number of cases considered in each stratum is more than one. Likewise, it may be also extended if an experiment involves more than one blocking structure simultaneously. As a result, treatment differences may be shown up clearly, because they are based on the comparison of similar patients. The success of this design obviously depends on how well the blocking situation succeeds in bringing together inherently similar patients/persons. This design can offer substantial improvement in experimental sensitivity through reduction in error variation.

The ultimate similarity among the treatment groups arises when a subject is compared with himself or herself. In this situation, each patient forms an individual block, with the order of treatments decided on a random basis. A randomized block design of this type is known as crossover design. If possible, such an approach is highly sensitive. But, because of many practical constraints discussed later, this design might not be that much used.

9.4.1.3. Other advanced designs

It is understood that the use of several blocking structures may be helpful in substantial reduction of random variation. But, sometimes it may require a large number of patients in comparison to calculated minimum sample size, just to accommodate a larger number of blocking structures. For example, to compare four discrete doses of a drug using blocks in relation to disease stages (4 categories) and age groups (8 categories), at least 128 (4 × 8 × 4) patients or multiples of 128 will be required. This problem can be avoided through use of the Latin Square design, provided that the number of categories in each blocking structure (e.g., disease stage & age group) can be made equal to the number of treatments under comparison. In other words, rows (i.e., disease stages) and columns (i.e., age groups) under this design need to be the same. The treatments (e.g., T_1, T_2, T_3, T_4) are allocated randomly to the individual cells in the square, with only one treatment per cell. Each treatment must only occur once in each row and once in each column. This is important to ensure that all the treatments are assessed under comparable conditions. Accordingly, randomization can be achieved through a systematic arrangement as follows:

Disease stage blocks	Age group (years) blocks			
	30- 45	45-50	50-55	55-60
Stage I+II	T_1	T_2	T_3	T_4
Stage III+IV	T_2	T_3	T_4	T_1
Stage I+II	T_3	T_4	T_1	T_2
Stage III+IV	T_4	T_1	T_2	T_3

Thus, this design offers a useful way of controlling two sources of variation with relatively small number of patients. However, if necessary, this process can be repeated. But, this can be planned only when the number of blocking rows (e.g., disease stages) and columns (i.e., age groups) each equals the number of treatments involved. Because of these constraints, this design is not so user-friendly in RCTs.

None of the designs described above may be helpful in dealing with the simultaneous study of several factors. To overcome this problem, there is another design called "factorial experiment" that involves simultaneous study of several factors. In an RCT using a factorial design, two or more interventions may not only be evaluated separately, but also in combination and against a control. For instance, a factorial design to study the intervention influence on the condition of heart, one would like to investigate two issues: involvement of physical exercise and non-fried dietary habit. Combining these two factors in a factorial experiment and also each factor at two levels, may give rise to four possibilities, that is, people doing physical exercise and eating non-fried meals; people doing physical exercise but eating fried meals; people not doing physical exercise but eating non-fried meals; and people neither doing physical exercise nor eating non-fried meals. Accordingly, this design means that patients will be allocated randomly to one of these four groups. This design allows the researchers to compare the experimental interventions with the control (that is, physical exercise versus placebo), compare the experimental interventions with each other (that is, physical exercise versus eating non-fried meals), and investigate possible interactions between them (that is, comparison of the sum of the effects of people doing physical exercise alone and eating non-fried meals alone with the effects of the combination). The efficacy of each intervention regarding one or more outcomes may be ensured. The factorial design is the only method that allows evaluation of interactions between interventions. Likewise, studies involving combinations of three or more interventions may also adopt factorial design. Many trials have used a factorial design, e.g., in evaluation of the effect of aspirin in preventing myocardial infarction and the effect of beta-carotene in preventing cancer. However, this design can be used only if there is involvement of at least two factors. Further, its utility in a clinical trial involving two/ more treatments may not be sometimes practical. Also, keeping in view the probable difficulties in doing this study, the ethical committees may not permit such studies.

Like in case of interventions, sometimes comparison among more than one treatment (e.g., radioactive iodine dose and laser therapy) may be of an added interest. In such a situation, rather than setting up separate studies to look at each treatment, it is more efficient and informative to combine the various treatments in a single experiment using factorial design. In case of two treatments, each having two levels, a 2×2 factorial design may be used. For example, in treating thyroid cancer patients after surgery, one might decide to investigate two treatments, namely, the radioactive iodine dose (with two levels – higher & lower) and the laser therapy (with two levels — weekly & monthly). Combination of these two treatments in a single factorial experiment results in four unique treatment combinations. The real advantage of an integrated factorial approach is, thus, not only to see whether radioactive iodine dose or the laser therapy affects outcome of interest, but also to see whether the two influence or "interact" with each other. There will be an interaction when the relative effectiveness of the levels of radioactive iodine dose is influenced by, or depends on, the presence or level of the laser therapy. The real power of a factorial experiment is in its ability to explore the possibility of interactions between different treatments.

9.4.2. Crossover Design

In crossover design, unlike parallel design, each of the study participants receives each of the treatments/ interventions under study in successive periods. Thus, participants are given two or more treatments in sequence. The time during which an intervention/ treatment is administered and evaluated is called a trial period. For example, if a patient receives an experimental treatment and is observed for improvement after six months of the start of the treatment, trial period with this drug will be six months. After a trial period with the first treatment, the participants are "crossed-over" to the other intervention. While doing so, because the same patient receives two treatments, one should try to avoid the presence of the effect of one treatment during the evaluation of another treatment, or what is called **carry-over effect**. For example, in a patient receiving standard available pain killer drug followed by a newly proposed pain killer drug, the presence of the effect of the standard available pain killer drug during evaluation of the effect of the newly proposed pain killer drug is known as carry-over effect. Its presence can be avoided when the duration of the effect of the drug is well known. Accordingly, to overcome this problem, the trial periods may be separated by a time period of sufficient length that will make the participants free of the influence of the treatment previously used by the time they receive the next treatment. This period of time is known as a **washout period**.

Under this design, the order in which the participants receive each of the study treatments has to be determined at random just to rule out the probable presence of treatment-period interaction. When the same group of patients receives two or more treatments and if any observed difference between the effects of the treatments can be explained by the order in which the treatments are given to the participants, this is known as **treatment-period interaction**. Its presence may obviously make the ongoing trial totally meaningless. To rule out this, if two treatments are involved in the study, participants are randomized to either Group I or Group II, which determines the order of the treatments. In this case, Group I may receive Drug A first, followed by Drug B, and Group II may receive Drug B first, followed by Drug A. There is also a need to take into account the probable presence of the period effects that are the differences between the trial periods that may be caused by progression, regression, or fluctuation of the disease. In summary, the order effects (i.e., carry over and period effects) need to be assessed and removed from the comparisons between the treatments.

In contrast to parallel designs (described in section 9.5.1) that produce between-participant comparisons, this design allows within-participant comparisons. In view of the fact that each participant acts as his or her own control, in comparison to parallel design, this design is likely to produce statistically and clinically more efficient results with the same number of participants. Further, for a given power, this design may require less number of patients. However, each of the treatments should ideally have rapid onset and short duration. Further, due precaution is required to rule out the presence of order effects that include period effects as well as carry-over effects. Sometimes, first treatment may permanently change the course of the disease and this design cannot be an appropriate choice. This design is more appropriate in case of a chronic and incurable disease. Also, this design may also be used in diseases involving recurrent conditions. For example, the crossover design may be useful in comparing various anti-hypertensive drugs regarding management of hypertensive patients. Also, the comparison of pain killers among the patients suffering from cancer and comparison of drugs among diarrhea patients may be carried out using crossover design.

9.5. Other Aspects of the RCTs

In addition to statistical experimental designs of RCTs, there are various other components also that play critical role in avoiding the above-mentioned problems, bias and confounding. Their understandings may go a long way in designing an RCT in a clear and lucid manner that may help in carrying out a conclusive RCT. These issues are described in following major sections.

9.5.1. Definition of Study Participant

To conduct an RCT, in addition to clearly defined treatments/ interventions, the study participants must also fulfill well-defined inclusion criteria and good performance status. One may plan to exclude the patients who received prior treatments/therapy for their problem (disease) or enroll only those patients who had prior treatments/therapy. Such studies that are designed to assess response rate require disease that is measurable (i.e., capable of being objectively assessed for improvement or worsening over time). To avoid any ambiguity, in addition to inclusion criteria, exclusion criteria may also be invariably listed, which consist of conditions that preclude entrance of participants into an RCT even if they meet the inclusion criteria. Ideally, inclusion criteria should not be modified after initiating the study.

9.5.2. Use of Co-treatments/Interventions

If otherwise feasible, the use of the co-treatments/interventions should be avoided that are sometimes given to some of the study participants as per their requirements in addition to the planned treatments under study, which might be applied differently to the treatment and control groups. If use of co-treatment is unavoidable, this may be a serious problem, especially when double blinding is absent. For example, in carrying out an RCT on remnant ablation among thyroid cancer patients, some of the participants who receive conventional higher dose of radioactive iodine may or may not need another dose whereas those receiving proposed lower dose of radioactive iodine may sometimes need another dose(s). In the same way, instead of considering additional dose of the main treatment as a co-treatment, one may involve different treatments all together as co-treatments. As such, imbalance in use of co-treatments among the study groups may complicate the understanding of the results under an RCT. However, if co-treatments/interventions are needed to be given in a balanced manner in both the groups, it should be pre-defined in the protocol and must be adhered to.

9.5.3. Size of Randomized Controlled Clinical Trials

Uncommon to other study designs (e.g., cohort studies; case-control studies), a small sample size is one of the most common problems seen in RCTs, because of non-availability of required patients within stipulated time and/or involvement of costly kits, etc. However, sample size is one of the major factors associated with power of the RCT. If no difference between treatments is seen, it could be because there was not enough power to detect a true difference. Even if a study is designed with adequate power to evaluate the primary outcome, the sample size may be inadequate for secondary outcomes or subgroup comparisons. An increase in the number of considered patients may directly increase the sensitivity of an experiment. This helps through decrease in the standard error and, hence, increases our ability to detect true treatment difference. In the absence of minimum required sample size, the experiment with a poor chance of detecting true treatment differences may simply be a waste of time and money. Thus, determination of the appropriate number of patients to be used in an RCT is an important and unavoidable task. In general, RCT involves the problem of testing of hypothesis, that is, comparison of proportions or means between treatment groups. In view of specific objective of the trial, using best available probable information (e.g., group specific cure rate) on the topic under investigation, the required minimum sample size may be calculated at pre-determined level of confidence (e.g., 95%), power of the study (e.g., 90%) and relative precision (e.g., 10%). Further, keeping in view the objective under study, a case of one-tail (one-sided) or two-tail (two-sided) test may be considered. The methods of calculating minimum sample size have been discussed in detail for various study designs including RCTs with design specific worked examples in Chapter 10.

9.5.4. Random Allocation of Patients

Patients should invariably be randomly allocated to the treatment groups to ensure unbiased comparison of the treatments under RCTs (either blind or open). Under randomization, the process of allocating treatments to subjects becomes totally outside the control of the investigator that enables unbiased comparison. Randomization is the usual method of allocating treatments to two or more groups of subjects in a clinical trial. It should, however, be noted that random allocation does not mean haphazard allocation. The randomization process is documented so that it is reproducible. Further, the principal reason for using a "randomization" technique is to avoid predictability in the treatment assignment, i.e., neither the patient nor the investigator knows or controls the treatment assignment before it is made. Successful randomization eliminates selection bias on the part of the study subject or the investigator, thus ensuring that characteristics of the patients do not influence the treatment that is assigned. Successful randomization also tends to create comparison groups that are more or less balanced in terms of both known and unknown factors that may be related to outcome. However, because of the random nature of treatment allocation, imbalances in baseline factors may still exist. The procedures of randomizations under various designs are explained under respective sections.

9.5.5. Blinded Study (i.e., Masked Study)

This is an RCT in which observer(s) and/or study participants are kept ignorant of the study group (i.e., treatment/intervention) to which the study participants are assigned. In case of ignorance of only participants, this may be called as a single blind RCT. Where both observer and subjects are kept ignorant, the RCT is termed as a double blind RCT. If the statistician involved in planning/analysis is also ignorant of the group to which participants belong, the RCT is sometimes described as triple blind. The purpose of "blinding" is to eliminate sources of bias mainly on the part of participants and observers.

9.5.6. Concealment

In case desired blinding is not feasible in a RCT, it is better if there is involvement of at least concealment in that study. This means, neither participant nor observer knows about the intervention/treatment group of a participant until a participant is randomly allocated to a group. As obvious, concealment helps to preserve the original randomization. This is ideally required to be maintained always irrespective of involvement of blinding in the study. This also helps in avoiding some sources of bias. In case of using spot randomization, rarely preferred, no concealment is required.

9.5.7. Ethical Clearance

It is mandatory to design an RCT carefully so that it can protect the participants and maintain their privacy and also answer the question(s) under investigation. The RCT generally needs clearance from either of the two committees: (i) Institutional Ethics Committee (IEC); or (ii) Institutional Review Boards (IRB). The process of ethical clearance helps in ensuring adherence to various important norms, for example, scientific validity, social values, independent reviews, right to know the existing knowledge about experimental and standard treatments, informed consent, fair selection of the participants, and respect for eligible and enrolled participants. Among them, consent is the most important component of ethical clearance. Patients entering in the RCT (specially phase III) must be counseled in detail about their prognosis and the expected benefits from participation in the study. They should also be told about benefits that could be expected from experimental treatment or standard treatments. Their known side effects should also be conveyed. Also, it should be made clear to the study participants that despite prior phase I and II testing, unexpected side effects may occur. The expected length of the study and follow-up measures should also be made clear. After completion or

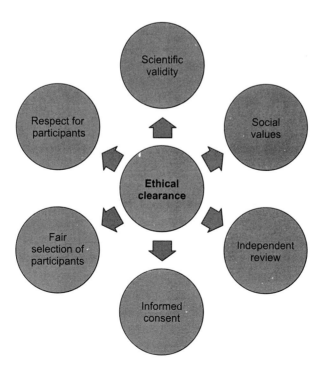

Fig. 9.2: Functions of ethical clearance

discontinuation of treatment, follow-up of patients may typically last for a longer time or until other treatment is initiated. Close observation of patients for both acute and chronic toxicity is necessary; unusual or chronic toxicities may be observed only in the large number of patients on phase III new regimen arms. Some of the measures, like tumor measurement, may require a detailed history and physical examination, blood tests, x-rays, scans, and sometimes repeated surgical biopsies. Patients must be informed of the nature of the diagnostic monitoring required by the study prior to their giving informed consent. Sometimes, the requirement for large number of study participants and lengthy follow-up makes phase III studies expensive and difficult to run. To overcome this problem, such trials have to be conducted as a multi-centric clinical trial that involves a number of study centers and may require additional planning strategy (not under purview of this book).

The detailed guidelines on ethical issues relevant to Indian context may be seen on the website of the Indian Council of Medical Research at www.icmr.nic.in. Further, a host of literature is available on the ethical guidelines on the net, e.g., NIH of US has an online material followed by a brief test for those who propose to carry out clinical trials and Ethics Committee Members. After clearing this test, a certificate is also issued. More details can be seen at www.cancer.gov/clinicaltrials/learning/page3 .

9.5.8. Compliance

This is a measure of the extent to which study participants have followed the instructions given by the investigators. It is also known as adherence. It is easier to achieve high compliance when the administration of the treatments/interventions is completely controlled by the investigators and/or other health professionals, who are not acting as investigators but are supportive of the services under the study. The compliance becomes difficult when the investigators do not administer the treatments/interventions, but it is done by the participants themselves, especially when the study has a long duration and the interventions have to be administered several times a day (e.g., in an RCT evaluating the effects of nutritional supplements among larynx cancer patients). The compliance may also be linked to related side effects and other problems. In such cases, inclusion of those patients may be preferred who have already shown high compliance in other studies but sometimes may introduce bias. An RCT involving very poor adherence by the participants may be a futile exercise.

9.6. Collection of Data

To make an RCT successful and conclusive, the criteria that are explicit and specified well in advance through written protocol must be strictly followed for data collection. To be more specific, it is essential that the same measurement methods, schedule, and criteria be applied to all patients in all treatment groups. After obtaining the consent, baseline characteristics of patients should be measured before patients are randomized so that knowledge of the treatment assignment cannot influence reporting of baseline characteristics. It is important to monitor all patients with respect to the randomly assigned treatments. Some of the patients may not stick to the assigned treatments because of refusal, partial compliance or total non-compliance. Such patients must be monitored with respect to the treatments, which they finally received. However, as stated earlier, efforts should be made to minimize the non-compliance.

The assessment of treatment efficacy is entirely based on the pre-determined outcome. In order to determine whether a new treatment is better/equally good, the criterion in terms of the primary outcome on which it will be judged, must be specified in advance. For example, a new drug that has 10% less positive response may be preferred in view of other factors (e.g., side effects; cost). Hence, other desirable and undesirable effects need to be measured in order to gain a more complete picture of the benefits and risks of the new treatment. Further, the primary outcome in an RCT is a measure that is easy to assess in all patients. In general, the outcome measures that are well defined and can be observed directly are preferred, such as death or survival, remnant ablation, recurrence of disease, and change in blood pressure. More subjective outcome measures, such as pain reduction, quality of life, and psychological status may be equally important but are more likely to be biased when the patient or the doctor/investigator knows which treatment the patient received. This may be true even in case of their feelings about such knowledge. In principle, the primary outcome should also be clinically relevant. For example, slight (say, one mm/hg) but statistically significant change in blood pressure may not be of much clinical relevance.

Similar criteria must be adopted to measure the outcome in each of the treatment groups. This means that all patients should be followed in the same way, with the same tests, and at the same intervals after treatment. Explicit criteria for determining outcome status must be specified well in advance. It is not enough to design a study to just see whether a new treatment reduces the blood pressure. It is necessary to specify the criteria for considering blood pressure to have decreased that have clinical relevance, i.e., the degree of change (percent change or absolute change) from baseline level that will be considered a success.

It may be worthwhile to remember that variables should not be categorized at the time of data collection. If necessary, categories of a covariate may be decided after some exploratory analysis, which may help us to have the correct idea about frequency distribution in various categories of a particular variable. At the same time, modification of categories of a particular variable should be carried out taking into account theoretical (topic specific relevance) aspects also in addition to simple statistical considerations. This means that finalization of the categories of variables should not add to distortion of the meaning, that is, distortion in existing relationship between the variables. Also, for easy understanding and interpretation, data collected on interval/ratio scale may be considered in the form of nominal/ordinal scale. This exercise should, however, be done carefully to have a meaningful understanding and interpretation. It may, however, be noted that whatever steps we take in transformation of data collected on interval/ratio scale in form of nominal/ordinal scale, there will be loss of some information. For example, smoking status may be considered in either of three forms: (i) simply smokers, non-smokers; (ii) smokers, ever smokers, never smokers; and (iii) appropriate form based on available data on ever/current smoking, duration and average smoking. As obvious, priority of the consideration of the appropriate form of this variable has to be in reverse order, that is, from (iii) to (i). Further, even if all other covariates are retained in the same form, change in one covariate's form may result in change in results. Hence, this consideration requires careful thinking instead of an ad-hoc approach.

9.7. Analysis of Data

An appropriate data analysis is one of the important steps in carrying out RCTs that yield accurate results and proper interpretation leading to useful policy implications. Ideally, as described earlier, the data collection has to be carried out in keeping with the objectives of the study and methods planned well in advance. However, there might have been methodological changes over a period of time because of the problems beyond the control of the investigators. This may also include substantial imbalance due to group-specific dropouts and/or missing data. Strictly speaking, such RCTs do not make much sense. Before data analysis, understanding all such problems present in the collected data through exploratory analysis is necessary in order to decide on appropriate methods of data analysis and for careful interpretation of the results. Also, exploratory analysis may sometimes provide important clues to remedial measures to overcome some of these problems. Although these issues are of utmost importance, their detailed coverage is not under the purview of the present book. Once we have got reliable and complete data in our hand, to carry out appropriate analysis of data, we have to follow certain steps under the data analysis. For meaningful data analysis and its interpretation, one has to address objectives under the RCT.

In view of the specific design used under the study, one has to decide appropriate methods of data analysis that are required to do meaningful interpretation of the results. There are certain methodologies, which are commonly used in data analysis irrespective of design of the study (e.g., descriptive data analysis). However, there are some methodologies which are used for a specific design of the study (e.g., deciding appropriate type of analytical tools like parametric/non-parametric analysis of variance; one way/multiway analysis of variance; survival analysis). Keeping in view these issues and also type of outcome variable, the analytical methods are summarized in the following sub-sections.

9.7.1. Analytical Methods for Quantitative Outcome Variable

As described in Chapter 5, if quantitative parameters are to be compared between two or more than two groups, there are specific procedures to be used after making certain assumptions. For example, if we want to compare means of a particular variable between two groups, we use unpaired *t*-test under the assumptions that data follow normal distribution and variances of two groups are comparable. If these assumptions do not seem to be true in a given case, we have to change the method of data analysis. For example, if the sample is relatively larger, we can further explore the possibility of using a parametric test like unpaired *t*-test through transformation of the variables. As we know, the purpose of transformation of the data is three-fold: (i) to minimize the variance, (ii) to normalize the data and (iii) to linearise the relationship with the other variable. If assumptions are not fulfilled even after the transformation of the data and also sample size is relatively small, we do not have a choice other than that of using a non-parametric Test. For example, in case of two groups, we use Wilcoxon's Rank Sum Test in place of unpaired *t*-test. Likewise, if we have follow-up data on same group at two points of time, we use paired *t*-test under certain assumptions. Otherwise, we go for a non-parametric test, viz., Wilcoxon's Signed Rank Test. It may be noted that while using non-parametric test, we compare medians instead of means.

If we have more than two groups in case of comparing means, because of theoretical reasons, we have to go for analysis of variance (ANOVA) instead of using unpaired/ paired *t*-tests. Obviously, here also there is involvement of similar assumptions. Otherwise, we have to go for appropriate non-parametric tests, e.g., in case of three or more independent groups, we can use Kruskal Walli's Test, whereas in case of repeated measures we can use Friedman's Test. In case of significant result under parametric/non-parametric analysis of variance, we have to go for appropriate Multiple Comparison Test. This is necessary to identify the pairs of groups having significantly different level of the study variable.

The above-described methods not only help us to see the relationship between the variables/categories, but also help us to understand our data in a better way and plan the future analysis appropriately. If our outcome variable is a quantitative variable (continuous/discrete), the analytical methods may be summarized in the following manner (Table 9.1).

Table 9.1: Analytical methods when outcome variable is a quantitative variable

Desired analysis	Type of data to be analyzed	
	Rank, score, or measurement (from Gaussian population)	Rank, score, or measurement (from non- Gaussian population)
Describe one group	Mean, SD	Median, Interquartile range
Compare one group to a hypothetical value	One-sample *t*- test	Wilcoxon's test
Compare two unpaired groups	Unpaired *t*- test	Wilcoxon's rank sum test/Mann-Whitney 'U' test
Compare two paired groups	Paired *t*- test	Wilcoxon's signed rank test
Compare three or more unmatched groups	One-way ANOVA	Kruskal-Wallis test
Compare three or more matched groups	Repeated-measures ANOVA	Friedman's test
Quantify association between two variables	Pearson's correlation coefficient	Spearman's rank correlation coefficient
Predict value from another measured variable	Simple linear regression or Nonlinear regression	Nonparametric regression
Predict value from several measured or binomial variables	Multiple linear regression or Multiple nonlinear regression	No equivalent analysis is available

Some of the above mentioned methods have been explained with examples in earlier chapters (Chapters 5 & 6). More details of these methods and their applications may be obtained from other publications (e.g., Altman[1], 1991; Armitage and Berry[2], 1987; Pocock[3], 1983).

9.7.2. Analytical Methods for Binomial Outcome Variable

As mentioned in Chapter 5, sometimes outcomes of our interest may be of binomial form. In case of qualitative data, for the purpose of comparison, we generally use Chi-square Test. If assumptions of Chi-square Test (e.g., mutually exclusive categories of covariates in the form of contingency table and expected frequency in a cell not less than five) are not fulfilled, we use alternative methods like Fisher's Exact Test. These tests are also used in case we want to compare proportion of interesting events between two or more than two categories (groups). Analytical methods used in such a case are summarized in Table 9.2.

Table 9.2: Analytical methods for binomial outcome variables

Desired analysis	Type of data to be analyzed
	Binomial(Two possible outcomes)
Describe one group	Proportion
Compare one group to a hypothetical value	Chi-square or Binomial test
Compare two unpaired groups	Chi-square for large samples (Fisher's exact test for small samples)
Compare two paired groups	McNemar's Chi-squared test
Compare three or more unmatched groups	Chi-square test
Compare three or more matched groups	Cochrane's Q
Quantify association between two variables	Contingency coefficients
Predict value from another measured variable	Simple logistic regression
Predict value from several measured or binomial/non-binomial variables	Multiple logistic regression

Some of the above mentioned methods have been explained with examples in earlier chapters (Chapters 5 & 6). For more details of these methods and their applications, other publications may also be referred (e.g., Altman[1], 1991; Armitage and Berry[2], 1987; Pocock[3], 1983; Collett[4], 2003a; Kleinbaum and Klein[5], 2002; Wright[6], 1986).

9.7.3. Analytical Methods for Outcome Variable as Time to Event

Most of the RCTs involve outcome in the form of survival data (i.e., time to a desired event, e.g., survival period after the surgery of a particular cancer patient; period of recurrence of disease and so on). The analytical methods applicable in such cases may be summarized in Table 9.3.

Table 9.3: Analytical methods for time to event outcome variable

	Type of data to be analyzed
Desired analysis	*Time to event*
Describe one group	Kaplan Meier survival curve
Compare two unpaired groups	Log-rank test or Mantel-Haenszel test
Compare two paired groups	Conditional proportional hazards regression
Compare three or more unmatched groups	Cox proportional hazard regression
Compare three or more matched groups	Conditional proportional hazards regression
Predict value from another measured variable	Cox proportional hazard regression(hazard or survival models)
Predict value from several measured or binomial variables	Cox proportional hazard regression (hazard or survival models)

Some of the above mentioned methods have been explained with examples in Chapter 8. More details of these methods and their applications are described in other publications (e.g., Altman[1], 1991; Armitage and Berry[2], 1987; Pocock[3], 1983); Collett[7], 2003b; Kleinbaum[8], 1996).

9.7.4. Analysis of Crossover Design

The designs of crossover trials are described in Section 9.5.2. A relatively straight forward analysis of quantitative outcome is to use paired t-test for paired differences. But this analysis makes two main assumptions. The first is that there is no systematic period effect (Armitage et al.[2], 2002) — no tendency among the patients to obtain better relief in one period (getting drug A followed by drug B) than that in the other period (getting drug B followed by drug A). The second assumption is that there is no treatment-period interaction (Jones and Kenward[9], 2003) – no change in average response between the treatments as observed in first group (getting drug A followed by drug B) than that in the second group (getting drug B followed by drug A). To test the period effect, comparison between two groups — first group getting drug A followed by drug B; and another group getting drug B followed by drug A — is carried out through unpaired t-test for comparing mean paired difference obtained in the first group with that obtained in the second group. If there is evidence of a period effect, one feels somewhat uneasy about interpreting any overall treatment difference within patients. To test carry-over effects and other interactions between treatment and period, the statistical test for interaction is again unpaired t-test for comparing mean of combined response to drug A and drug B in Group 1 versus Group 2. If a significant interaction is found, one's best policy is to abandon the above within patient analysis of the whole set of data.

For a better understanding, the analysis of a crossover trial can be illustrated with a trial comparing depin, an anti-hypertensive drug, and placebo in the management of hypertensive patients. The data on systolic blood pressure are shown in Tables 9.4 and 9.5 separately for the groups having depin followed by placebo and placebo followed by depin.

Table 9.4: Group A — treatment with Depin followed by placebo (n=10)

S. No.	D	P	$d_1 = D-P$	$a_1 = (D+P)/2$	P-D
1.	135	140	-5	137.5	5
2.	140	145	-5	142.5	5
3.	160	155	5	157.5	-5
4.	140	150	-10	145.0	10
5.	130	140	-10	135.0	10
6.	140	145	-5	142.5	5
7.	130	135	-5	132.5	5
8.	150	160	-10	155.0	10
9.	140	150	-10	145.0	10
10.	150	155	-5	152.5	5
Mean	141.5	147.5	-6	144.5	6
S.D.	9.44	7.9	4.59	8.39	4.59

Table 9.5: Group B – treatment with placebo followed by Depin (n=10)

S. No.	P	D	$d_2 = P-D$	$a_2 = (D+P)/2$	P-D
1.	145	135	10	140	10
2.	140	145	-5	142.5	-5
3.	150	145	5	147.5	5
4.	155	155	0	155.0	0
5.	140	130	10	135.0	10
6.	135	130	5	132.5	5
7.	145	150	-5	147.5	-5
8.	155	150	5	152.5	5
9.	150	145	5	147.5	5
10.	160	150	10	155.0	10
Mean	147.5	143.5	4	145.5	4
S.D	7.91	8.83	5.68	7.89	5.68

The change (d_i) in measurement on systolic blood pressure for each patient can be calculated using the observation listed under each period for each of the patients in both groups. Likewise, the average (a_i) of the observations in the two periods can also be worked out for each group. The descriptive statistics, namely, mean and standard deviation can be worked out for each of the period, differences and averages under each of the two groups of patients.

In doing a simple comparison of the treatments, ignoring the design of the study will not be correct. Before doing so, the possibility of a period effect needs to be ruled out through carrying out two-sample *t*-test to compare the differences between the periods in the two groups of patients. It is expected that the mean differences between the periods in the two groups would be of the same size but having opposite signs, especially in the absence of the possibility that patients do comparatively better in one of the two groups. Accordingly, the test for a period effect can be carried out using two-sample *t*-test comparing. In the above mentioned example, regarding period effect, at 18 degrees of freedom, the observed p-value is 0.39, which is statistically not significant. It suggests absence of the period effect in this data set.

In the absence of a treatment-period interaction, a patient's average response to the two treatments would be the same regardless of the order in which they were received. Accordingly, the test for such interaction may also be carried out using two-sample *t*-test comparing. In the above-mentioned example, regarding treatment-period interaction, at 18 degrees of freedom, the observed p-value is 0.78, which is statistically not significant. It suggests absence of treatment-period interaction in this data set.

The analysis of a crossover trial becomes simple, especially when there is no period effect and no treatment-period interaction. Both a marked period effect and treatment-period interaction may not be appropriate, which indicate that the observed magnitude of the treatment effect depends on the order in which the treatments were given. Comparatively, treatment-period interaction is a more serious problem because it leads to biased estimate of the treatment effect.

The treatment effect can be tested by performing a one-sample *t*-test of 20 within subject differences between the two treatments. Sometimes, the two crossover groups may not be of the same size; hence, it is preferable to consider the average effect in the two periods, which is equivalent to performing a two-sample *t*-test comparing. In the above mentioned given data set, at 18 degrees of freedom, the observed p-value is 0.004, which is statistically significant. As is evident from pooled results in the last column of each group, average reduction in systolic blood pressure because of using depin comes out to be 5 mmHg. However, because of small sample size, 95% confidence interval may indicate uncertainty regarding true benefit of depin.

9.7.5. Interim Analysis

For ethical & economic reasons, a series of interim analyses are usually planned during the course of the trial at different periods. This helps in applying appropriate statistical techniques, depending upon the nature of data gathered.

9.7.5.1. Guidelines for the interim analysis

(a) For the interim analysis, it is not necessary to select all the response and prognostic variables. Since long-term response variable may show up only at the end of the trial, only short-term response variables need to be included under interim analysis. If the most important response variable appears only after a long period, interim analysis of other response variables may not be of much use as far as termination of the trail is concerned. Interim analysis may be done only for some academic reasons in such situations.

(b) The decision to stop the trial should be taken only on statistical grounds - significant treatment effect differences or equivalent effects with the standard treatments with adequate pre-determined Power of the test. It may also be based on financial and practical considerations.

(c) Strict confidentiality of the results from the interim analysis should be maintained till the final analysis is done to avoid any possible biases and change of protocol.

(d) Type-I error at each interim analysis should be decided based on the statistical requirements and computations. The formula for computing the type-I error is:

ZiK=CK Sq Root (K)/Sq Root (i), where i = 1 to K

where CK is the critical value for a total of 'K' interim analyses.

Value of K can be obtained from the following Table:

K	O'Brien Critical Value[10]
1.	1.96
2.	1.978
3.	2.004
4.	2.024
5.	2.040

If K = 3 (three interim analyses)
For I = 1, Z1K = 3.47; i = 2, Z2K = 2.45; i = 3, Z3K = 2.004

9.7.6. Intention to Treat Analysis (ITT)

Under this method of data analysis in an RCT, individual outcomes are analyzed according to the group to which they were randomized; even if they never received the treatment they were assigned or assigned treatment was changed to another due to serious side effects, general negligence, etc. Ideally, this situation is to be avoided, but in practice it may not be possible. It affects the balance of randomization and introduces bias in the treatment comparisons. To avoid this, analysis may be done as per the original grouping itself. This analysis is called **intention to treat analysis (ITT)**. It may not sound logical to do the analysis as per ITT. Normally, it is not recommended for all clinical trials, but, in certain situations, as indicated above, this procedure may have to be adopted to keep up randomization at the cost of logic. When treatment A is not effective and for ethical reasons another treatment has to be given for the benefit of the patient, this type of analysis may be recommended. Coronary by-pass surgery & medication for unstable angina pectoris — medication may not be effective in some patients and for ethical reasons and keeping the treatment for the benefit of the patient, coronary by-pass surgery may have to be done in such patients.

This method provides a better measure of effectiveness than efficacy. The basic idea behind this approach is to retain the original randomization that was assigned to the patient. Further, ideally, the two methods of analysis as per randomization "de facto" and "de jure" providing similar results may reflect the strength of RCT. Since there are conflicts and difference of opinions among the clinicians and statisticians on ITT analysis, it would always be better to do the analysis by both ways -'intention to treat' and 'as per protocol' and compare the results before making the final interpretation of results of the clinical trial.

9.7.7. Number Needed to Treat (NNT)

In the fast developing clinical research and decision making process, a new paradigm has emerged in the recent past - **Evidence Based Medicine (EBM)**. This is based on intuition, systematic as well as unsystematic clinical experience and pathophysiologic rationale as grounds for clinical decision making. EBM stresses on examination of evidence from clinical research —mainly by literature search — and applying formal scientific & statistical methods in evaluating it. Because of easy access to the computer and Internet facilities, literature search has become much easier and faster. This is a method which helps the clinicians in taking decisions about the care of individual patients using the current best evidence consciously, explicitly & judiciously.

One of the important statistical method commonly used in EBM is the risk analysis .The concept of "Number Needed to Treat" (NNT), which is computed from the risk analysis, has gained a lot of popularity now because of its simple and fashionable translation which has attracted the clinicians. Perhaps, the term itself was coined mainly for the sake of clinicians. NNT gives the number of patients who need to be treated to achieve one additional favourable outcome (say, cure) or to avoid one additional bad outcome (say, death). When clinicians and policy makers are presented with research results in different formats like NNT, ARR (Attributable Risk Ratio) and RRT (Relative Risk Ratio), it is found that they take more conservative decisions when presented with NNTs than those when they are presented with ARR or RRR. This topic has been discussed in detail in Chapter 8.

9.7.8. Issues Related to Multivariable Analysis

This aspect of data analysis has already been discussed in detail in Chapter 7. But, for completeness of this chapter, brief aspects are summarized again here.

It is often noticed that we are tempted to carry out multivariable analysis without looking into our objectives, type of the data in our hand, especially number of variables, and sample size. Sometimes, analysis of a well-designed RCT may not involve multivariable analysis. However, if necessary, we should take due consideration of sample size in view of the number of variables. As mentioned earlier, after a series of exploratory analyses, we should finalize the form of the variables to be considered in data analysis, including multivariable analysis. While doing so, we should explore the possibility that the relationships between the variables do not get distorted because of change in scale of measurements or categories of a variable.

The next important issue under multivariable analysis is to define our outcome/dependent variable clearly. In view of the specific form of the dependent variable, we decide the method to be used in multivariable analysis. For example, if the dependent variable is continuous, we generally explore the possibility of carrying out multiple linear regression analysis; if the dependent variable is dichotomous (diseased/non-diseased), multiple logistic regression analysis is used; and so on. Sometimes, form of the independent variable also plays a role in deciding the method of data analysis. In summary, the method of data analysis should be decided taking into account all the necessary issues/assumptions.

Once the forms of variables and methods of data analysis are finalized, the next important question is to select sub-group of variables to be finally included in multivariable analysis. Sometimes, we give excessive importance to statistical significance and take the sub-set of independent variables in multivariable analysis only if these are significantly related with the dependent variable. However, to have a better strategy for multivariable modeling, we should also include those variables that are statistically insignificant, but are clinically important. Also, we should consider the known confounders (e.g., age and sex) irrespective of their significance. Moreover, for multivariable analysis, we should prefer a higher level of significance (preferably 25%) to have an appropriate modeling. There are various issues involved in multivariable analysis even after selection of sub-group of independent variables to be included in data analysis. We should explore the presence of collinearity among the covariates and also explore and explain interaction effects of the variables. Amongst various strategies, we should prefer the step-wise regression analysis approach to obtain results comparable to those obtained through all possible regression approach. Efforts should be made to rule out each of the other explanations regarding treatment differences so that effect of each of the treatment may be judged and reported without any ambiguity.

9.8. Interpretation and Reporting of Results

This issue of interpretation and reporting the results is equally important once we have results in our hand. Needless to mention, we have to interpret results in view of our question, design of study, sample size, methodology used in data analysis, and so on. In summary, we can conclude the results of an RCT only if we have got data through a scientifically well planned study, which ideally takes into account aspects like the question under investigation, defined population, sample size, sampling method, method of data collection, design of study, accuracy of data and appropriate analysis. Otherwise, the results may be described only in a suggestive manner with a suggestion for need of another well-planned scientific study.

Table 9.6: Items to include when reporting a randomized trial

Topic	Item	Descriptor	Reported on Page #
TITLE & ABSTRACT	1	How participants were allocated to interventions (*e.g.*, "random allocation", "randomized", or "randomly assigned").	
INTRODUCTION Background	2	Scientific background and explanation of rationale.	
METHODS Participants	3	Eligibility criteria for participants and the settings and locations where the data were collected.	
Interventions	4	Precise details of the interventions intended for each group and how and when they were actually administered.	
Objectives	5	Specific objectives and hypotheses.	
Outcomes	6	Clearly defined primary and secondary outcome measures and, when applicable, any methods used to enhance the quality of measurements (*e.g.*, multiple observations, training of assessors).	
Sample size	7	How sample size was determined and, when applicable, explanation of any interim analyses and stopping rules.	
Randomization-Sequence generation	8	Method used to generate the random allocation sequence, including details of any restrictions (*e.g.*, blocking, stratification)	
Randomization-concealment Allocation	9	Method used to implement the random allocation sequence (*e.g.*, numbered containers or central telephone), clarifying whether the sequence was concealed until interventions were assigned.	
Randomization-implementation	10	Who generated the allocation sequence, who enrolled participants, and who assigned participants to their groups.	
Blinding (masking)	11	Whether or not participants, those administering the interventions, and those assessing the outcomes were blinded to group assignment. If done, how the success of blinding was evaluated.	
Statistical methods	12	Statistical methods used to compare groups for primary outcome(s); Methods for additional analyses, such as subgroup analyses and adjusted analyses.	
RESULTS Participant flow	13	Flow of participants through each stage (a diagram is strongly recommended). Specifically, for each group report the numbers of participants randomly assigned, receiving intended treatment, completing the study protocol, and analyzed for the primary outcome. Describe protocol deviations from study as planned, together with reasons.	
Recruitment	14	Dates defining the periods of recruitment and follow-up.	
Baseline data	15	Baseline demographic and clinical characteristics of each group.	
Numbers analyzed	16	Number of participants (denominator) in each group included in each analysis and whether the analysis was by "intention-to-treat". State the results in absolute numbers when feasible (*e.g.*, 10/20, not 50%).	
Outcomes and estimation	17	For each primary and secondary outcome, a summary of results for each group, and the estimated effect size and its precision (*e.g.*, 95% confidence interval).	
Ancillary analyses	18	Address multiplicity by reporting any other analyses performed, including subgroup analyses and adjusted analyses, indicating those pre-specified and those exploratory.	
Adverse events	19	All important adverse events or side effects in each intervention group.	
DISCUSSION Interpretation	20	Interpretation of the results, taking into account study hypotheses, sources of potential bias or imprecision and the dangers associated with multiplicity of analyses and outcomes.	
Generalizability	21	Generalizability (external validity) of the trial findings.	
Overall evidence	22	General interpretation of the results in the context of current evidence.	

9.8.1. Reporting a Randomized Controlled Trial

This is now a well-known fact that reporting of a RCT should have transparency regarding why the study was undertaken and how it was conducted and analyzed, which may be necessary to comprehend the results of an RCT without ambiguity. To make authors' task easier, a group of investigators and editors of journals have prepared a checklist of items and flow diagram [Begg et al.[11]]. As a convention, this is known as CONSORT (Consolidated Standards of Reporting Trials) statement. To improve the quality of reporting of RCT further, Moher et al.[12] (for the CONSORT Group) revised the checklist of items as well as a flow diagram (Fig. 9.3). The revised checklist provides complete information that is essential to judge the reliability or relevance of the findings. For completeness, the revised checklist of items is reproduced in Table 9.6.

9.8.2. Flow-Diagram

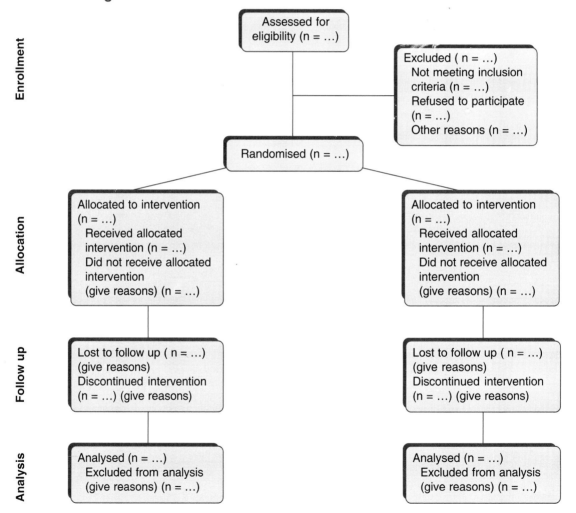

Source: The CONSORT Statement: revised recommendations for improving the quality of reports of parallel-group randomized trials: Moher, David, Altman D.G. et al., *Lancet.* 2001; 357: 1191-94.

Fig. 9.3: Flow diagram

The revised diagram provides information at each of four major stages of the trial (i.e., enrolment, intervention allocation, follow-up, and analysis). The information on the number of participants for each treatment group those were included in the primary data analysis further reveals status about intention to treat analysis. For completeness, the revised flow-diagram is reproduced above. Recently, Piaggio et al.[13] published similar guidelines (an extension of the CONSORT statement) related to reporting of non-inferiority and equivalence randomized trials.

An RCT is considered to be completed as an RCT only if it is carried out in the manner in which it had to be carried out methodologically as written in the protocol. As a matter of fact, such studies that are completed using well-planned scientific methodologies may only be used to generate definite conclusions. Otherwise, conclusive statements should invariably be avoided. All efforts should be made to describe the RCTs as desired under revised checklist of items and also the revised flow diagram.

Multiple Choice Questions

Choose the correct answers in the following multiple choice questions. The correct answers are listed on p. 344.

Q.1. **The number of phases in a typical clinical trial is:**
    a. One   b. Two
    c. Three   d. Four

Q.2. **Randomized controlled trial (RCT) is a typical clinical trial of:**
    a. Phase one   b. Phase two
    c. Phase three   d. Phase four

Q.3. **When each of the participants receive each treatment under the clinical trial, the design is called:**
    a. Parallel design   b. Balanced design
    c. Cross-over design   d. Block design

Q.4. **The term wash out period is used in:**
    a. Parallel design   b. Balanced design
    c. Cross-over design   d. Block design

Q.5. **Kaplan-Meir method is used in clinical trial for:**
    a. Sensitivity analysis   b. Cross-over design data analysis
    c. Survival analysis   d. Risk analysis

Q.6. **To test the statistical significance of the difference in survival experiences in patients between two treatment groups, the statistical test usually applied is:**
    a. Student's t-test   b. Chi-square test
    c. Anova   d. Log rank test

Q.7. **If the analysis of data is done as per the original treatment allocation the analysis is called:**
    a. Interim analysis   b. Intention to treat analysis
    c. As per protocol analysis   d. Hazard analysis

Q.8. **NNT (number needed to treat) is computed based on:**
    a. Odds ratio   b. Risk ratio
    c. Absolute risk reduction   d. Attributable risk ratio

Q.9. **Trials which are conducted for prevention of disease are called:**
    a. Clinical trial   b. Laboratory trial
    c. Prophylactic trial   d. Hospital based trial

Q.10. **When each of the participants in a clinical trial receives only one treatment, the design is called:**
    a. Cross-over design   b. Block design
    c. Parallel design   d. Balanced design

References

1. Altman DG. *Practical Statistics for Medical Research*. New Delhi: Chapman and Hall, India; 1991: 514-517.
2. Armitage P, Berry G, Matthews JNS. *Statistical Methods in Medical Research*. 4th ed. London: Blackwell Science Ltd.; 2002.
3. Pocock Stuart J. *Clinical Trials: A practical Approach*. New York: John Wiley & Sons; 1983.
4. Collett David. *Modelling Binary Data*. 2nd ed. London: Chapman & Hall/ CRC; 2003.
5. Kleinbaum DG, Klein M. *Logistic Regression: A Self Learning*. 2nd ed. London: Springer; 2002
6. Wright Susan. *Social Science Statistics*. Allyn and Bacon; 1986.
7. Collett David. *Modelling Survival Data in Medical Research*. 2nd ed. London: Chapman & Hall/ CRC; 2003.
8. Kleinbaum DG. *Survival Analysis: A Self-learning Text*. New York: Springer; 1996
9. Jones Byron, Kenward Michael G. *Design and Analysis of Cross-Over Trials*. 2nd ed. New York: Chapman Hall/ CRC; 2003.
10. Chow Shein Chung, Liu Jen Pei. *Design and Analysis of Clinical Trials*. New York: John Wiley; 2004
11. Begg Colin, Cho Mildred et al. Improving the quality of reporting of randomized controlled trials: The CONSORT Statement. *JAMA*. 1996; 276 (8): 637-39.
12. Moher David, Altman DG et al. The CONSORT Statement: revised recommendations for improving the quality of reports of parallel-group randomized trials. *Lancet*. 2001; 357: 1191-94
13. Piaggio Gilda, Elbourne Diana R, Altman Douglas G, Pocock Stuart J, Evans Stephen J W. Reporting of noninferiority and equivalence randomized trials: an extension of the CONSORT Statement. *JAMA*. 2006; 295: 1152-1160.

10 | Estimation of Sample Size

- Importance of sample size in research design
- Methods of calculating minimum sample size
- Estimation of mean, comparison of two means
- Estimation of proportion, comparison of two proportions
- Cluster surveys, expanded programme on immunization, nutritional anthropometry surveys
- Estimating an odds ratio with specified relative precision, tests of significance for odds ratio
- Estimating relative risk with specified relative precision, tests of significance for a relative risk
- Tests of equivalence of two treatments, equivalence of two means, equivalence of two proportions
- Comparison of two survival curves, comparison of two survival rates, comparison of two median survival times
- Comparison of a population proportion with a given proportion

Everything should be made as simple as possible, but not simpler.

Albert Einstein

10.1. Importance of Sample Size in Research Design

To carry out any scientific study, two commonly asked general questions are: what should be the minimum sample size? And which method of sampling should be used to draw the desired sample out of the study population? Methods of sampling have already been discussed in Chapter 2. This chapter is aimed at addressing the first question posed above. Moher, Dulberg and Wells[1] reviewed the reporting of minimum sample size calculation while planning the studies with special reference to clinical trials and came out with the observation that hardly one-fourth of the studies reported this aspect. Too small a sample is one of the most common problems, which is especially seen in randomized controlled clinical trials. Larger sample size is known to increase the power of the study. If no difference between treatment effects is seen, it could be because the sample was so small that it did not have enough power to detect a true difference. Even in a study with adequate power to evaluate the primary outcome, the sample size may be inadequate for secondary outcomes or subgroup comparisons. The ultimate goal of achieving optimum sensitivity in terms of power and confidence in an experiment requires consideration of the optimum number of subjects included (i.e., minimum sample size).

The studies with smaller or larger sample sizes than actually required (minimum sample size for a specified power and confidence) have several disadvantages. We are very often unaware of the disadvantages and consider the sample size as per our convenience or because of various constraints. Studies small in size fail to detect actual differences in the outcome of interest between the groups, or may estimate those outcomes too imprecisely. A study that is unnecessarily large in size may be a waste of scarce resources and may even lead to loss in accuracy, as it is often more difficult to maintain data quality and high coverage rates in a larger study than in a smaller one. But, a study with small sample size may not have its desired power, which may lead to inaccurate results leading to contradictory implications. Therefore, it is a wise step to decide about the required minimum sample size in a scientific manner at the planning stage itself. This will decrease the standard error and, hence, increase our ability to detect true treatment difference. In the absence of required minimum sample size, the experiment has a poor chance of detecting true treatment differences and would be inconclusive. A similar view is true in case of other study designs also. Thus, determining the minimum sample size required for a scientific study is an important component of a research design. This necessitates inclusion of a separate section on calculation of minimum sample size in research proposals/reports and research articles.

The minimum required sample size has to be calculated taking into account various inputs based on specific objectives. The investigator must consider whether the type of considered outcome variable is quantitative (i.e., continuous such as birth weight of a new born) or qualitative (i.e., dichotomous such as death/alive, a condition being present/absent). A rough idea about the outcome index is one of the important inputs for the sample size calculation. This has to be decided by the investigator on the basis of his own previous work or review of the literature on the subject. In case of outcome variable being quantitative, generally mean and standard deviation would be the required summary measures, while for a qualitative outcome variable, proportions and standard deviation would be needed.

An investigator may plan a study with research question that response to new treatment B may be different from that to the standard treatment A. This statement would be framed as an alternative hypothesis, while the null hypothesis would be that the difference between the responses to the two treatments is not significant statistically or the difference between outcome measures in the two groups is due to chance alone. Another input inversely related to the sample size is the amount of difference to be regarded as clinically important. In addition, desired relative/ absolute allowable error of the estimate is also required.

Two other inputs, which are based on statistical considerations, are level of confidence and/ or power of the study. Such studies that involve testing of hypothesis (e.g., clinical trials generally involve testing of hypothesis) have involvement of both — level of confidence as well as power of the study — in the minimum sample size calculation. On the other hand, a study involving only estimation (e.g., prevalence of a disease), involves only level of confidence, in minimum sample size calculation. These inputs may further be explained again as tabulated below:

Decision taken by the researcher	Truth	
	H_0	H_1
Treatment B # Treatment A (H_1)	Type-I Error	Correct Decision (Power of the study)
Treatment B = Treatment A (H_0)	Correct Decision (Level of Confidence)	Type-II Error

In a study, no investigator can be 100% sure that the decision taken is correct. Therefore, at the time of sample size calculation, considerable levels of the two types of possible errors are incorporated. First is to specify the amount of error one is prepared to tolerate in concluding that a difference exists when in fact there is no difference. This is known as chance or 'Type-I error'. As described earlier, the chance of committing Type-I error is denoted by α. While there is no hard and fast rule regarding choosing α level, conventionally it is taken as 0.05. Attempt is made to take α as small as possible (e.g., 0.01, 0.001) which helps in maintaining higher level of confidence (i.e., $1-\alpha$).

Secondly, the investigator has to specify the amount of error he is prepared to tolerate in concluding that the difference between the two groups does not exist when in fact the difference exists. In statistical terms, it has been labeled as chance of Type-II error that is denoted by β. Any investigator would like to maximize the probability of concluding that the difference in the two groups exits when the difference truly exists. This corresponds to the concept of power of the study $(1-\beta)$. Usually, β is selected to be 0.10 or 0.20, i.e., power of the study as 0.90 (90%) or 0.80 (80%), respectively.

The value of area under the normal curve (Z) at a considered level of significance depends on whether two-sided or one-sided tests are to be carried out. They are denoted by Z1-α/2 and Z1-α, respectively. Hence, sample size requirement for a two-sided test will be higher than that for a one-sided test. However, this remains the same in either of the cases at a considered power of the study and is denoted by Z1-β. These values corresponding to the commonly used values of significance level (α) and power $(1-\beta)$ that are necessary statistical inputs for sample size calculation are listed below:

		Z-Value	
		Two-sided test	One-sided test
		Z1-α/2	Z1-α
Significance level	0.01	2.576	2.326
	0.05	1.960	1.645
	0.10	1.645	1.282
		Z1-β	
Power	0.80	0.842	
	0.90	1.282	
	0.95	1.645	
	0.99	2.326	

Some of the commonly used methods of minimum sample size calculation are described below. To clarify the involved issues further, for each of them, a worked example is also given.

10.2. Methods of Calculating Minimum Sample Size

10.2.1. Estimation of Mean

To calculate sample size requirement for estimating mean of a quantitative variable in a study population, required inputs are:
  (a) Expected mean of the variable in the study group = $\bar{x}$
  (b) Expected standard deviation of the variable in group = s
  (c) Expected absolute allowable error in the mean = d (e.g., for 10% relative allowable error as 10% of $\bar{x}$)
  (d) Value of the normal deviate at considered level of confidence = Z1-α/2
  Accordingly,
  Sample size (n) = $[\{Z1-\alpha/2\}^2 s^2] / d^2$ (10.1)

Example 1:
To estimate hemoglobin level (g/dl) among pregnant women of a community, it was expected that the mean and standard deviation of hemoglobin in pregnant women from the considered community were about 10.3 and 2.3 (g/dl), respectively. Then, at $\alpha = 0.05$ and relative allowable error 10%, how many pregnant women from the community should be studied?
  Calculation: Given inputs are:

Mean ($\bar{x}$) = 10.3, standard deviation (s) = 2.3,
Z1-α/2 = Z1-(0.05/2) = 1.96, d = (10/100)*10.3 = 1.03
Therefore, the required sample size is:
Sample size (n) = [{Z1-α/2}^{2} s^2] / d^2
$$= [(1.96)^2 * (2.3)^2] / (1.03)^2$$
$$= 19$$
Thus, a total of at least 19 pregnant women need to be studied.
Accordingly, after rounding off, 20 pregnant women may be included in the study.

10.2.2. Comparison of Two Means

To calculate sample size requirement for comparing means of a quantitative variable between treatment and control groups, required inputs are:
(e) Mean of the variable in group 1 = $\bar{x}_1$
(f) Mean of the variable in group 2 = $\bar{x}_2$
(g) Standard deviation of the variable in group 1 = s_1
(h) Standard deviation of the variable in group 2 = s_2
(e) Value of the normal deviate at considered level of confidence = Z1-α/2 (Two-sided test)
$$= Z1\text{-}\alpha \text{ (One-sided test)}$$
(f) Value of the normal deviate at considered power of the study = Z1-β

(i) For a two-sided test:

$$Sample\ size\ (n) = (s_1^2 + s_2^2) \frac{[Z1 - \alpha/2 + Z1 - \beta]^2}{(\bar{x}_1 - \bar{x}_2)^2} \qquad (10.2)$$

(ii) For a one-sided test:

$$Sample\ size\ (n) = (s_1^2 + s_2^2) \frac{[Z1 - \alpha + Z1 - \beta]^2}{(\bar{x}_1 - \bar{x}_2)^2} \qquad (10.3)$$

Example 2:
A study to see the effect of iron supplements for a specific period on hemoglobin level among pregnant women of a community has to be carried out. Under a preliminary study or as reported in the literature, it was observed that the standard deviation of hemoglobin in pregnant women from a similar community with an intervention was 2.3 (g/dl), while that without intervention was 3.4 (g/dl). If α = 0.05 and β = 0. 20, how many pregnant women from each group should be studied if one wants to detect a difference of 2.0 (g/dl) in hemoglobin in the two groups?

Calculation: Given inputs are:
($\bar{x}_1$-$\bar{x}_2$) = 2.0, s_1 = 2.3 and s_2 = 3.4
Z1-α/2 = Z1-(0.05/2) = 1.96, Z1-α = Z1-0.05 = 1.64,
Power of the test (1-β) = 80%, i.e., Z1-β = 0.842.
Therefore, the required sample size is:

(a) For a two-sided test:

$$n = (s_1^2 + s_2^2) \frac{[Z1 - \alpha/2 + Z1 - \beta]^2}{(\bar{x}_1 - \bar{x}_2)^2}$$

$$= (5.29 + 11.56) * [\{1.96 + 0.842\}^2] / (2)^2 = 33$$

(b) For a one-sided test:

$$n = (s_1^2 + s_2^2) \frac{[Z1 - \alpha + Z1 - \beta]^2}{(\bar{x}_1 - \bar{x}_2)^2}$$

$= (5.29 + 11.56) * [\{1.64 + 0.842\}^2 / (2)^2 = 26$

Therefore, for a two-sided test, a minimum of 33 pregnant women from each group and in the case of a one-sided test, a minimum of 26 pregnant women from each group would be required to be included in the study. Hence, sample size for a two-sided test may be fixed as 35 from each group, whereas that for one-sided test may be fixed as 30 from each group. It may be noted that the required sample size is smaller in the case of one-tailed test compared to that for two-tailed test.

10.2.3. Estimation of Proportion (i.e., Prevalence Study)

To calculate sample size requirement for estimating prevalence of a qualitative event in a population, required inputs are:

    (i)   Expected prevalence of the event in the study group = p
    (j)   Expected absolute allowable error in the p = d (e.g., for 10% relative allowable error as 10% of p)
    (k) Value of the normal deviate at considered level of confidence = Z1-α/2

Accordingly, the required sample size will be,

$$n = z_{1-\alpha/2}^2 \, p(1-p)/d^2 \tag{10.4}$$

Example 3:

The current prevalence of malaria in a community is expected to be around 40%. Hence, to estimate the current prevalence of malaria in that community, how many persons should be included in the study at 5% level of significance and absolute allowable error as 10%?

Calculation: Given inputs are:

$p = 0.40$, $Z_{1-\alpha/2} = Z_{1-(0.05)/2} = 1.96$, absolute allowable error (d) = 0.10.
Therefore, the required sample size is:

$n = z_{1-\alpha/2}^2 \, p(1-p)/d^2$
$\quad = [(1.96)^2 * 0.40 * 0.60]/(0.10)^2 = 92$

Thus, a minimum of 92 people should be included in the study. Accordingly, 95 persons may be included in the study.

10.2.4. Comparison of Two Proportions

To calculate sample size requirement for comparing proportions of a qualitative event between two groups (e.g., treatment and control groups), required inputs are:

    (a) Anticipated prevalence of event in group 1 = p_1
    (b) Anticipated prevalence of event in group 2 = p_2
    (c) Value of the normal deviate at considered level of confidence = Z1-α/2 (two-sided test)
                                              = Z1-α (one-sided test)
    (d) Value of the normal deviate at considered power of the study = Z1-β

Accordingly, minimum sample size may be calculated as:

(i) For a two-sided test:

$$n = \frac{\left[Z1 - \alpha/2.\sqrt{\{2p(1\text{-}p)\}} + Z1 - \beta\sqrt{\{p_1(1-p_1) + p_2(1-p_2)\}}\right]^2}{(p_1 - p_2)^2} \tag{10.5}$$

where p = $(p_1 - p_2)^2$

(ii) For a one-sided test:

$$n = \frac{\left[Z1-\alpha. \sqrt{\{2p(1-p)\}} + Z1-\beta \sqrt{\{p_1(1-p_1)+p_2(1-p_2)\}} \right]^2}{(p_1-p_2)^2} \tag{10.6}$$

where $p = (p_1 + p_2)/2$

Example 4:

Children attending public schools have expected dental problem among them as 80%. In another group of children attending government/municipal corporation schools, 70% are expected to have this problem. How many children should be included from each group to determine whether this difference is significant at 5% level if we wish to have 80% chance of detecting the difference if it is real?

Calculation:

(a) For a two-sided test:

Known inputs are:

$p_1 = 0.8$, $p_2 = 0.7$, $p = (0.8+0.7)/2 = 0.75$,

$z_{1-\alpha/2} = z_{1-(0.05)/2} = 1.96$, power $(z_{1-\beta}) = 0.842$.

Therefore, the required sample size is:

$$n = \frac{\left[Z1-\alpha/2. \sqrt{\{2p(1-p)\}} + Z1-\beta \sqrt{\{p_1(1-p_1)+p_2(1-p_2)\}} \right]^2}{(p_1-p_2)^2}$$

$$= [1.96\sqrt{\{2(0.75)(1-0.75)\}} + 0.842\sqrt{\{(0.8)(1-0.8)+(0.7)(1-0.7)\}}]^2/(0.8-0.7)^2$$

$$= 294$$

Therefore, at least 294 children should be included from each group. Accordingly 295 children from each group may be included in the study.

(i) For a one-sided test:

Known inputs are:

$p_1 = 0.8$, $p_2 = 0.7$, $p = (0.8+0.7)/2 = 0.75$,

$z_{1-\alpha/2} = z_{1-0.05} = 1.64$, power $(z_{1-\beta}) = 0.842$.

Therefore, the required sample size is:

$$n = \frac{\left[Z1-\alpha. \sqrt{\{2p(1-p)\}} + Z1-\beta \sqrt{\{p_1(1-p_1)+p_2(1-p_2)\}} \right]^2}{(p_1-p_2)^2}$$

$$= [1.64\sqrt{\{2(0.75)(1-0.75)\}} + 0.842\sqrt{\{0.8)(1-0.8)+(0.7)(1-0.7)\}}]^2/(0.8-0.7)^2$$

$$= 233$$

Hence, a minimum of 233 children should be included from each group. Thus, 235 children from each group may be included in the study.

10.2.5. Cluster Surveys

The above-mentioned methods of sample size calculation provide required minimum sample size in case simple random sampling method is used. However, because of unavoidable reasons, sometimes other methods like cluster random sampling are preferred. As a result of this, as described in Chapter 2, same precision may not be achieved as under simple random sampling method. Hence, to overcome this problem, calculated sample size has to be adjusted in view of the design effect (DEFF) that may be calculated as ratio of expected variance under used sampling design to that under simple random sampling method. The earlier calculated sample size has to be multiplied by the design effect. Accordingly, we can get modified form of the formulae used in sample size calculation. For example, section 10.2.2.1 may be modified as:

$$n = \left[z_{1-\alpha/2}^2 p(1-p)/d^2 \right] * DEFF \qquad (10.7)$$

As reported by Sullivan et al.[2] (1995), in most of the surveys including immunization and nutrition surveys, design effect is usually taken as around two. However, if there is a large difference in the proportion of events from one cluster to another, say 90% in some clusters and 10% in others, then the design effect may be more than two. Accordingly, the earlier calculated sample size has to be multiplied by the design effect that usually varies between 2 and 4 (Sullivan et al., 1995). In example 3, considering design effect as two because of cluster sampling, there will be need to cover twice the earlier suggested sample size, that is 190 persons.

Further, in case of unknown p, 0.5 (or 50%) is used which produces largest sample size for given values of z and d. Further, if p is expected to be between two values, e.g., 15% & 30%, the value closest to 50% may be preferred, e.g., 30% here.

10.2.5.1. *Standard surveys*
Example 5:
As described by Sullivan et al.[2] (1995), the sample size traditionally used in EPI and nutritional anthropometry surveys are based on the following considerations:
(i) Expanded programme on immunization
For this, following considerations are made:
p = 50%
At 95% confidence, Z = 1.96
d = 10% (Relative allowable error as 20% of 50%)
DEFF = 2
Accordingly, n = 193
If 30-clusters are to be considered, as in case of EPI survey, one has to cover approximately:
(193/ 30) = 7 children per cluster
(ii) Nutritional anthropometry surveys:
For this, the following considerations are made:
p = 50%,
At 95% confidence, Z = 1.96
d = 5% (Relative precision as 10%)
DEFF = 2
Accordingly, n = 768
If 30-clusters are to be considered, as in the case of nutrition survey, one has to cover approximately: (768/ 30) =26 children per cluster.
However, 30 children per cluster are usually covered.

10.2.6. Estimating an Odds Ratio with Specified Relative Precision

To carry out a case control study described in Chapter 8 with an objective to estimate an odds ratio, any two of the following should be known:
(i) Anticipated probability of "exposure" for cases (i.e., people with the disease) = p_1
(ii) Anticipated probability of "exposure" for controls (i.e., people without the disease) = p_2
(iii) Anticipated odds ratio = OR = $[p_1/(1-p_1)]/[p_2/(1-p_2)]$
From this, one can obtain (Lwanga and Lemeshow, 1991) the following relationship:
$$p_2 = p_1 /[OR(1-p_1] + p_1)$$

And the following:

(iv) Value of the normal deviate at considered level of confidence = Z1-α/2

(v) Relative allowable error = d_1

Then, required minimum sample size may be calculated as:

$$n = z^2_{1-\alpha/2}\{1/[p_1(1-p_1)]+1/[p_2(1-p_2)]\}/[\log_e(1-d_1)]^2 \qquad (10.8)$$

Example 6:

An anticipated probability of being smoker among patients of coronary heart disease is 70%. To estimate an anticipated odds ratio as 2.5 in comparison to controls, calculate required minimum sample size at 95% confidence level, if the desired relative allowable error has to be within 25% of the true odds ratio.

Calculation:

Known inputs are:

p_1, = 0.70, OR= 2.5, relative allowable error (d_1) = 0.25

$z_{1-\alpha/2} = z_{1-(0.05)/2} = 1.96$

$p_2 = p_1/[OR(1-p_1) + p_1]$

= 0.70/[2.5(1–0.70) + 0.70] = 0.4827

Therefore, the required sample size is:

$$n = z^2_{1-\alpha/2}\{1/[p_1(1-p_1)]+1/[p_2(1-p_2)]\}/[\log_e(1-d_1)]^2$$
$$= (1.96)^2\ \{1/[0.70(1–0.70)] + 1/[0.48(1–0.48)]\}/[\log_e(1–0.25)]^2$$
$$= 407$$

Thus, a minimum of 407 cases and 407 controls should be included in the study. Accordingly, 410 cases and equal number of controls may be covered in the study.

10.2.7. Test of Significance for an Odds Ratio

To carry out a case-control study described in Chapter 8 with an objective to test an odds ratio, as in case of estimation of odds ratio, any two of the following should be known:

(i)   Anticipated probability of "exposure" for cases (i.e., people with the disease) = p_1

(ii) Anticipated probability of "exposure" for controls (i.e., people without the disease) = p_2

(iii) Anticipated odds ratio = OR = $[p_1/(1-p_1)]/[p_2/(1-p_2)]$

From this, one can obtain (e.g., Lwanga and Lemeshow, 1991) the following relationship:

$p_2 = p_1/[OR(1-p_1) + p_1]$

And the following:

(iv) Value of the normal deviate at considered level of confidence = Z1-α/2 (Two-sided test)

= Z1-α (One-sided test)

(v) Value of the normal deviate at considered power of the study =Z1-β

Then, minimum sample size may be calculated as:

(i) For two-sided test:

$$n = \left\{z_{1-\alpha/2}\sqrt{\left[2p_2\left(1-p_2\right)\right]} + z_{1-\beta}\sqrt{\left[p_1\left(1-p_1\right) + p_2\left(1-p_2\right)\right]}\right\}^2 / \left(p_1 - p_2\right)^2 \qquad (10.9)$$

(ii) For one-sided test:

$$n = \left\{z_{1-\alpha}\sqrt{\left[2p_2\left(1-p_2\right)\right]} + z_{1-\beta}\sqrt{\left[p_1\left(1-p_1\right) + p_2\left(1-p_2\right)\right]}\right\}^2 / \left(p_1 - p_2\right)^2 \qquad (10.10)$$

Example 7:

Available information indicates that about 60% of the HIV positive people indulge in oral sex. Further, an odds ratio for indulging in oral sex is anticipated as 4 among HIV positive people in comparison to healthy controls. To test its significance at 5% level and with 80% power, how many cases (i.e., HIV positive) and controls (i.e., HIV negative) should be included in the study?

Calculation:

Known inputs are:

$p_1 = 0.60$, OR= 4.0

$z_{1-\alpha/2} = z_{1-(0.05)/2} = 1.96$, $z_{1-\alpha} = z_{1-0.05} = 1.64$, $z_{1-\beta} = 0.842$

$p_2 = p_1/[OR(1 - p_1) + p_1)$

$= 0.60/[4.0(1 - 0.60) + 0.60] = 0.2727$

(i) For a two-sided test:

$$n = \left\{ z_{1-\alpha/2} \sqrt{\left[2p_2\left(1 - p_2\right) \right]} + z_{1-\beta} \sqrt{\left[p_1\left(1 - p_1\right) + p_2\left(1 - p_2\right) \right]} \right\}^2 / \left(p_1 - p_2\right)^2$$

$$= \left\{ 1.96\sqrt{\left[2*0.27\left(1 - 0.27\right) \right]} + 0.842\sqrt{\left[0.60\left(1 - 0.60\right) + 0.27\left(1 - 0.27\right) \right]} \right\}^2 / \left(0.60 - 0.27\right)^2$$

$$= 29$$

Thus, in case of two-sided test, a minimum of 29 cases and 29 controls should be included in the study. Accordingly, 30 cases and 30 controls may be included in the study.

(i) For a one-sided test:

$$n = \left\{ z_{1-\alpha} \sqrt{\left[2p_2\left(1 - p_2\right) \right]} + z_{1-\beta} \sqrt{\left[p_1\left(1 - p_1\right) + p_2\left(1 - p_2\right) \right]} \right\}^2 / \left(p_1 - p_2\right)^2$$

$$= \left\{ 1.64\sqrt{\left[2*0.27\left(1 - 0.27\right) \right]} + 0.842\sqrt{\left[0.60\left(1 - 0.60\right) + 0.27\left(1 - 0.27\right) \right]} \right\}^2 / \left(0.60 - 0.27\right)^2$$

$$= 23$$

Thus, in case of one-sided test, a minimum of 23 cases and 23 controls should be included in the study. Accordingly, 25 cases and 25 controls may be included in the study.

10.2.8. Estimating a Relative Risk with Specified Relative Precision

To carry out a cohort study described in Chapter 8 with an objective to estimate a relative risk, any two of the following should be known:

(i)   Anticipated probability of disease/ event in people exposed to the factor of interest = p_1

(ii) Anticipated probability of disease/ event in people not exposed to the factor of interest = p_2

(iii) Anticipated relative risk = $RR = p_1/p_2$

And the following:

(iv) Value of the normal deviate at considered level of confidence = Z1-α/2

(vi) Relative allowable error = d_1

Then, required minimum sample size may be calculated as:

$$n = z^2_{1\alpha/2} \, [(1 - p_1)/p_1 + (1 - p_2)/p_2]/[\log_e (1 - d_1)]^2 \qquad (10.11)$$

Example 8:

As per a newspaper report, in general, 5% males in Delhi are found infertile. There is need to carry out an epidemiological study to estimate the relative risk of infertility among males due to an exposure of keeping mobile phones inside pockets of the trousers. At 95% confidence level, what sample size would be needed in each of the two groups, exposed and not exposed, to estimate the relative risk within 50% of the true value that is anticipated to be 2?

Calculation:

Known inputs are:

$p_2 = 0.05$ (expected same as in general male population), RR = 2, relative precision (d_1) = 0.5

$z_{1-\alpha/2} = z_{1-(0.05)/2} = 1.96$

We can calculate,

p_1 [RR* $p_2 = 2*0.05 = 0.1$

Therefore, the required sample size is:

$n = z^2_{1\alpha/2} [(1 - p_1)/p_1 + (1 - p_2)/p_2]/[\log_e (1 - d_1)]^2$

$= (1.96)^2 [1 - 0.1)/0.1 + (1 - 0.05)/0.05]/[\log_e (1 - 0.5)^2 = 224$

Thus, a minimum of 224 persons from exposed and 224 from unexposed population should be included in the study. Accordingly, 225 persons from each group should be included in the study.

10.2.9. Test of Significance for a Relative Risk

To carry out a cohort study described in Chapter 8 with the objective to test a relative risk, any two of the following should be known:

(i) Anticipated probability of disease/ event in people exposed to the factor of interest = p_1

(ii) Anticipated probability of disease/ event in people not exposed to the factor of interest = p_2

(iii) Anticipated relative risk = $RR = p_1/p_2$

And the following:

(iv) Value of the normal deviate at considered level of confidence = Z1-α/2 (two-sided test)

= Z1-α (one-sided test)

(v) Value of the normal deviate at considered power of the study =Z1-β

Then, required minimum sample size may be calculated as:

(i) For a two-sided test:

$$n = \left\{ z_{1-\alpha/2} \sqrt{\left[2\bar{p}(1-\bar{p}) \right]} + z_{1-\beta} \sqrt{\left[p_1(1-p_1) + p_2(1-p_2) \right]} \right\}^2 / (p_1 - p_2)^2 \qquad (10.12)$$

(ii) For a one-sided test:

$$n = \left\{ z_{1-\alpha} \sqrt{\left[2\bar{p}(1-\bar{p}) \right]} + z_{1-\beta} \sqrt{\left[p_1(1-p_1) + p_2(1-p_2) \right]} \right\}^2 / (p_1 - p_2)^2 \qquad (10.13)$$

Example 9:

After exposure of a group of population to toxic gas, an epidemiological cohort study is required to see whether this exposure significantly increases the risk of chest disease after one year. The reported probability of chest disease among unexposed population is 20%. If the exposure is known to double the relative risk of suffering from chest disease (i.e., RR = 2), how many individuals should be included from each of the two groups (i.e., exposed and unexposed) so that one can be 80% confident of correctly rejecting the null hypothesis (i.e., RR = 1), the null hypothesis being tested at 5% level of significance?

Calculation:

Known inputs are:

$p_2 = 0.2$, RR = 2.0

$z_{1-\alpha/2} = z_{1-(0.05)/2} = 1.96$, $z_{1-\alpha} = z_{1-0.05} = 1.64$, $z_{1-\beta} = 0.842$

$p_1 = RR * p_2 = 2.0*0.2 = 0.4$, $\bar{p} = \dfrac{(p_1 - p_2)}{2} = \dfrac{(0.4 + 0.2)}{2} = 0.3$

Therefore, the required sample size is:
(i) For a two-sided test:

$$n = \left\{ z_{1-\alpha/2} \sqrt{\left[2\bar{p}(1-\bar{p}) \right]} + z_{1-\beta} \sqrt{\left[p_1(1-p_1) + p_2(1-p_2) \right]} \right\}^2 / (p_1 - p_2)^2$$

$$= \left\{ 1.96 \sqrt{2*0.3(1-0.3)} + 0.842 \sqrt{\left[0.4(1-0.4) + 0.2(1-0.2) \right]} \right\}^2 / (0.4 - 0.2)^2$$

$$= 82$$

Thus, in case of two-sided test, a minimum of 82 people from exposed group and 124 from unexposed group should be included in the study. Accordingly, 85 people from exposed group and 85 from unexposed group may be included in the study.

(ii) For a one-sided test:

$$n = \left\{ z_{1-\alpha} \sqrt{\left[2\bar{p}(1-\bar{p}) \right]} + z_{1-\beta} \sqrt{\left[p_1(1-p_1) + p_2(1-p_2) \right]} \right\}^2 / (p_1 - p_2)^2$$

$$= \left\{ 1.64 \sqrt{2*0.3(1-0.3)} + 0.842 \sqrt{\left[0.4(1-0.4) + 0.2(1-0.2) \right]} \right\}^2 / (0.4 - 0.2)^2$$

$$= 64$$

Thus, in case of one-sided test, a minimum of 64 people from exposed group and 64 from unexposed group should be included in the study. Accordingly, 65 people from exposed group and 65 from unexposed group may be included in the study.

10.2.10. Testing Equivalence of Two Treatments

As described in Chapter 9, sometimes one may be interested in showing that the new treatment is equivalent in efficacy to the standard treatment. It is always not necessary to establish superiority through comparison of means/ proportions, especially when the standard treatment is invasive, expensive and/ or toxic. Also, the new treatment may have lesser side effects, may be cheaper and / or easy to adopt. Further, equivalence does not mean to find a non-significant difference in the means/ proportions. Also, one can calculate the confidence interval at a considered level of confidence that will cover the true difference in means/ proportions. However, for equivalence, one needs to specify a limit of difference between means/ proportions within which two means/ proportions will be considered equivalent, and to specify power of the study at which the confidence limit will not exceed this specified value. To be more specific, under testing of equivalence, there is involvement of an additional parameter "d" that indicates the maximum clinical difference allowed for an experimental treatment to be considered equivalent with a standard treatment.

In other words, under equivalence, attempt is made only to demonstrate that the new treatment is not significantly worse than the standard treatment. Accordingly, one does not try to prove that the new treatment is better than the standard treatment. Hence, this supports consideration of one-sided tests. Also, under such circumstances, there may not be serious error in consideration of increased level of significance because of its only consequence to keep the patients on the standard treatment (Machin and Campbell, 1987).

10.2.10.1. Equivalence of two means

To calculate sample size requirement in order to test the equivalence of means of a quantitative variable between two groups (e.g., standard treatment and new treatment), required inputs are:

    (i)   Anticipated mean of the variable in standard treatment group = m_1
    (ii) Anticipated mean of the variable in new treatment group = m_2
    (iii) Anticipated variance of the variable in standard treatment group = v_1

(iv) Anticipated variance of the variable in new treatment group = v_2

(v) Considered maximum difference between means within which two means will be considered equivalent = d

(vi) Value of the normal deviate at considered level of confidence = Z1-α (one-sided test)

(vii) Value of the normal deviate at considered power of the study = Z1-β

Accordingly, minimum sample size may be calculated as:

$$n = \frac{\left(z_{1-\alpha} + z_{1-\beta}\right)^2 \left[v_1 + v_2\right]}{\left[d - \left(m_1 - m_2\right)\right]^2}$$

(10-14)

Example 10:

Average change in blood sugar level of a group of diabetic patients through standard treatment is 20.5 mg%, with standard deviation of 5.0 mg%. Another group of similar patients through new treatment is expected to show an average change of 15.0 mg%, with standard deviation of 5.5 mg%. The maximum clinical difference allowed for new treatment to be considered equivalent with the standard treatment is 7.0 mg%. How many patients should be covered for each group in the study with an objective of equivalence of new treatment with standard treatment at 95% confidence level and 80% power of the study?

Calculation:

Given inputs are:

$m_1 = 20.5$, $m_2 = 15.0$, $v_1 = 25$, $v_2 = 30.25$, $d = 7$

$z_{1-\alpha/2} = z_{1-0.10} = 1.282$, $z_{1-\beta} = 0.842$

Therefore, the required sample size is:

$$n = \frac{\left(z_{1-\alpha} + z_{1-\beta}\right)^2 \left[v_1 + v_2\right]}{\left[d - \left(m_1 - m_2\right)\right]^2}$$

$$= \frac{\left(1.282 + 0.842\right)^2 \left[25 + 30.25\right]}{\left[7 - \left(20.5 - 15\right)\right]^2}$$

$$= 111$$

Thus, a minimum of 111 patients should be included in each treatment group of the study. Accordingly, 115 patients may be included in each treatment group.

10.2.10.2. Equivalence of two proportions

To calculate sample size requirement for testing equivalence of proportions of an event between two groups (e.g., standard treatment and new treatment), required inputs are:

(i) Anticipated event rate during a fixed period in standard treatment group = p_1

(ii) Anticipated event rate during a fixed period in new treatment group = p_2

(iii) Considered limit of difference between proportions within which two proportions will be considered equivalent = d

(iv) Value of the normal deviate at considered level of confidence = Z1-α (one-sided test)

(v) Value of the normal deviate at considered power of the study = Z1-β

Accordingly, minimum sample size may be calculated as:

$$n = \frac{\left(z_{1-\alpha} + z_{1-\beta}\right)^2 \left[p_1\left(1 - p_1\right) + p_2\left(1 - p_2\right)\right]}{\left[d - \left(p_1 - p_2\right)\right]^2}$$

(10-15)

Example 11:

The general understanding is that higher the iodine radioactive dose, higher will be the remnant ablation achieved among thyroid cancer patients. In view of the fact that higher dose will require hospitalization of the patients and may also lead to side effects, one wants to assess equivalence of lower dose with higher dose. It is anticipated that higher dose will result in ablation among 80%, whereas lower dose will result in ablation among 74%. The lower dose would be considered equivalent to higher dose if the achieved ablation in this group is at most 10% less than that under higher dose. To test this equivalence, how many patients are required in each group if $\alpha = 0.10$ (one-sided) and $\beta = 0.20$?

Calculation:

Known inputs are:

$p_1 = 0.80$, $p_2 = 0.74$, d = 0.10

$z_{1-\alpha} = z_{1-0.10} = 1.282$, $z_{1-\beta} = 0.842$

Therefore, the required sample size is:

$$n = \frac{\left(z_{1-\alpha} + z_{1-\beta}\right)^2 \left[p_1\left(1-p_1\right) + p_2\left(1-p_2\right)\right]}{\left[d - \left(p_1 - p_2\right)\right]^2}$$

$$= \frac{(1.282 + 0.842)^2 \left[0.80(1-0.80) + 0.74(1-0.74)\right]}{\left[0.10 - (0.80 - 0.74)\right]^2}$$

$$= 994$$

Thus, for an equivalence trial involving proportions, a minimum of 994 patients in standard treatment group and 994 in the new treatment group should be included in the study. Accordingly, 995 patients for each group may be selected in the study.

10.2.11. Comparison of Two Survival Curves

In contrast to simple comparison of two proportions described in section 10.2.4, sometimes under cohort studies and /or clinical trials, comparison of median survival time or time to an event in different groups may be preferred for planning purpose. For example, an objective criterion of success/failure of a treatment may involve presence or absence of an event after a fixed period of treatment. However, consideration of individual survival experience of all the study patients /persons till desired time may be more appropriate because of consideration of complete records including censored one. Under such circumstances, the number of observed events becomes more important than the number of study subjects. The minimum sample size may be calculated in the following ways (Machin and Campbell[3], 1987).

10.2.11.1. Comparison of two survival rates

To carry out a study with an objective of testing a hazard ratio of the risks of vital event (e.g., death) in the two groups at some chosen point of time described in Chapter 8, any two of the following should be known:

    (i)   Anticipated survival rate in people exposed to the factor of interest (or treatment group) = p_1

    (ii) Anticipated survival rate in people not exposed to the factor of interest (or control group) = p_2

    (iii) Anticipated hazard ratio, that is, ratio of the risks of vital event (e.g., death, recurrence of disease) in the two groups, and if this does not change with time it may be estimated as:

        $h = \log p_1 / \log p_2$

        And the following:

(iv) Value of the normal deviate at considered level of confidence = Z1-α/2 (two-sided test)

= Z1-α (one-sided test)

(v) Value of the normal deviate at considered power of the study = Z1-β

Then, required minimum sample size may be calculated as:

$$n = \frac{2N_E}{(2 - p_1 - p_2)}$$

Where, N_E is the minimum number of desired events and may be estimated as,

$$N_E = \frac{(z_{1-\alpha} + z_{1-\beta})^2 (h+1)}{2(h-1)}$$

Accordingly,

(i) For a two-sided test:

$$n = \frac{(z_{1-\alpha/2} + z_{1-\beta})^2 [\log p_1 + \log p_2]^2}{[\log p_1 - \log p_2]^2 (2 - p_1 - p_2)} \tag{10.16}$$

(ii) For a one-sided test:

$$n = \frac{(z_{1-\alpha} + z_{1-\beta})^2 [\log p_1 + \log p_2]^2}{[\log p_1 - \log p_2]^2 (2 - p_1 - p_2)} \tag{10.17}$$

Example 12:

A double blind randomized controlled trial has to be conducted regarding treatment of asthma patients with a newly developed drug in comparison to placebo. If it is expected that after one year of treatment the placebo group may show relief among 30% patients whereas 60% will get cured in the treatment group, how many patients need to be included in each group if power has to be maintained as 80% and level of significance as 5%.

Calculation:

Known inputs are:

$p_1 = 0.30$, $p_2 = 0.60$

$z_{1-\alpha/2} = z_{1-(0.05)/2} = 1.96$, $z_{1-\alpha} = z_{1-0.05} = 1.64$, $z_{1-\beta} = 0.842$

(i) For a two-sided test:

$$n = \frac{(z_{1-\alpha/2} + z_{1-\beta})^2 [\log p_1 + \log p_2]^2}{[\log p_1 - \log p_2]^2 (2 - p_1 - p_2)}$$

$$n = \frac{(1.96 + 0.842)^2 [\log(0.30) + \log(0.60)]^2}{[\log(0.30) - \log(0.60)]^2 (2 - 0.30 - 0.60)}$$

$$= 44$$

Thus, for comparison of survival rates under a two-sided test, a minimum of 44 patients in placebo group and 44 in the treatment group should be included in the study. Hence, 45 patients may be included in each of the treatment groups.

(ii) For a one-sided test:

$$n = \frac{\left(z_{1-\alpha} + z_{1-\beta}\right)^2 \left[\log p_1 + \log p_2\right]^2}{\left[\log p_1 - \log p_2\right]^2 \left(2 - p_1 - p_2\right)}$$

$$n = \frac{\left(1.64 + 0.842\right)^2 \left[\log\left(0.30\right) + \log\left(0.60\right)\right]^2}{\left[\log\left(0.30\right) - \log\left(0.60\right)\right]^2 \left(2 - 0.30 - 0.60\right)}$$

$$= 34$$

Thus, for comparison of survival rates under a one-sided test, a minimum of 34 patients in placebo group and 34 in the treatment group should be included in the study. Hence, 35 patients may be included in each of the treatment groups.

10.2.11.2. Comparison of two median survival times

Sometimes one may prefer to consider treatment differences in terms of median survival times rather than survival rates. Further, in contrast to non-parametric approach used in case of survival rates in section 10.2.11.1, parametric approach may be used considering the underlying form of the survival distributions. For the purpose of planning, the commonly used form of survival distribution is exponential distribution that requires fewer study subjects than those suggested under non-parametric approach. As in section 10.2.11.1, in this case also, any two of the following should be known:

(i) Anticipated median survival time in people exposed to the factor of interest (or treatment group)
$$= m_1$$
(ii) Anticipated median survival time in people not exposed to the factor of interest (or control group)
$$= m_2$$
(iii) Anticipated hazard ratio, which is the smallest ratio of medians that is of interest. Since exponential distribution has a constant hazard rate, the risk of failure per unit time, it may be estimated as:
$$h^* = m_2 / m_1$$
And the following:
(iv) Value of the normal deviate at considered level of confidence = Z1-α/2 (two-sided test)
$$= Z1\text{-}\alpha \text{ (one-sided test)}$$
(v) Value of the normal deviate at considered power of the study =Z1-β

Then, required minimum number of events "N_E" may be calculated as:

$$N_E = \frac{2\left(z_{1-\alpha} + z_{1-\beta}\right)^2}{\left(\log h^*\right)^2}$$

Where, $h^* = m_2/m_1$ is the smallest ratio of medians that it is of interest.

Accordingly, required minimum number of events may be calculated as:

(i) For a two-sided test:

$$n = \frac{2\left(z_{1-\alpha/2} + z_{1-\beta}\right)^2}{\left(\log m_2 - \log m_1\right)^2} \tag{10.18}$$

(ii) For a one-sided test:

$$n = \frac{2\left(z_{1-\alpha} + z_{1-\beta}\right)^2}{\left(\log m_2 - \log m_1\right)^2} \tag{10.19}$$

Example 13:

A double blind randomized controlled trial has to be conducted regarding treatment of breast cancer patients with a newly developed drug in comparison to the standard drug. If median survival period of the new drug group is expected to be 8.5 years in comparison to that for standard drug group as 7.0 years, how many events need to be included in each group, if power has to be maintained as 80% and level of significance as 5%.

Calculation:

Known inputs are:

$m_1 = 8.5$, $m_2 = 7.0$

$z_{1-\alpha/2} = z_{1-(0.05)/2} = 1.96$, $z_{1-\alpha} = z_{1-0.05} = 1.64$, $z_{1-\beta} = 0.842$

(i) For a two-sided test:

$$n = \frac{2\left(z_{1-\alpha/2} + z_{1-\beta}\right)^2}{\left(\log m_2 - \log m_1\right)^2}$$

$$n = \frac{2\left(1.96 + 0.842\right)^2}{\left[\log(7.0) - \log(8.5)\right]^2}$$

$$= 2206$$

Thus, for comparison of median survivals under a two-sided test, a minimum of 2206 events in new treatment group and 2206 in the standard treatment group should be included in the study. Accordingly, based on the expected incidence of the disease and period of follow up, number of patients in each treatment group should be decided in such a way that 2210 events are observed in each group.

(ii) For a one-sided test:

$$n = \frac{2\left(z_{1-\alpha} + z_{1-\beta}\right)^2}{\left(\log m_2 - \log m_1\right)^2}$$

$$n = \frac{2\left(1.64 + 0.842\right)^2}{\left[\log(7.0) - \log(8.5)\right]^2}$$

$$= 1733$$

Thus, for comparison of median survivals under a one-sided test, a minimum of 1733 events in new treatment group and 1733 in the standard treatment group should be included in the study. Accordingly, based on the expected incidence of the disease and period of follow-up, number of patients in each treatment group should be decided in such a way that 1735 events are observed in each group.

10.2.12. Comparison of a Population Proportion with a Given Proportion

Sometimes one may be interested in testing the hypothesis that the proportion of individuals in a population suffering from a particular disease is equal to a particular value. To calculate required minimum sample size, the desired inputs are:

(i)   Anticipated proportion of the event in the study group = p

(ii) Expected value of the above-mentioned proportion = p^*

(iii) Value of the normal deviate at considered level of confidence = Z1-α/2 (two-sided test)

= Z1-α (one-sided test)

(iii) Value of the normal deviate at considered power of the study = Z1-β

Accordingly, required minimum number of events may be calculated as:

(i) For a two-sided test:

$$n = \left\{ z_{1-\alpha-2} \sqrt{\left[p(1-p) \right]} + z_{1-\beta} \sqrt{\left[p^*(1-p^*) \right]} \right\}^2 / (p - p^*)^2 \tag{10.20}$$

(ii) For a one-sided test:

$$n = \left\{ z_{1-\alpha} \sqrt{\left[p(1-p) \right]} + z_{1-\beta} \sqrt{\left[p^*(1-p^*) \right]} \right\}^2 / (p - p^*)^2 \tag{10.21}$$

Example 14:

As per a review of existing literature, the prevalence of hearing problem among school going children is 20%. In a study for assessing the change in the prevalence, how many children should be included if it is required to be 80% sure of detecting a rate of 15% at the 5% level of significance?

Calculation:

Known inputs are:

$p = 0.20$, $p^* = 0.15$

$z_{1-\alpha/2} = z_{1-(0.05)/2} = 1.96$, $z_{1-\alpha} = z_{1-0.05} = 1.64$, $z_{1-\beta} = 0.842$

(i) For a two-sided test:

$$n = \left\{ z_{1-\alpha/2} \sqrt{\left[p(1-p) \right]} + z_{1-\beta} \sqrt{\left[p^*(1-p^*) \right]} \right\}^2 / (p - p^*)^2$$

$$n = \left\{ 1.96 \sqrt{\left[0.20(1-0.20) \right]} + 0.842 \sqrt{\left[0.15(1-0.15) \right]} \right\}^2 / (0.20 - 0.15)^2$$

$$= 470$$

Thus, for a two-sided test, a minimum of 470 school going children should be included in the study.

(ii) For a one-sided test:

$$n = \left\{ z_{1-\alpha} \sqrt{\left[p(1-p) \right]} + z_{1-\beta} \sqrt{\left[p^*(1-p^*) \right]} \right\}^2 / (p - p^*)^2$$

$$n = \left\{ 1.64 \sqrt{\left[0.20(1-0.20) \right]} + 0.842 \sqrt{\left[0.15(1-0.15) \right]} \right\}^2 / (0.20 - 0.15)^2$$

$$= 366$$

Thus, for a one sided test, a minimum of 366 school going children should be included in the study. Accordingly, 370 school going children may be included in the study.

This chapter describes commonly used methods for calculation of required minimum sample size. However, the readers are encouraged to go through the references listed under Further Reading at the end of the Book.

A study generally has a single or primary outcome measure of interest. Other outcome measures, if any, should be considered as secondary outcomes. However, there may be situations when more than one outcome measures are of equal importance. In this case, separate sample size calculations may be done for each of the outcome measures and the largest required sample size should be used in the study. The calculated sample size may be further adjusted in view of the anticipated problems (e.g., no response, drop out, etc.). Also, if necessary, sample size may be adjusted in view of the size of study population. However, if there is no constraint of time and money, coverage of larger sample size than the calculated sample size is recommended.

Multiple Choice Questions

Choose the correct answers in the following multiple choice questions. The correct answers are listed on pp. 344-345.

Q.1. The expected proportion of people suffering from a disease in the population is 50%. An investigator is interested in estimating the prevalence of that disease within a range of 45 to 55% with 95% confidence. What minimum sample size will be required for the study?
a. 100   b.   200
c. 300   d.   400

Q.2. In the estimation of sample size in a cross-sectional study on the prevalence of a disease, the information required are:
a. Only a rough estimate of the prevalence of the disease
b. Only the amount of error the investigator would like to accept in the estimate
c.   Both a and b
d.   Both a and b together with the confidence required in the estimation

Q.3. If in an investigation to estimate the prevalence of smoking in college students, a sample of 100 students was taken with an assumed prevalence of 20%. What is the error margin for which this sample size is adequate, with 95% confidence?
a. 10%   b.   20%
c. 8%   d.   Cannot be determined

Q.4. Required sample size for testing a hypothesis will be highest , if we consider:
a. Higher level of significance   b.   Higher level of power
c. Both (a) and (b)   d.   None of the above

Q.5. If the expected mean of systolic BP in the community is 120 units with standard deviation of 10 units, what sample size is needed to estimate the mean level of BP within 5% of the assumed mean with 99% confidence?
a. 19   b.   45
c.   7   d.   27

Q.6. In a clinical trial to test the efficacy of a new drug in comparison to the standard drug in the treatment of a disease, it was found from a previous study that 60% of the patients who had received the standard drug showed improvement while 80% of the patients who had received the new drug showed improvement. What will be the minimum sample size required (in each arm?) for a new clinical trial being planned by an investigator if he wants the sample which will give 95% confidence and 80% power:
a. 65   b.   85
c. 163   d.   135

Q.7. In a previous epidemiological study, it was reported that 70% of the lung cancer cases were smokers, while only 50% of those who didn't have lung cancer were smokers. What will be the minimum sample size required (in each arm?) for a new study being planned by an investigator if he wants the sample which will give 95% confidence and 90% power:
a. 95   b.   140
c. 125   d.   75

Q.8. Mean birth weight of babies born to women with good nutrition was found to be 3.0 kg with an SD of 0.5 kg. The corresponding mean value and SD of birth weight of babies born to women having poor nutritional status were 2.5 kg and 0.7 kg, respectively. What will be the minimum sample size required (in each arm) for a new study being planned by an investigator if he wants a sample that will give 95% confidence and 90% power?
a. 31   b.   25
c. 18   d.   23

Q.9. From a previous study it was found that percentage of subjects having diabetics in those who were doing exercise daily was 5% and the corresponding percentage of subjects having diabetics in those who were not doing any exercise was 15%. What will be the minimum sample size required (in each arm) for a new study being planned by an investigator if he wants the sample that will give 95% confidence and 90% power?

a. 150

b. 190

c. 140

d. 110

Q.10. In a clinical trial, comparing the efficacy of a new drug with that of the standard drug, apart from the rough estimates of the efficacy with the new drug and the standard drug from previous studies, estimation of minimum sample size depends also on:

a. Type I error alone

b. Type II error alone

c. Both type I and II errors

d. None of the above

References

1. Moher David, Dulberg Corinne S, Wells George A. Statistical power, sample size, and their reporting in randomized controlled trials. *JAMA*. 1994; 272:122-124.

2. Sullivan KM, Houston R, Gorstein J, Cervinskas J. *Monitoring Universal Salt Iodization Programmes*. Geneva: WHO; 1995.

3. Machin D, Campbell MJ. *Statistical Tables for the Design of Clinical Trials*. Oxford, London: Blackwell Scientific Publications; 1987.

11 | Diagnostic Tests - Principles and Methods

- Accuracy of a diagnostic test
- Predictive values: Limitations of predictive values
- Bayes' theorem
- Likelihood ratios: LR of a positive test, LR of a negative test, post-test odds when the test outcome is positive, post-test odds when the test outcome is negative
- Tree method of obtaining post-test probabilities
- Interpretation of post-test probability of disease
- Diagnostic tests involving quantitative measurements
- Receiver operating characteristic curve (ROC curve): Choosing a cut-off point
- Multiple tests: Serial and parallel tests

Often in their practice, clinicians have to make a guess about an individual patient's status as to be diseased or not. We know that the diagnosis of an individual physician is seldom certain, no matter how vast his/her experience and clinical acumen are. With the available information based on clinical history, physical examination and result(s) of relevant laboratory investigation(s), the individual physician tries to make a best guess. The tests or laboratory investigations that aid in this process of diagnosing a condition are called diagnostic tests. For example, the level of Prostate Specific Antigen (PSA) of a man might give a lead to a urologist whether that particular man could have prostate cancer. Similarly, an ophthalmologist might be able to guess about a person whether he/she could have glaucoma, based on the intra-ocular pressure (IOP) measurement. Generally, this type of tests form the first level of investigations in a doctor's armour and depending on the need, he might order further specific confirmatory investigations. While such tests might help in taking decisions at the initial stages, as mentioned earlier, there is a chance that they are not correct. So an understanding of the accuracy of a diagnostic test is important while taking clinical decisions based on it. Critical evaluation of any diagnostic procedure is necessary so that it can be justified, especially when the resources are limited and the costs of medical care are mounting. In this chapter, we shall present the various measures to assess the performance of a diagnostic test.

11.1. Accuracy of a Diagnostic Test

To begin with, an assessment of a diagnostic test requires some comparative decisions based on 'truth'. We understand that the 'truth' – whether the disease is present or absent in an individual — is based on the result of a well established, known confirmatory method like a culture for some infection or a biopsy for a particular cancer and so on. Usually, these confirmatory tests are time-consuming, expensive or may not be always feasible and so other diagnostic tests need to be employed. A confirmatory test is generally referred to as 'gold standard' and the test under consideration is compared to this gold standard.

The simplest measure of the quality of a diagnostic procedure or test is the fraction of cases in which the test result agrees with the 'truth'. This fraction is called the accuracy of the diagnostic test. Naturally, the higher this fraction, the better a test is.

Though it appears that the accuracy is a simple and good measure of the quality of a diagnostic test, it can be very misleading. For example, if we are screening for a rare condition whose prevalence in the community is 1%, we can be very accurate even after ignoring any evidence and declare all the subjects as unaffected by the condition. In other words, even if one declares blindly that the disease is absent in a subject, he/she is right 99% of the time. So, the accuracy of a diagnostic test has limited utility as an index of how a diagnostic test performs, as it is dependent on the prevalence of the disease/condition.

In the light of its dependence on the prevalence, one is tempted to conclude that accuracy can be a useful index for comparing two or more tests in diagnosing a condition in a given population, because the prevalence is fixed in that given population. Unfortunately, this is also not correct. Two diagnostic tests can have similar accuracies in diagnosing a condition, but their performance may be very different. Two tests A and B both can have 90% accuracy, but is possible that all the 10% inaccurate decisions by test A could be due to missing true cases (false negatives) and those in test B could be due to missing normal individuals (false positives). Therefore, the utility of the two tests A and B could be very different for patient management. For instance, in the diagnosis of prostate cancer by prostate specific antigen, a false positive may mean an unnecessary biopsy and a false negative result may mean missing a cancer case.

So the accuracy of a diagnostic test, though a simple measure, should be interpreted cautiously.

11.2. Sensitivity and Specificity

Because of the limitations of the accuracy, we need indices, which are independent of the prevalence of the condition and which also separate the various types of right and wrong conclusions.

The possible situations in any diagnostic test, when the outcome is binary (Yes or No type), can be summarized in a 2×2 table as shown in Table 11.1 below. With the help of this 2×2 Table, we can easily understand the various concepts.

Table 11.1: Possible situations in a diagnostic test when the outcome is binary

Prediction by the diagnostic test	Truth		Total
	Disease present	Disease absent	
Disease present	a	b	$a + b$ (predicted as diseased)
Disease absent	c	d	$c + d$ (predicted as disease free)
Total	$a + c$ (truly diseased)	$b + d$ (truly disease free)	N

As we can see from the Table above, the test can lead to a conclusion that the disease is present when the disease is truly present as well as when it is truly absent. Similarly, the test result can lead to a negative conclusion when there is truly no disease and also when the disease present. Obviously, there is scope for an error, whatever decision we take based on the diagnostic test.

In particular, one might ask questions, such as: i) how likely a person with the disease is shown as positive by the diagnostic test; and ii) what is the chance that an individual who does not have the disease is shown as negative by the test also? If both these probabilities are high, we can be assured that the test is very useful. Now to assess these probabilities we can select two groups of subjects, namely, with and without the disease and perform the diagnostic test under consideration on the selected individuals in both these groups. The results of this comparison can be shown as in Table 11.1.

The rows of the Table 11.1 indicate the result from the diagnostic test under consideration while the columns indicate the same based on the gold standard. The frequency a will indicate the number of diseased persons who had a positive result by the diagnostic test and, therefore, the remaining (c) diseased persons' test results are negative. Similarly, d indicates the number of normal (no disease) individuals who showed a negative result by the test and b is the number of normal persons showing a positive test result.

Coming back to the two questions that we have raised above, the proportion $a / (a+c)$ will answer the first question – the chance or probability of a diseased individual shown as diseased by the diagnostic test also. The second question of the probability of a normal person showing non-diseased by the test will be answered by the proportion $d / (d+b)$. The proportion $a / (a+c)$ is called the **Sensitivity** and the proportion $d / (d+b)$ is called the **Specificity** of the test. Thus, sensitivity of the diagnostic test is the probability of picking up the disease when it is present and specificity is probability of showing a normal result when the disease is absent. We shall show these by probability notations.

We denote the presence and absence of disease by D+ and D- respectively. Similarly, the positive and negative results of a diagnostic test are denoted by T+ and T- respectively.

Sensitivity = Probability (test result is positive, given that the disease is truly present)

$$= P (T+|D+) \tag{11.1}$$

Sensitivity is the True Positive Fraction (TPF) of the total positives declared by the test and is analogous to the 'power' or $(1 - \beta)$ of a statistical test of hypothesis (probability of a declaring a significant difference between two treatments by the statistical test, when in fact a significant difference exists).

Specificity = Probability (test result is negative, given that truly there is no disease)

$$= P (T-|D-) \tag{11.2}$$

Specificity is the True Negative Fraction (TNF) of the total negatives declared by the test.

In terms of the frequencies,

Sensitivity = $a / (a+c)$ $\tag{11.3}$

Specificity = $d / (b+d)$ $\tag{11.4}$

As can be seen, both Sensitivity and Specificity are conditional probabilities.

Let us explain these two concepts further with an example. Suppose the CD4 count has been made in 200 persons who are proven cases of HIV (by a confirmatory test like ELISA/ Western blot, etc.) and also in 200 persons who are proven to be free of HIV. Taking a CD4 count $\leq$ 300 as an indication of the presence of HIV in an individual, the Table 11.2 below summarizes the results.

Table 11.2: Diagnostic accuracy of CD4 in detecting HIV infection

CD4	ELISA		Total
	HIV+	*HIV-*	
$\leq$ 300 (HIV+)	130	50	180
> 300 (HIV-)	70	150	220
Total	200	200	400

Out of the 200 confirmed HIV cases, 130 were also positive by the CD4 criteria ($\leq$ 300). Therefore, Sensitivity of the CD4 criteria will be 130/200 = 65%. In other words, if an individual is truly infected, his/ her chance of having CD4 count $\leq$ 300 is 65%. Similarly, out of the 200 uninfected individuals, 150 were also shown to be normal by the CD4 (> 300) and this means our diagnostic criterion has a Specificity of 150/200 = 75%. So the chance of a truly uninfected individual having a CD4 count > 300 is 75%.

To get a better idea of these measures and to account for the role of chance in observing the results, we can construct the 95% confidence intervals for both Sensitivity and Specificity. Using the principles explained in Chapter 5 (Inference Statistical Methods), we know that the standard error of a proportion $p = \sqrt{\dfrac{(p * q)}{n}}$, where n is the number of subjects studied and $q = 1 - p$. For the Sensitivity, we have $n = 200$ (truly diseased), $p = 0.65$ and $q = 0.35$ and so the standard error will be $\sqrt{\dfrac{(0.65 * 0.35)}{200}} = 0.0337$. The 95% confidence interval for the calculated Sensitivity will then be $p \pm 1.96 * SE$, which is equal to (58.4% - 71.6%). The confidence interval indicates that though we obtained an estimate of the Sensitivity as 65%, it could vary between 58.4% and 71.6%, over repeated samples of the same size, 95% of times.

Similarly, we can obtain the 95% confidence interval for the Specificity and it will be equal to (69.0% - 81.0%). To have ample confidence in the results that we obtain (narrow interval of probable range), it is imperative that the testing is done on adequate number of individuals.

Recall that the accuracy is the fraction of the study subjects that have been classified correctly by the test. It is the weighted sum of the Sensitivity and Specificity, the weights being the fractions of truly positive and truly negative subjects in the population, respectively.

Accuracy = (Sensitivity * fraction of diseased subjects in the population)

+

(Specificity * fraction of normals in the population) (11.5)

In terms of the frequencies in Table 11.1,

Overall accuracy = $(a+d) / n$ (11.6)

In the example, the overall accuracy of the diagnostic test with the gold standard is $(130+150) / 400 = 70.0\%$, with a 95% CI (65.5% - 74.5%).

At this stage we can define two more probabilities that can also help in assessing the performance of a diagnostic test. Looking at the example above, we note that out of the 200 true cases of HIV, 70 individuals were shown to be negative by the test criteria. Therefore, these 70 were false negatives. Similarly, of the 200 true negatives we notice that 50 were declared as positive by the test. These are false positives. So we can use these two quantities also to assess a diagnostic test.

False Positive Fraction (FPF): It is the relative frequency of normal subjects being declared as diseased and is equal to the complement of Specificity or True Negative Fraction (TNF).

False Positive Fraction = $(1 - \text{Specificity}) = 1 - [d / (b+d)] = b / (b+d)$ (11.7)

In the example it is = 50/200 = 25.0%. It may be mentioned here that FPF is analogous to the 'p value' or Type-I error of a statistical test of hypothesis (probability of declaring a significant difference between two treatments by the statistical test, when in fact there is no difference between the two).

False Negative Fraction (FNF): It is the relative frequency of diseased subjects being declared as non-diseased and is equal to the complement of Sensitivity or True Positive Fraction (TPF).

False Negative Fraction = $(1 - \text{Sensitivity}) = 1 - [a / (a+c)] = c / (a+c)$ (11.8)

In the example, False Negative Fraction is = 70/200 = 35.0%. FNF is analogous to Type-II error or 'β' of a statistical test of hypothesis (probability of declaring no difference between two treatments/groups by the statistical test, when in fact there is a difference between the two). For an accurate diagnostic test, both False Positive Fraction and False Negative Fraction should be as small as possible.

True Negative Fraction (TNF) is Specificity itself and so TNF + FPF = 1

True Positive Fraction (TPF) is Sensitivity itself and so TPF + FNF = 1

It is easy to visualize that the result of a diagnostic test is more likely to be abnormal in a subject with more advanced stage of the condition being investigated. So, it should be noted that Sensitivity (hence False

Negative Fraction) of a diagnostic test is influenced by the severity of the disease. In the example we discussed above, the CD4 count is more likely to be ≤ 300 in an individual who has been a more chronic case of HIV as compared to an individual who has just acquired the HIV infection. Just as Sensitivity is dependent on the severity of the disease, so is Specificity (hence the False Positive Fraction) dependent on the general state of health in the non-diseased individuals. In view of this, due consideration must be given to include an appropriate mix of disease characteristics in the sampled population as the results or conclusions are applicable only to the sample population.

11.3. Predictive Values

In the previous section, we proceeded from the truth to the result shown by the test under consideration and arrived at the measures – Sensitivity, Specificity, FPF and FNF. These measures will tell us about the properties of a diagnostic test and, hence, whether to use such a test in a given situation or not. But once the test is applied on a suspected subject, what is more relevant to a clinician is whether that particular subject is diseased or normal. In particular, he/she would like to know i) the probability of a person shown positive by the test having the disease and ii) probability of a person shown as negative by the test to be truly disease free. In other words, we need to assess how predictive is the test's result, when it declares an individual as a positive or a negative. These are called the predictive values of a positive test and a negative result respectively. To arrive at these measures, we proceed from the test result to the truth.

Using the notations introduced earlier, we can define them as:

Predictive value of a positive test (PV+) = Probability (disease present given that the test result is positive)

$$PV+ = P\ (D+|T+) \tag{11.9}$$

Predictive value of a negative test (PV–) = Probability (disease absent given that the test result is negative)

$$PV- = P\ (D-|T) \tag{11.10}$$

In terms of frequencies,

$$PV+ = a\ /\ (a+b) \tag{11.11}$$

$$PV- = d\ /\ (c+d) \tag{11.12}$$

As the case with the Sensitivity and Specificity, both the predictive values are also conditional probabilities. In the example, the positive predictive value of CD4 count (≤ 300) will be:

Out of the 400 suspected individuals examined, 180 were declared as diseased by the CD4 criteria and among these, only 130 had the disease by the confirmatory test ELISA.

∴ PV+ = 130 / 180 = 0.7222 or 72.22%

In other words, if a patient has a positive test result, his chance of having disease is 72.2%.

Similarly, out of the 220 declared as negative by the CD4 count (> 300), only 150 were truly negative.

∴ PV- = 150 / 220 = 0.6818 or 68.18%

So, if a patient has a negative test result, his chance of having no disease is 68.2%

If the results presented in Table 11.2 are taken as the likely picture in the type of patients being considered, a new patient who comes to the physician is likely to be a HIV positive in 200 out of 400, i.e., 50% probable because the prevalence is 50% in the community. Now if the test result by way of the CD4 count indicates that the same patient is positive, his/her chance of being diseased is represented by the positive predictive value of the test, which is 72.2%. In other words, the prior probability or pretest probability of having disease (50%) is revised to 72.2% after the test result is known to be positive. Similarly, if the test shows a negative result, the prior probability of being diseased will have to be revised to that of the complement of negative predictive value of the test. In the CD4 count example, a negative test result will revise our prior or pretest probability of 50% to 31.82% for a person to be diseased. The revised assessments after the test result is available are called posterior probabilities or post-test probabilities. So, for any diagnostic test to be of practical relevance, post-test probability should increase if the test is positive and decrease if the test result is negative.

11.3.1. Limitation of Predictive Values

Though the predictive values of a positive and a negative test have useful interpretations in assessing the accuracy of a diagnostic test, unfortunately the values of these two measures depend on the prevalence of the disease or condition being investigated in the community. We shall try to explain this by an example.

Consider a diagnostic test, which has both Sensitivity and Specificity of 90% for diagnosing a certain condition. If we perform 1000 tests in a population where the prevalence of the condition being diagnosed is 2%, the likely scenario can be as shown below in Table 11.3.

Table 11.3: Predictive values for a diagnostic test with 90% sensitivity and 90% specificity for a condition with 2% prevalence in the population

Prediction by the diagnostic test	Truth		Total
	Disease present	Disease absent	
Disease present	18	98	116 (predicted as diseased)
Disease absent	2	882	884 (predicted as disease free)
Total	20 (truly diseased)	980 (truly disease free)	1000

Since the prevalence is 2%, there will be 20 true cases out of the 1000 examined and so the remaining 980 will be normal individuals. Since the test has 90% Sensitivity, out of the 20 true cases, on the average 18 will be declared as positive by the test and the remaining 2 will be false negatives. Similarly, with 90% Specificity, we can expect 980 * 0.9 = 882 declared as negatives by the test and so the remaining 98 will be false positives. The positive and negative predictive values for the test under these conditions will be equal to 18/116 = 15.5% and 882/884 = 99.8%, respectively.

Now the same diagnostic test for the same specific condition is applied in a population where the prevalence of the condition being diagnosed is 10% instead of 2%, the resulting picture for 1000 examinations (assuming the 90% Sensitivity and Specificity as earlier) will be as under in Table 11.4.

Table 11.4: Predictive values for a diagnostic test with 90% sensitivity and 90% specificity for a condition with 10% prevalence in the population

Prediction by the diagnostic test	Truth		Total
	Disease present	Disease absent	
Disease present	90	90	180 (predicted as diseased)
Disease absent	10	810	820 (predicted as disease free)
Total	100 (truly diseased)	900 (truly disease free)	1000

From these results, we obtain a positive predictive value of 50% (90/180) and a negative predictive value of 98.8% (810/820). Notice that the PV+ has increased from 15.5% when the prevalence is 2% to 50.0% when the prevalence is 10%, though Sensitivity and Specificity remained same. Thus, the predictive values of a diagnostic test depend on the prevalence of the condition being diagnosed.

These results also indicate that while testing for rare conditions, most of positive test results may turn out to be false positives and, hence, the physicians should be prepared for additional tests on their patients. Similarly, while testing for a condition, which is highly prevalent, most negatives could be false negatives.

11.4. Bayes' Theorem

We know that the predictive values (hence the post-test probabilities) of a diagnostic test depend on the pre-test probability or prevalence of the condition. But most often we do not know the extent of prevalence of the condition in the community. So, as a more practical guide to the performance of a test, we provide the post-test probabilities for different possible values of the prevalence of the condition being diagnosed.

One way of determining the predictive values/post-test probabilities is by way arranging the data in a 2×2 Table as shown above. The same can also be achieved without a 2×2 table, so that for a given prevalence of the condition, we can obtain the posttest probabilities easily. A mathematical relation involving the probabilities, called the Bayes' theorem due to Thomas Bayes, an English mathematician, is used for this purpose. This theorem gives a method for recalculating a probability based on the available new evidence, i.e., the outcome of the diagnostic test.

In general, Bayes' rule states that,

$$P(B \mid A) = \frac{[P(A \mid B) * P(B)]}{[P(A \mid B) * P(B)] + [P(A \mid B^c) * P(B^c)]} \tag{11.13}$$

where $P(B^c)$ is the probability of the event other than B, and other terms are as defined earlier.

If event A is the positive result of a diagnostic test and B is the presence of the disease, $P(B|A)$ is same as $P(D+|T+)$, which is the positive predictive value. Therefore, the positive predictive value of a test can be defined as,

$$P(D+ \mid T+) = \frac{[P(T+ \mid D+) * P(D+)]}{[P(T+ \mid D+) * P(D+)] + [P(T+ \mid D-) * P(D-)]} \tag{11.14}$$

Most often, we will have $P(T+|D+)$ and $P(T+|D-)$ from earlier studies and $P(D+)$, the prevalence, may vary from place to place. So by substituting different values of $P(D+)$ in equation 11.14, we can obtain the corresponding predictive values of a positive test.

In the diagnostic terminology, the Bayes' theorem can be expressed as:

$$P(D+ \mid T+) = \frac{(\text{Sensitivity} * \text{Prevalence})}{(\text{Sensitivity} * \text{Prevalence}) + [(1 - \text{Specificity}) * (1 - \text{Prevalence})]} \tag{11.15}$$

Similarly, the posttest probability of a negative test can be obtained as,

$$P(D+ \mid T-) = \frac{[P(T- \mid D+) * P(D+)]}{[P(T- \mid D+) * P(D+)] + [P(T- \mid D-) * P(D-)]} \tag{11.16}$$

$$P(D+ \mid T-) = \frac{(1-\text{Sensitivity}) * \text{Prevalence}}{[(1-\text{Sensitivity}) * \text{Prevalence}] + [\text{Specificity} * (1 - \text{Prevalence})]} \tag{11.17}$$

Referring to Table 11.2 above, we have $P(D+) = 200/400 = 0.5$ and so $P(D-) = 0.5$

$P (T+|D+) = 130/200 = 0.65$, which is nothing but the Sensitivity

$P (T+|D-) = 50/200 = 0.25$, which is the False Positive Fraction.

Substituting the values in 11.14, the post-test probability when the test results in a positive outcome

$= (0.65 * 0.5) / [(0.65 * 0.5) + (0.25 * 0.5)]$

$= 0.325 / (0.325 + 0.125)$

$= 0.7222$ or 72.22%, same as the Positive Predictive Value (PV+) we obtained from the tabular presentation.

Post-test probability for a negative test will be,

$[(1-0.65) * 0.5] / [\{(1-0.65) * 0.5\} + (0.75 * 0.5)]$

$= (0.35 * 0.5) / [(0.35 * 0.5) + (0.75 * 0.5)]$

$= 0.175 / (0.175 + 0.375)$

$= 0.175 / 0.55$

$= 0.3182$ or 31.82%, which is same as the complement of Negative Predictive Value PV.

We can show that the denominator of equation 11.14 is nothing but the probability of finding a positive result by the test in total population $P(T+)$.

$$[P(T+|D+] * P(D+)] + [P(T+|D-) * P(D-)] = P(T+) \tag{11.18}$$

Therefore, Bayes' theorem in a simple form can be expressed as,

$$P(D+|T+) = P(D+)\frac{P(T+|D+)}{P(T+)} \tag{11.19}$$

It should be noted from equation 11.19 that the Bayes' theorem merely recalculates the odd or pre-test probability based on the new evidence of the test result. It can also be viewed as that the prior probability of disease is multiplied by a factor $P(T+|D+) / P(T+)$, to recalculate disease probability after the test result is positive. If this factor $P(T+|D+) / P(T+)$ is greater than one, the new probability $P(D+|T+)$ will be greater than the prior probability $P(D+)$. This is possible when there is good association between the presence of disease and the test result, and the result is positive more often when the disease is present than in the general population. Similarly, if the factor $P(T+|D+)/P(T+)$ is close to or less than one, it implies that the test results in a positive outcome less or equally often when the disease is present as compared to test in a general population, indicating a poor or no association between the disease and the test result.

11.5. Likelihood Ratios

Bayes' theorem, no doubt, helps us to quantify the uncertainty in the light of the available evidence under different pre-test probabilities, but it is difficult to evaluate these post-test probabilities without a pen and paper or a calculator. In view of this, one may use another simple method of obtaining post-test probabilities based on the use of 'odds' instead of probabilities.

The odds of an event are defined as the ratio of the probability of that event occurring to the probability of its not occurring. It is an easy way to calculate the effect of new information on the uncertainty.

$$\text{Odds of an event} = \frac{\text{Probability of the event occurring}}{\text{Probability of the event not occurring}} \tag{11.20}$$

If we call the probability that the event will occur as P, then the odds of the event are,

$$\text{Odds of the event} = \frac{P}{(1-P)} \tag{11.21}$$

For example, if the probability of an event is 0.6, the odds of that event occurring are 0.6 / 0.4 = 1.5 or 3:2.

Using these concepts, the pre-test probability of a subject being diseased can be expressed as the pre-test odds and similarly the post-test probability can be expressed as post-test odds.

The discriminating ability of a test between diseased individuals and normal individuals can be measured by an index called the Likelihood Ratio (LR). Like the predictive values, LR is calculated separately for positive test and negative tests.

11.5.1. LR of a Positive Test (LR+)

It is defined as the ratio of True Positive Fraction (Sensitivity) to the False Positive Fraction (1-Specificity).

$$LR+ = \text{Sensitivity} / (1\text{-Specificity}) = [a / (a+c)] \div [b / (b+d)] \tag{11.22}$$

In the example data of Table 11.2, Sensitivity $a / (a+c) = 130/200 = 65.0\%$ and the FPF or (1 – Specificity) = 25.0%. Therefore, LR+ = 65/25 or 2.6.

Therefore, if the test results in a positive outcome for an individual subject, he/she is 2.6 times more likely to be diseased than non-diseased. LR+ can also be viewed as the ratio of a 'desirable' quantity to an 'undesirable' quantity. Naturally, the more this ratio, the better the test will be. We also note here that both the Sensitivity and the FPF are independent of the prevalence of the disease/condition being diagnosed.

11.5.2. LR of a Negative Test (LR-)

It is defined as the ratio of False Negative Fraction (1-Sensitivity) to the True Negative Fraction (Specificity).

$$LR- = (1 - \text{Sensitivity}) / \text{Specificity} = [c / (a+c)] \div [d / (b+d)] \tag{11.23}$$

In the example data of Table 11.2, Sensitivity $a / (a+c) = 130/200 = 65.0\%$ and so the FNF = 35.0%. Similarly, Specificity is 75%. Therefore, LR- = 35/75 or 0.4667.

It implies that if the test result is negative, the individual subject is 53.3% (100 – 46.67%) less likely to be truly non-diseased. Unlike LR+, the LR- is the ratio of an 'undesirable' quantity to a 'desirable' quantity. Therefore, the smaller this ratio, the better the test will be. Like we noted with LR+, both the Specificity and the False Negative Fraction are independent of the prevalence of the disease/condition being diagnosed.

The clinical finding can be characterized by the two LRs, one corresponding to the positive finding (LR+) and the other corresponding to a negative finding (LR-). Both these LRs obviate remembering two numbers (TPF and FPF) as against only one now to evaluate the post-test uncertainty.

11.5.3. Post-test Odds when the Test Outcome is Positive

The post-test odds of disease when the test result is positive can be obtained as the product of the pre-test odds and the LR+.

$$\text{Post-test odds when the test outcome is positive} = \text{Pre-test odds} * LR+ \tag{11.24}$$

In the example data of CD4 counts, we have,

$$\text{Pre-test Odds of HIV} = \frac{\text{Probability of a Subject having HIV}}{\text{Probability of a Subject not having HIV}}$$

$$= 0.5 / (1 - 0.5) = 1$$

The Likelihood ratio of a positive test (CD4 ≤ 300) = 2.6. Therefore, the Post-test Odds = 1 * 2.6 = 2.6 or 2.6 : 1.

Recall that Bayes' rule gives us the post-test probabilities and not post-test odds. To convert the odds into probabilities, a simple relation between the two is used.

$$\text{Probability } p = \frac{\text{Odds of Disease}}{1 + \text{Odds of Disease}} \qquad (11.25)$$

Therefore, Post-test Probability of Disease = Post-test Odds of disease / (1 + Post-test Odds)

P (D+|T+) = 2.6 / (1+2.6) = 2.6 / 3.6 = 0.7222 or 72.22%, which is exactly same as we obtained from the Bayes' rule earlier.

11.5.4. Post-test Odds when the Test Outcome is Negative

The post-test odds of disease when the test result is negative or normal can be obtained as the product of the pretest odds and the LR-.

Post-test Odds when the test outcome is negative = Pre-test Odds * LR-   (11.26)

In the example data of CD4 counts, we have,

Pre-test Odds of HIV = 1

The Likelihood ratio of a negative test (CD4 > 300) = 0.4667

Therefore, the Post-test Odds = 1 * 0.4667 = 0.4667 or 1 : 2.14

To convert the post-test odds of HIV, when the CD4 count > 300 into post-test probability,

P (D+|T-) = 0.4667 / (1+0.4667) = 0.3182 or 31.82%, which is same as we obtained by the Bayes' theorem earlier.

Use of Likelihood Ratios makes the task of evaluating the post-test uncertainty of the disease easier as we have to remember only one number instead of two. This task of evaluating the post-test probability/odds can be made further simple by having nomograms for a positive test and a negative test separately. It is easy to construct such nomograms for any given value of a LR+ or LR- and a given pretest probability of disease. TJ Fagan[1] has developed one such nomogram, which can be used as a ready reckoner by practicing clinicians.

11.6. Tree Method for Obtaining Post-test Probabilities

So far we have seen three methods, namely, the 2 × 2 Table, Bayes' theorem and LR method for evaluating the post-test probabilities of disease. Another method, which is also easy to understand, is based on construction of a Tree diagram (Fig. 11.1).

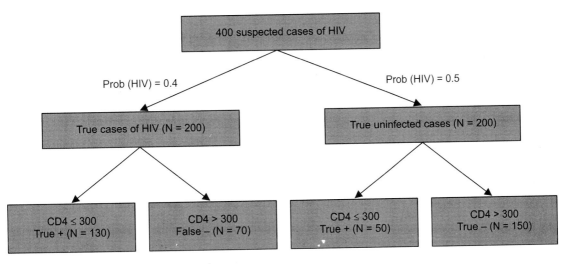

Fig. 11.1: Tree diagram for the calculation of post-test disease probabilities

To start with, we imagine that there are a large number of suspected cases on whom we wish to apply the diagnostic test. Using the disease prevalence, divide the total into two branches of the Tree. Each branch is further divided into two sub-branches depending on the nature of the test result as positive or negative. These details can be shown in a Tree diagram as in the figure below for the CD4 data of Table 11.2.

Using the assumed prevalence or the pre-test probability, we divide the total into two parts as the truly diseased and truly non-diseased. Now multiplying the number of truly diseased with the known value of TPF, we can get the number of true positives and the remaining of truly diseased will be the false negatives. Similarly, multiplying the number of truly non-diseased with the known FPF, we can obtain the number of false positives and the remaining of true non-diseased will be the number of true negatives.

To calculate the post-test probability of disease if the test result is positive, we have 130 true positives out of the total of 180 positives (130+50). Therefore, the post-test probability is 130/180 = 72.22%. Similarly, the post-test probability of disease when the test result is negative will be 70/220 as the proportion of false negatives to the total number of negatives, which is equal to 31.82%.

11.7. Interpretation of Post-test Probability of Disease

We have seen 4 methods of obtaining the post-test probability of disease when the test result is positive and negative. Though the probabilities help us upgrade our assessment in the light of the evidence by the diagnostic test, a proper understanding of them is essential.

Consider a diagnostic tool, which has a TPF of 90% and a FPF of 9%. Table 11.5 below shows the post-test probability of a positive test result for various pre-test probabilities of disease. Since the TPF is 0.9 and FPF is 0.09, we have the LR+ as 10 for this diagnostic test.

Table 11.5: Post-test probabilities for a positive result of a given diagnostic test under various pre-test probabilities

Pre-test prob. (%)	Pre-test odds	LR+	Post-test odds	Post-test prob. (%)
1.0	0.0101	10	0.1010	9.2
5.0	0.0526	10	0.5263	34.5
10.0	0.1111	10	1.1111	52.6
20.0	0.25	10	2.50	71.4
30.0	0.4286	10	4.2857	81.1
40.0	0.6667	10	6.6667	87.0
50.0	1.00	10	10.00	90.9
60.0	1.50	10	15.00	93.8
70.0	2.3333	10	23.3333	95.9
80.0	4.00	10	40.00	97.6
90.0	9.00	10	90.00	98.9
95.0	19.00	10	190.00	99.5
99.0	99.00	10	990.00	99.9

From Table 11.5, notice that initially the post-test probability increases rapidly as the pre-test probability increases, but this increase is very marginal with higher pre-test probabilities. For example when the pre-test probability increased from 5.0% to 10.0%, the post-test probability increased from 34.5% to 52.6%. But the increase in post-test probability is marginal (98.9% to 99.5%) only, when the pre-test probability increased from 90.0% to 95.0%. At low pre-test probabilities, the post-test probabilities are much higher than the pre-test probabilities and as the pre-test probability approaches 1, the post-test probability is only marginally more than the pre-test probability.

Similarly, for the same test, the post-test probabilities of a negative result can also be worked out as shown in Table 11.6. Since the TPF is 90% and FPF is 9%, the FNF and TNF are 10% and 91%, respectively. So the LR- will be 0.1/0.91 = 0.1099.

Table 11.6: Post-test probabilities for a negative result of a given diagnostic test under various pre-test probabilities

Pre-test prob. (%)	Pre-test odds	LR–	Post-test odds	Post-test prob. (%)
1.0	0.0101	0.1099	0.0011	0.11
5.0	0.0526	0.1099	0.0058	0.57
10.0	0.1111	0.1099	0.0122	1.21
20.0	0.25	0.1099	0.0275	2.67
30.0	0.4286	0.1099	0.0471	4.50
40.0	0.6667	0.1099	0.0733	6.83
50.0	1.00	0.1099	0.1099	9.90
60.0	1.50	0.1099	0.1648	14.15
70.0	2.3333	0.1099	0.2564	20.41
80.0	4.00	0.1099	0.4396	30.54
90.0	9.00	0.1099	0.9891	49.73
95.0	19.00	0.1099	2.0881	67.62
99.0	99.00	0.1099	10.8801	91.58

It can be seen that for a negative test also the post-test probabilities depend on the level of the pre-test probability. But the influence of the magnitude of pre-test probability on the post-test probabilities is not as much as we saw with a positive test result, since the post-test probability increased slowly with the increase in the pre-test probability and becomes high when the pre-test probability is also high.

Thus, it is evident that the post-test probability and, hence, the interpretation of the test result depends on the pre-test probability or what we know already. Further, when we are certain about the diagnosis before the test (pre-test probability is either very low or very high), the gain or additional information by way of the test result is minimal. This also raises a question as to the need and utility of a diagnostic test when we are already certain about the diagnosis.

The points that we discussed in the previous sections make us realize that the estimates of probability of disease depend on the experience and judgment of an individual clinician as well as representative estimates of the test characteristics. It is not always possible to obtain the test characteristics such as TPF, FPF and LRs every time and in every setting. One has to search the relevant literature, which may be tedious and time consuming. Sox et al.[2] compiled the characteristics of about 100 common diagnostic tests. Using these details and his/her estimate of pretest probability, a practicing clinician may be able to assess quickly the uncertainty of disease in a given patient.

11.8. Diagnostic Tests Involving a Quantitative Measurement

Sometimes a diagnostic test involves measurement of a quantity and the clinician needs to interpret the result as to the individual being a positive or negative, based on the level of this measurement. The individual will be classified as abnormal or normal depending on his/her level of the measure exceeds a certain value. For example, if the intra-ocular pressure (IOP) exceeds 21 mm/Hg, an ophthalmologist suspects that the eye could be glaucomatous. This cut-off value of 21 mm/Hg seems to be arbitrary and theoretically any cut-off could be used. Similarly, the 24 hour thyroid uptake values or blood serum assays lead to values that have an overlap of true positive and true negative patients for any cut-off value and no single threshold can separate the population exactly. For each threshold or cut-off value chosen, we can evaluate the Sensitivity and Specificity, comparing the decisions with a gold standard diagnosis.

Fig. 11.2 shows the conditional probabilities of each decision (equal to the area under the curve on one side of the threshold) when two possible threshold values of a quantity are chosen on which decisions are based. As can be seen in the upper panel of the figure, choosing a higher threshold value will decrease both the True Positive Fraction as well as False Positive Fraction. At the same time it increases the True Negative Fraction as well as False Negative Fraction. On the other hand, choosing a lower threshold value will increase both the True Positive Fraction as well as False Positive Fraction and decrease the True Negative Fraction as well as False Negative Fraction (lower panel of Fig. 11.2). It can be realized easily that both TPF and FPF must increase or decrease together and so must TNF and FNF. In view of this, a threshold value must be chosen so that it yields an appropriate compromise among these gains and losses.

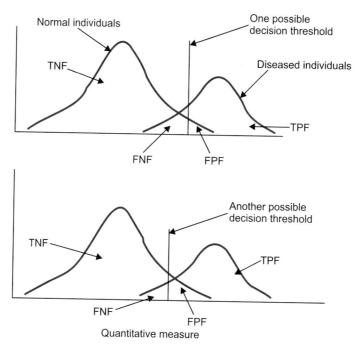

Fig. 11.2: Effect of altering the cut-off value for an abnormal test result

11.9. Receiver Operating Characteristic Curve (ROC Curve)

In the situations such as the one described above, the question that arises is: how to decide which is the best cut-off? Towards this objective, we borrow a technique called Receiver Operating Characteristic Curve (ROC Curve) from the signal detection theory. To draw this curve, we use the TPF (Sensitivity) and FPF (1-Specificity) for each cut-off value. Taking TPF on the vertical axis (Y-axis) and the corresponding value of FPF on the horizontal axis (X-axis), all the pairs of values are plotted for each cut-off. Joining the points on the graph will give us a convex curve called the ROC curve. Each point on this curve indicates the TPF and FPF at a particular threshold value of the quantitative test. It is called Receiver Operating Characteristic Curve because the receiver of the test information can operate at any point on the curve by using an appropriate decision threshold.

Fig. 11.3 below shows three possible operating points that correspond to a very strict threshold (case is called positive only if it is definitely positive), a moderate threshold and a lax threshold (case is called positive even by a suspicion).

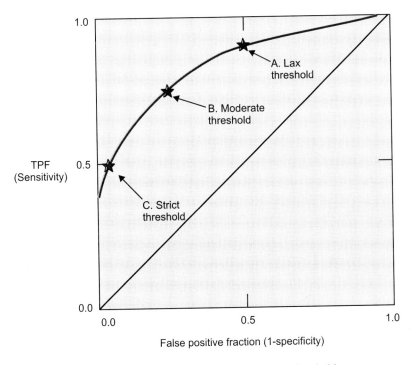

Fig. 11.3: An ROC curve with three decision thresholds

The ROC curve must inevitably pass through the lower left corner (FPF = 0, TPF = 0) of the graph because all the individuals tested can be called negative and through the upper right corner (FPF = 1, TPF = 1) of the graph because all the subjects tested can be positive. If the diagnostic test is of any help to the decision maker, the points in between (0,0) and (1,1) must lie above the diagonal line joining the two points (0,0) and (1,1). This is so because if the test is useful, a positive decision should be more probable when a case is actually positive than when a case is actually negative. Therefore, the more the area under the ROC curve, the better the overall discriminating ability of the diagnostic criteria.

The area under the ROC curve has another interesting meaning.[3] If there are n_1 truly diseased and n_2 truly non-diseased subjects of the total number we test, we can form $n_1 * n_2$ number of random pairs of subjects in which one is truly diseased and the other truly non-diseased. If the diagnostic criterion has any ability in discriminating the diseased from the non-diseased, it should assign a higher probability of having the disease in truly diseased subjects as compared to the truly non-diseased. Naturally, the higher the number of such pairs, the more the discriminating ability of the test criterion. The area under the ROC curve corresponds to the proportion of the total number of possible pairs of truly diseased and truly non-diseased subjects, in which the truly diseased subject has been assigned a higher probability of having the disease. For example, if we test 50 suspected subjects for a condition and supposing there were 30 truly diseased and 20 truly non-diseased subjects, we can form $30 * 20 = 600$ random pairs of subjects in which one is a diseased subject and the other non-diseased. If the area under the ROC curve for this diagnostic test is 0.8 or 80%, it means out of the 600 possible pairs, in 80% or 540 pairs the probability of having disease is higher in truly diseased than those not having the disease. In other words, 80% of the total subjects have been diagnosed correctly by the diagnostic test.

Recall from Section 11.3.1 that when we are dealing with a rare condition or whose prevalence is low, we must keep the number of false positives to be small; otherwise, almost all positives will be false positives. When there are many false positives, their diagnoses and consequently further treatment and follow-up, etc., will unnecessarily burden heath care system. If the consequences of a false positive decision involve risky procedures such as a radiotherapy or surgery, then also it is imperative to keep the false positives to be minimal. In such situations, the decision maker must operate on the lower left part of the ROC (for example threshold C in Fig. 11.3) to keep FPF small, though it may mean a low TPF and correspondingly high FNF. We realize that at threshold C, only 50% of the diseased can be detected as positive by the test, but very few (less than 5%) false positives will occur.

Alternatively, when the disease prevalence is high or it is important to catch positive cases, the decision maker should choose a threshold higher on the curve so that a higher FPF is acceptable to keep the TPF high and FNF low. This is a lax criterion corresponding to the threshold A in Fig. 11.3. At this threshold, we can expect that 90% of the diseased could be picked-up but at the same time 50% false positives also could occur. Other situations might fall in between with a moderate threshold such as B in Fig. 11.3.

The ROC curve describes the various compromises that we can make between the TPF (consequently FNF) and FPF (consequently TNF) as we vary the decision threshold. Since both TPF and FPF are independent of the prevalence of the condition being diagnosed, the ROC curve is independent of the prevalence and also the effect of the decision threshold. We should remember here that this holds true when the distribution of the severity of disease in the tested subjects is similar to that in the population for which the diagnostic test is intended.

The ROC curve has another property: the slope of the straight line drawn from the origin (0,0) to any point on the ROC curve is equal to the likelihood ratio at that cut-off. The total area under the ROC curve is a measure of the ability of the diagnostic criteria to discriminate between presence and absence of disease, independent of both the cut-off and disease prevalence.[3]

11.9.1. Choosing a Cut-off Point

To choose an appropriate threshold or cut-off value, knowledge of the prevalence of the disease being diagnosed in the target population will help, because the pre-test or prior probability is the fraction of the subjects affected by the condition in the target population for whom the diagnostic test is likely to be applied. As we know, for any decision threshold chosen, there are costs associated with errors in diagnosis. These costs can be divided into health related and monetary related costs. Health costs can be based on morbidity and mortality and can be assessed in terms of person-years of life, healthy person-years of life, etc. Financial costs can include medical and other expenditure paid by the patient and the additional costs to the society (insurance, support to the family, etc.) due to the disability or premature death of the patient. Both the health costs and financial costs can be used in determining the optimum cut-off.

To start with, if we consider the health costs, we would like to minimize the differences in healthy person-years of life between our diagnosis and the diagnosis based on the gold standard.

Denoting the additional cost in person-years associated with a false negative diagnosis as AC_{FN} and that associated with a false positive diagnosis as AC_{FP}, the optimum operating point on the ROC curve will be the point where the slope of the ROC curve equals[4]

$$\frac{AC_{FP}}{AC_{FN}} \frac{P(D-)}{P(D+)} \tag{11.27}$$

where *P (D-)* and *P (D+)* are the pretest probabilities of being normal and diseased respectively as defined earlier.

If the average cost of missing a true case is high and that of treating a false positive is low, intuitively we should operate near threshold A in Fig. 11.3. Under such a condition, AC_{FN} / AC_{FP} in equation 11.27 above will be small, so that the slope of the ROC changes very slowly, which is near threshold A of Fig. 11.3. On the other hand, if the health costs of treating a false positive are high and the therapeutic results of treating the disease are only marginal, we should operate near the threshold C in the Fig. 11.3. In this situation the AC_{FN} / AC_{FP} in equation 11.27 above will be high corresponding to the steep slope near threshold C. Likewise, if the pre-test probability of the disease (prevalence) is very low, $P(D-)$ / $P(D+)$ in equation 11.27 will be high corresponding to the threshold towards the lower left of the ROC curve.

If we are interested in financial costs, AC_{FN} and AC_{FP} in equation 11.27 will be replaced by the additional financial costs associated with a false negative diagnosis and a false positive diagnosis respectively and the same principles apply. It should be noted that the optimal cut-off chosen is appropriate for the measure of costs chosen. The cut-off chosen on financial costs could be different from the one based on health costs.

Most often we will not have accurate estimates of the additional costs associated with the errors and so a cut-off is chosen such that it minimizes our mistakes. This position on the ROC occurs when the slope is equal to *P (D-)* / *P (D+)*.[5] This point, which minimizes the errors, could be different from the two thresholds that are based on health costs and financial costs.

To demonstrate the construction of an ROC plot, we take an artificial data of the Intra-Ocular Pressure (IOP) measurements and the gold standard diagnosis for 100 suspected cases of glaucoma. There are 72 true cases of glaucoma as determined by perimetry and field analysis. The raw data is not shown but the analysis results are shown below.

From the Table 11.7 we can see that every observed value of the IOP is taken as a cut-off, so that all subjects whose IOP is more than or equal to the cut-off will be declared as cases of glaucoma. The least value of the IOP observed in the sample is 9 mm, so naturally all the subjects will be declared as glaucoma cases at the cut-off of 9 mm leading to 100% Sensitivity and 0% Specificity. The fourth column of the output indicates the proportion of subjects that have been classified correctly with each cut-off value. For example, with the cut-off of 9 mm, 72% of the sampled subjects were diagnosed correctly. As the cut-off increases, notice that the Sensitivity comes down while the Specificity goes up. At a cut-off of 48 mm, the Specificity is 100% while the Sensitivity is very low (20.8%). The fifth and the sixth column indicate the likelihood ratio of a positive and negative test respectively, at each cut-off. If we assume equal costs associated with false positive and false negative results, the threshold at which the sensitivity and specificity are equal would be the best cut off. In our example data, it is 25 mm.

The last rows in Table 11.7 indicate the total area under the ROC curve, which is an indication of the proportion of total persons (normal as well as diseased) classified correctly by the diagnostic criteria. In the example, it is about 82% indicating a moderately high correct decision. The 95% confidence interval for the area under the ROC curve is also reported to get an idea of the fluctuations over repeated testing in different samples of the same size.

Based on the results of Table 11.7, the ROC curve drawn is depicted in Fig. 11.4. The smoothness of the ROC curve depends not only on the sample size, but also on the spread of different values of the parameter being measured.

Table 11.7: ROC analysis of the IOP data

Cut point	Sensitivity	Specificity	Correctly Classified	LR+	LR−
(> = 9)	100.00%	0.00%	72.00%	1.0000	
(> = 10)	100.00%	3.57%	73.00%	1.0370	0.0000
(> = 11)	100.00%	10.71%	75.00%	1.1200	0.0000
(> = 12)	98.61%	14.29%	75.00%	1.1505	0.0972
(> = 13)	97.22%	21.43%	76.00%	1.2374	0.1296
(> = 14)	95.83%	21.43%	75.00%	1.2197	0.1944
(> = 15)	94.44%	21.43%	74.00%	1.2020	0.2593
(> = 16)	94.44%	25.00%	75.00%	1.2593	0.2222
(> = 17)	93.06%	35.71%	77.00%	1.4475	0.1944
(> = 18)	90.28%	42.86%	77.00%	1.5799	0.2269
(> = 20)	84.72%	50.00%	75.00%	1.6944	0.3056
(> = 21)	83.33%	60.71%	77.00%	2.1212	0.2745
(> = 22)	81.94%	67.86%	78.00%	2.5494	0.2661
(> = 23)	81.94%	75.00%	80.00%	3.2778	0.2407
(> = 24)	79.17%	75.00%	78.00%	3.1667	0.2778
(> = 25)	77.78%	78.57%	78.00%	3.6296	0.2828
(> = 26)	75.00%	82.14%	77.00%	4.2000	0.3043
(> = 27)	72.22%	82.14%	75.00%	4.0444	0.3382
(> = 28)	69.44%	82.14%	73.00%	3.8889	0.3720
(> = 29)	68.06%	82.14%	72.00%	3.8111	0.3889
(> = 30)	66.67%	82.14%	71.00%	3.7333	0.4058
(> = 31)	63.89%	85.71%	70.00%	4.4722	0.4213
(> = 32)	62.50%	85.71%	69.00%	4.3750	0.4375
(> = 33)	58.33%	85.71%	66.00%	4.0833	0.4861
(> = 34)	56.94%	89.29%	66.00%	5.3148	0.4822
(> = 35)	52.78%	89.29%	63.00%	4.9259	0.5289
(> = 36)	50.00%	92.86%	62.00%	7.0000	0.5385
(> = 37)	45.83%	92.86%	59.00%	6.4167	0.5833
(> = 38)	44.44%	92.86%	58.00%	6.2222	0.5983
(> = 39)	41.67%	92.86%	56.00%	5.8333	0.6282
(> = 40)	40.28%	92.86%	55.00%	5.6389	0.6432
(> = 41)	36.11%	92.86%	52.00%	5.0556	0.6880
(> = 42)	34.72%	92.86%	51.00%	4.8611	0.7030
(> = 43)	30.56%	92.86%	48.00%	4.2778	0.7479
(> = 44)	27.78%	92.86%	46.00%	3.8889	0.7778
(> = 45)	26.39%	96.43%	46.00%	7.3889	0.7634
(> = 46)	23.61%	96.43%	44.00%	6.6111	0.7922
(> = 47)	22.22%	96.43%	43.00%	6.2222	0.8066
(> = 48)	20.83%	100.00%	43.00%	0.7917	
(> = 49)	19.44%	100.00%	42.00%	0.8056	
(> = 50)	18.06%	100.00%	41.00%	0.8194	
(> = 51)	13.89%	100.00%	38.00%	0.8611	
(> = 54)	11.11%	100.00%	36.00%	0.8889	
(> = 55)	6.94%	100.00%	33.00%	0.9306	
(> = 56)	2.78%	100.00%	30.00%	0.9722	
(> 56)	0.00%	100.00%	28.00%	1.0000	

Obs	ROC Area	Std. Err.	−Asymptotic Normal−− [95% Conf. Interval]	
100	0.8172	0.0469	0.72535	0.90907

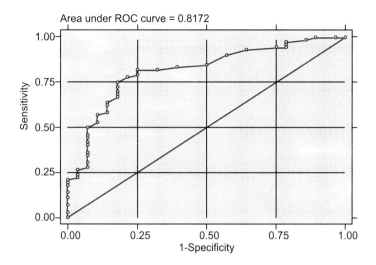

Fig.11.4: Receiver operating characteristic curve for the IOP data

11.10. Multiple Tests

As is evident from the concepts that have been presented in the earlier sections, it is obvious that no single test can be 100% sensitive and 100% specific. Because of this inherent limitation, one has to resort to two or more diagnostic tests before arriving at a decision. For example, in diagnosing pulmonary tuberculosis, chest X-ray and sputum culture are two tests that are employed. Multiple tests can be employed either in serial order or parallel to each other.

11.10.1. Serial and Parallel Testing

In the **serial testing method**, an individual is subjected to the first diagnostic test and put on the second test only if the first test resulted in a positive finding. Similarly, the third test in sequence is employed only when the second test leads to a positive result. As soon as one diagnostic test results in a negative finding, further testing is stopped and the subject is said to be disease free or negative. A positive finding of disease presence is taken only when all the tests employed lead to a positive finding.

The order or sequence of the various tests is determined as per their properties. The first diagnostic test will be the most specific followed by the one that has the next highest Specificity and the last of the sequence will naturally have the highest Sensitivity but the least Specificity. This strategy leads us to very specific results.

In **parallel testing** strategy, all the tests are employed simultaneously or parallelly and the individual subject is said to be positive if any of the test results in a positive outcome. This strategy enhances the Sensitivity of the decision made, but the Specificity will be compromised. DiMagno[6] et al. (1977) employed 4 different tests in the diagnosis of pancreatic cancer and compared them with a gold standard diagnosis. Various strategies are evaluated in the diagnosis and the article is a must for any serious reader who wishes to have a fuller understanding of multiple testing.

Multiple Choice Questions

Choose the correct answers in the following multiple choice questions. The correct answers are listed on p. 345.

Q.1. **Percentage of cases correctly classified as cases by the test is called:**
a. Positive predictive value
b. Negative predictive value
c. Specificity
d. Sensitivity

Q.2. **Sensitivity is defined as:**
a. The percent of those who have the disease and are so indicated by the test
b. The percent of those who do not have the disease and are so indicated by the test
c. The percent of those who have the disease, and are not so indicated by the test
d. The percent of those who do not have the disease and are not so indicated by the test

Q.3. **Specificity is defined as:**
a. The percent of those who have the disease, and are so indicated by the test
b. The percent of those who do not have the disease and are so indicated by the test
c. The percent of those who have the disease and are not so indicated by the test.
d. The percent of those who do not have the disease and are not so indicated by the test

Q.4. **A drug company is developing a new pregnancy test kit for use on an outpatient basis. The company uses the pregnancy test on 100 women who are known to be pregnant and out of 100 women, 99 showed positive. Upon using the same test on 100 non-pregnant women, 90 showed negative. What is the sensitivity of the test?**
a. 90%   b. 99%
c. 10%   d. 100%

Q.5. **What is the specificity of the test for the results given in Q.4?**
a. 90%   b. 99%
c. 10%   d. 90.8%

Q.6 **Likelihood ratio of positives (LR+) for the results given in Q.4 is:**
a. 0.1   b. 9.9
c. 0.01   d. 1.1

Q.7. **Likelihood ratio of negatives (LR-) for the results given in Q.4 is:**
a. 1.1   b. 0.01
c. 9.9   d. 0.1

Q.8. **In a study 90% of the confirmed cases were truly classified as cases by a new relatively simpler and less expensive test. That value (90%) is called:**
a. Predictive value of the positives
b. Specificity
c. Sensitivity
d. Accuracy

Q.9. **To assess the utility of alpha-fetoprotein (AFP) values in diagnosing liver cancer, a hepatologist found that out of the 100 suspected cases 40 were cancer cases by histo-pathological diagnosis. It is also noted that 20 out of the 40 true cases and 20 non-diseased persons had elevated AFP levels. The positive predictive value (PV+) of AFP in diagnosing liver cancer will be:**
a. 50%   b. 66.7%
c. 33.3%   d. 40%

Q.10. **The threshold value of a measurable variable to diagnose a condition/disease can be computed from:**
a. Frequency curve
b. Histogram
c. ROC curve
d. Scatter diagram

References

1. Fagan TJ. Nomogram for Bayes' Theorem. *N Engl J Med*. 1975; 293: 257.
2. Sox HC, Blatt MA, Higgins MC, Marton KI. *Medical Decision Making*. Stoneham, Massachusetts: Butterworth-Heinemann; 1988.
3. Hanley JA, McNeil BJ. The meaning and use of the area under a receiver operating characteristic (ROC) curve. *Radiology*. 1982; 143:29-36.
4. Swets John A, ed. *Signal Detection and Recognition by Human Observers*. New York: John Wiley; 1964.
5. McNeil BJ, Keeler E, Adelstein SJ. Primer on certain elements of medical decision making. *N Engl J Med*. 1975; 293: 211-215.
6. DiMagno EP, Malagelada JR, Taylor WF, Go VL. A prospective comparison of current diagnostic tests for pancreatic cancer. *N Engl J Med*. 1977; 297:737-742.

12 | Introduction to Medical Demography

The science of man is the most difficult of all sciences.

Alexis Carrel — Nobel Laureate

12.1. Introduction

The word "Demos" is derived from a rhetorical term used for the population of an ancient Greek state and together with the term "graphy" it signifies a statistical study or description of populations. Demography is a very general science that can be applied to any dynamic population, which tends to change over time or space. Thus, demography can be defined as the study of any population with respect to its size, composition, the spatial and/or temporal changes associated with birth, migration, aging and death, and the interaction of all these with social and economic conditions.

There is a close link between the principles of epidemiology and demography. Epidemiology is the study of distribution and determinants of disease frequency in a population and demography is the study of populations. Many diseases and conditions in a population depend on the composition of that population. For example, a population with a larger proportion of aged people may have a higher burden of cardio-vascular diseases as compared to a population with a smaller proportion of the same. Thus, the background knowledge of the population helps in a better understanding of the epidemiologic principles.

Medical demography is a part of demography that deals with the study of distribution of health, illness, healthcare quality and utilization and their relationship with various bio-social and socio-cultural characteristic within a population. In medical demography, various indicators are used to convey different demographic aspects, which have a bearing on health of a community or vice versa, i.e., health indices that have a bearing on the population. Thus, medical demography covers both aspects — the effects of population forces on the delivery of medical services as well as the effects of medical services on populations.

A proper understanding of various demographic terms is necessary to avoid any possible errors in collecting the data as well as in calculating the indices. As this book is of an introductory nature, some commonly used demographic terms along with their interpretations and some commonly used indices only are described here. Readers interested in detailed description of demographic techniques dealing with estimation of various health indicators and their relationship with biosocial and socio-cultural factors are advised to refer to the books suggested for further reading.

12.2. Basic Terminologies

12.2.1. Demography

Demographic factors. Factors such as age, sex, births and deaths, etc., that have a bearing on the population characteristics are collectively called demographic factors.

Demographic transition. Gradual change in the composition of a population with respect to different aspects like age, sex, etc., is referred to as demographic transition. In many countries, it is generally observed that a situation of relatively high fertility and mortality is slowly shifting towards a scenario of relatively low fertility and low mortality. Thus, a demographic transition or evolution is taking place. This transition might also give rise to a rapid growth in the population size, especially in the initial stages of the transition, as there will be a fall in the mortality before a fall in the fertility level takes place.

Historical demography. This generally means the study of the history of the population changes. Further, this also implies the study of the population history in the period prior to the availability of proper statistics.

Sources of demographic data. Those sources that make available demographic data in published and/or unpublished form are called sources of demographic data. The common sources of demographic data for any country are census, registration of records (e.g., births and deaths) and demographic surveys.

Vital events. All the events that may bring about changes in the composition of population are called vital events. For example, live births and deaths are the most important vital events. However, fetal deaths, marriages, divorces, legal separations and migrations are also called vital events.

Vital statistics. Demographic data concerning all the vital events are called vital statistics and they are expressed as some indices. They provide important clues to the policy planners.

12.2.2. Population Studies

Base population. The population on which different vital rates are calculated is called the base population.

Closed population. A population not exposed to flow of migration (either inward or outward) is called closed population. As a result, the change in population size may occur entirely due to births and deaths in a closed population. Some of the tribal populations in remote parts of India are considered as closed populations.

Component method of population projection. It is a population projection method in which projection is made for each age group using varying components (e.g., births, deaths, immigration, out migration) by taking the initial age-distribution of the population. This can also be done using gender or other variables.

Density of population. It is an index showing the relationship between a population and the physical extent of the area of a region. It is obtained by dividing the total population of a region by the area of that region in square kilometers and is expressed as the number of persons per square kilometer. The more the population density, the more crowded is the place.

Dependency ratio. The ratio of the economically dependent part of a population (or inactive population like persons above 65 years and below 15 years) to economically independent part of the population (or working population like those in the age-group 15 to 64 years) is called dependency ratio. The lower ratio indicates better economic condition of that population.

Exponential growth. In a continuously growing population over a period of time, a constant range of growth is called exponential growth. For instance, almost 2.0 percent growth in Indian population annually, continuously over a period of time may be described as an exponential growth.

Natural increase. The natural increase in population of a region means the surplus or deficit of births over deaths in population of that region in a given time period.

Open population. A population exposed to flow of migration (either in-migration or out-migration) is called an open population. Most of the modern societies are open populations.

Population at risk. It consists of all individuals for whom there is a chance of an occurrence of a specified event and is called a population at risk for that event. The use of this term 'risk' does not imply that the event in question is dangerous or in any way unwanted. For example, women in the age-group 15 years to 49 years are exposed to the 'risk' of pregnancy; and the entire population is exposed to the 'risk' of mortality.

Population distribution. The arrangement of the members of a population into various categories of a specific variable or characteristic is called the population distribution with respect to that characteristic. For example, sex distribution of the Indian population as per the 2001 census[1] is 937 females per 1000 males. Similarly, we can have the proportion of the population in each 5 year age-groups, which can be called the age distribution.

Population dynamics. It is defined as a change, movement or development of a population. It is a continuous process, because of the continuous occurrence of vital events such as births, marriages, divorces, deaths and migration.

Population explosion. Population explosion refers to a situation in which the size of a population tends to be very large in a finite interval of time. Rapid increases in population for a long time may also be termed as population explosion. This phenomenon can happen if the birth rate increases and/ or is very much higher than the death rate for a long time like in Indian population.

Population growth. The growth of population in a region means increase or decrease in population of that region. Positive or negative growth of population in a region may be attributed mainly to regional births, deaths and migration.

Population increase. It is an upward change in size of a population in a given period of time. This is the net result of births, deaths and migration in the population in that period of time.

Population momentum. It is a phenomenon that refers to the proportion of the population capable of giving birth to children and is yet to have their children. Such persons are scheduled to eventually have children, which would add to the population size. Naturally, the higher the proportion of such people, the larger the population growth will be. So, population will continue to grow, even if the fertility rate reaches a replacement level. High fertility levels in the past would have caused a large proportion of population capable of giving birth to children and yet to have their children.

The phenomenon of population momentum can lead to different growth rates between two populations with same initial size and fertility levels. This can be explained with an example. Suppose states A and B have a population size of 100000 each and the fertility rate of 2.5 children per woman. Let us further suppose that state A has 30% of the population under 18, while state B has only 10%.

State A has 30% of 100000, i.e., 30000 persons below 18 years. Assuming a sex ratio of 1:1, it implies 15000 couples, who will have 2.5 children each, on the average. It leads to 37500 new babies. Similar calculation on State B would give us 12500 new babies only (10% of $100000 \times \frac{1}{2} \times 2.5$).

It is clear that though both states have the same initial population sizes and similar fertility rates, because of a high proportion of child bearing population in State A, its growth is 3 times of that of State B.

Population policy. Population policy may be defined as deliberately constructed or modified institutional arrangements and/or specific programs through which governments influence, directly or indirectly, demographic change (see *Population Policy,* Paul Demeny[2]; Ministry of Health & Family Welfare[3]). The broad aim of such policy is to bring about quantitative changes in the population. Many countries in the world including India have their own population policies.

Population projection. The prediction of the population size for the future is referred to as population projection. Needless to say that such an exercise involves certain assumptions regarding the future trends in fertility, mortality and migration rates. Also, there are different methods of population projections. Usually, more than one prediction is made (e.g., low, medium and high), so that different possible scenarios about the future population can be understood.

Population pyramid. When the age distribution, say in 5 year age-groups, is represented diagrammatically, the shape of such a diagram appears like a pyramid and so is the name for such a diagram. In this diagram, we take the age-group on the vertical axis and the percentage of the population in each age-group is indicated on the horizontal axis. The percentage in each age-group is shown as a bar, whose length corresponds to the magnitude of the proportion. Male and female populations are shown simultaneously on each side of the vertical axis.

The shape of the population pyramid may be expansive for many developing countries like India. The pyramid has a broad base indicating a high proportion of children and a rapid rate of population growth. As the age increases, the length of the bars shrinks showing lesser and lesser proportion of older persons in the population. For some countries, the pyramid is constrictive, that is, it has a narrower base than the middle of the pyramid indicating a recent decline in fertility. Many of the Western and European countries have a stationary pyramid; the pyramid has a narrow base and roughly equal numbers in each age-group, but tapering off at the older ages indicating a moderate proportion of children and a slow or zero rate of growth.

Population studies. Studies of demographic phenomena in actual populations are called population studies.

Quasi-stable population. A population with almost constant fertility but with declining mortality may be called as a quasi-stable population. The age distribution of such a population generally experiences little change.

Stable population. When a closed population experiences a constant age-specific fertility and mortality rates for a sufficiently long period of time, its annual rate of increase tends to be a constant. Any closed population that achieves this stage is called a stable population. It obviously has an unchanging age composition.

Stationary population. A stable population with zero natural growth is called a stationary population, where age composition does not change. Obviously, in a stationary population, fertility and mortality are equal.

Working population. It is a group of all those persons who work for pay or profit. Housewives engaged in unpaid domestic duties, students and retired teachers, etc., are generally excluded from this category.

Young population. It is a population with a relatively high proportion of children, adolescents and young adults. Obviously, such population has a low median age, and a high potential for further growth.

Youth dependency ratio. The ratio of the number of people in the less than 15 years of age group to the number of people in age group 15-65 years is sometimes referred to as youth dependency ratio. It is generally expressed as percentage. Accordingly, a youth dependency ratio of 47 in India means there are 47 persons below 15 years of age for every 100 people in the age group of 15 years to 65 years.

Zero population growth. The zero population growth means a population in equilibrium with growth rate zero, which can be achieved when births plus immigration equal deaths plus emigration. A population could reach this equilibrium in various ways — births equaling deaths (as would happen in a population that reached the replacement level of fertility for a long time) and net migration is zero, or births exceeding deaths, but the surplus is balanced by net emigration; or deaths exceeding births, but the deficit is balanced by net immigration.

12.2.3. Census-related Terms

Census circles. When larger areas of a country are divided into smaller areas for census purposes, these smaller areas are called census circles. A census tract/circle may contain several administrative districts/wards.

Census. The complete coverage of every member of entire population of a given area is called census of that area. For example, decennial census conducted in India.

Civil registration system. Under civil registration system, each of the vital events like births, deaths and marriages or divorced cases needs to be registered with a civil/designated authority. This system exists in India for a long time and is generally called "Civil Registration System".

De-facto population. During the census enumeration of a place, we can find persons belonging to one place in another place as temporary visitors. De-facto population of a place refers to those who are found in that place during the census enumeration, irrespective of general place of stay/residence. In other words, it is the actual population of a given area that is present during the census enumeration. Hence, under this approach, visitors are also treated as residents in the area they are present during the census enumeration.

De-jure population. This is defined as all the people who habitually live in the concerned area. It consists of only the permanent residents who are present in the area on the census day, and also the temporary absentees who are absent from the area on that day. Accordingly, visitors are not included in this population.

Fertility survey. Surveys undertaken with a view to investigating mainly human fertility are known as fertility surveys. Examples are standard fertility surveys and world fertility survey conducted in some of the countries.

KAP surveys. The surveys with major focus on knowledge, attitude and practice (KAP) related to important issues like HIV/AIDS, family planning, etc., are called as KAP surveys. These surveys are helpful in programme development and implementation on topics of national importance.

Sample registration system. Unlike in civil registration system, sample registration system continuously records vital events like births, deaths, marriages and divorces, etc., only in randomly selected villages and towns, through local informants. Further, it is supplemented by independent semi-annual house-to-house surveys by the supervisors to detect omissions, if any. The problem of incompleteness under civil registration system necessitated this scheme during 1964 in India and it continues to provide more reliable estimates of the birth and death rates in the country since then.

Sample surveys. A sample survey is a special investigation for a specified objective(s) on a randomly selected population. It may be carried out at block/district/state/country level covering only one or many aspects of fertility, mortality, health, migration, etc. For instance, the National Family Health Survey (NFHS)[4] in India covered almost all states and union territories in the country. The third round of NFHS was completed in India during 2005-2006.

12.2.4. Cohorts

Age cohort. Age cohort is defined as a group of persons who have the same age in a specified period of time, usually a calendar year. For example, people belonging to a birth cohort.

Birth cohort. A group of persons born within a specified period of time, usually a calendar year, is called a birth cohort.

Cohort. It is defined as a group of people who share a common temporal demographic experience in a specified period of time. For example, all children in a primary school can be considered as a cohort, as they are likely to be in the same age group.

Generation. A generation is a group of persons born within a specified period of time, generally a calendar year. In other words, a birth cohort is also a generation. This term is also used to denote the descendants of a group of persons who are themselves a generation.

Radix. It is a cohort consisting of a group of individuals who might have experienced the same significant demographic event during a specified period of time, usually a year, and who may be identified as a group at successive later dates on the basis of this common demographic experience. For example, a radix of a life table is the number of births in a year constituting the original cohort, which is taken as a standard number, usually 100,000.

Synthetic cohort. A synthetic cohort is synonymous with a hypothetical cohort and is defined as a cohort imagined or assumed to exist.

12.2.5. Family & Marriage-related Terms

Age at first marriage. The age at marriage of a person getting married for the first time is called as age at first marriage.

Age at marriage. The age of a person at the time of his/her marriage is called his/her age at marriage. The two partners of a marriage may have different ages at their marriage and so there are age at marriage of males and age at marriage of females for any population. The younger the age at marriage in a population, the longer the span of fertility and so is the likelihood of high fertility. Besides, younger age at marriage, especially for females, may also lead to younger age at first child's birth associated with more maternal risks, etc.

Age distribution. The distribution of a population classified according to age is called 'age distribution'. For this, age may be considered by individual years of age or by suitable age groups. Graphically, a population pyramid may represent an age distribution, which is a histogram showing the population by age.

Age heaping. An accumulation of many persons having some preferred digits is called 'age-heaping'. The general tendency of people to quote their age to the nearest digit ending with a 0 or 5 makes a sudden increase in the numbers with age ending with these digits. For example, even if a person is aged 21 years, it is likely to be reported as 20. This phenomenon is also called digital preference.

Amenorrhea. The absence of menstruation in a woman during the usual menstrual cycle (after puberty and before menopause) is called 'amenorrhea'. When it occurs temporarily after a child birth, it is known as "post-partum amenorrhea (PPA)'. The related period is known as period of PPA and may vary from one woman to another as well as from one parity to another parity for the same woman. During this period, women are not susceptible to conception.

Coital frequency. The frequency of the sexual intercourse of a couple is called coital frequency. It is generally expressed as average frequency per week/month.

Consanguineous marriage. A marriage between persons closely related by blood (e.g., marriage between a woman and her cousin brother) is called a consanguineous marriage. In some primitive societies, marriages between brother and sister are also a common practice.

Couple. In general, two persons of opposite sexes living in stable union, whether legal or not, are called a couple. However, in Indian set up, a couple means a married couple.

Eligible couple. It means a couple where both partners are surviving and staying together and wife is in the reproductive age group of 15 to 49 years. In other words, generally a couple that fulfills inclusion criteria under fertility study is known as an eligible couple.

Family. A family is a social unit consisting of two or more persons united by blood, marital or equivalent ties. It may include members who do not share the household but are united to other members by blood, marital or equivalent ties. When a family includes a group of persons comprising members of various generations united by blood, marital or equivalent ties, it is called an extended family.

Household. A household consists of a group of individuals who live under the same roof and eat from the same kitchen. It is not necessary that these members be from the same family. It is a commonly used sampling unit in demographic studies.

Marital duration. The difference between present age and age at marriage of any partner of an eligible couple is defined as marital duration.

Marital status. The status of any person with regard to marriage is called marital status. The different categories of marital status are single (bachelor or spinster) that are never married, married, and widowed, divorced or separated who are ever married.

Marriage. A ceremony prescribed by law/custom involving rights and obligations that establishes a union between a male and a female as husband and wife is known as marriage or wedding or nuptiality.

Marriageable population. This is defined as the persons who are legally eligible for marriage out of the total. For example, in India, a total of all spinsters who have attained minimum age for marriage fixed as 18 years and all bachelors who have attained minimum age for marriage fixed as 21 years will constitute the marriageable population.

Menstrual cycle. The periodic appearance of menses in women is called menstrual cycle. It starts after attaining puberty and ends with menopause. Although the conventionally known cycle period is of 28 days, there may be variation in the duration of the cycle from one woman to another and also for the same woman from one period to another period.

Offspring. The totality of all the descendants of a common ancestor is defined as offspring.

Present age. It may also be called as 'age at last birthday' and coveys the completed age, usually in years. Thus, the age of all infants below one year is zero. If a person is going to complete 15 years after the day of data collection, strictly speaking, his/ her age will be recorded as 14 years. It is a basic characteristic of any person covered in a study.

Reproductive period. This is also known as child bearing period of a woman and is defined as the period between puberty and menopause. Usually, it is taken as 15 to 49 years.

Stable age distribution. If the proportion of persons in different age groups in a stable population is constant, then it is said to have a stable age distribution. Such a distribution is independent of the initial age distribution, but depends only on the prevailing fertility and mortality rates.

Widowhood. If a marriage is dissolved because of the death of either the husband or the wife, the surviving spouse is called a widower in case of male and a widow in case of female. This state is called widowhood. It is one of the categories of marital status of an individual.

12.2.6. Fertility-related Terms

Abortion. A fetus becomes usually capable of independent existence outside its mother (i.e., viable), when the duration of pregnancy is at least 20 weeks. If an expulsion of the fetus takes place before it is viable, it is called abortion. It may be spontaneous, induced, illegal or legal. It may occur due to several reasons (e.g., criminal, intentional, therapeutic, unintentional).

Birth control/family planning. The number of children and spacing between them may be controlled through adoption of various contraceptive methods that permit sexual intercourse with reduced likelihood of conception. Such restriction/limitation of births, either to achieve the desired interval between successive births or to prevent more births than desired, is called birth control/family planning.

Birth order. Birth order of a child is defined as the serial number of that child among children born alive to the same mother. Children here include the present child also. In other words, birth order of a child is its rank order of all live children born to a mother. This adds another dimension to analysis of child survival.

Closed birth interval. The interval between two live births is called a closed birth interval. An interval between marriage and first birth is also called a birth interval, but not the closed birth interval.

Completed fertility. The average cumulative fertility of a cohort (e.g., birth or marriage cohort), measured at the time when all its living members reach the end of the reproductive period, is called completed fertility.

Conception. It is the fertilization of the female ovum by a male spermatozoon leading to pregnancy.

Contraceptive method. Any measure taken to prevent sexual intercourse from resulting in conception is known as contraception. A method employed for contraception is known as contraceptive method (e.g., condom, intra-uterine device, sterilization).

Controlled fertility. It is the fertility experience of a population that is subjected to various birth control methods.

Differential fertility. Fertility is known to vary between various categories of a population. Such fertility variation between different groups is called differential fertility. To study this, specific fertility rates are used. For example, it can be reported in relation to varying age and/or sex groups.

Fecundability. The probability of conception in a menstrual cycle of a woman in an eligible couple, who are not on any contraceptives, is called fecundability.

Fecundity. The ability (i.e., physiological capacity) of a man, a woman or a couple to participate in reproduction (i.e., conception leading to a live birth) is called fecundity. Such persons/couples are known as fecund persons/couples.

Fertility. This is the most important factor in population dynamics. Fertility is defined as the child bearing performance of a woman or a group of women in terms of actual number of children born. It starts with the age at menstruation/marriage date and ends with menopause/secondary sterility. On an average, reproductive life span of a woman extends from the age 15 to 50 years. A change in fertility level causes change in both the size and composition of the population. Fecundity is capacity for reproductive performance, whereas fertility is actual performance itself.

Fetal death/intra-uterine mortality. Fetal death or fetal mortality means death of a product of conception prior to the complete expulsion or extraction from the mother's womb irrespective of the duration of the pregnancy. Accordingly, it includes both abortions and stillbirths.

Fetus. It is the product of the fertilization of the female ovum by a male sperm indicating the beginning of pregnancy.

Induced abortion. An abortion that is purposely (or intentionally) carried out is called an induced abortion. This is to be distinguished from an unintentional (or spontaneous) abortion, which is also known as miscarriage.

Live birth. It is the complete expulsion or extraction of a product of conception. After such separation, irrespective of the duration of pregnancy, he/she breathes or shows any other evidence of life, such as beating of the heart, pulsation of the umbilical cord, or definite movement of voluntary muscles. It is observed irrespective of whether or not the umbilical cord has been cut or the placenta is attached.

Mother's age at birth of last child. The age of a mother at the birth of her last child is called a mother's age at birth of the last child. Similarly, a mother's age at birth of the first child can also be defined. These give a measure of the period of time required on the average for family building.

Open birth interval. The interval between the last live birth prior to an enquiry and the date of same enquiry for a married woman in the reproductive period is called the open birth interval.

Parity progression ratios. The ratios of all women with a parity of zero and whose fertility is complete, to all women with parity of a value "n" in the same population, are known as parity progression ratios. These are useful as a kind of fertility index, as they reflect all prior childbearing. They may also be computed for women of a specified age or cohort.

Parity. The number of children previously born alive to a woman is called parity of women. For example, a woman of parity two is a woman who had two live children born to her up to then. A zero-parity woman is one who had no children born to her till then. This is to be distinguished from birth order. It adds another dimension to analysis of fertility and is applicable to any woman.

Puerperium. A specified period after delivery, during which the uterus usually regains its normal size and in which the probability of conception is low, is called puerperium. It is generally of about six week's period.

Replacement level fertility. It is a level of fertility at which a cohort of women, on an average, will have enough daughters just to replace themselves in the population. Sometimes, the total fertility rate is also used to indicate replacement level fertility. Once replacement level fertility is reached, births gradually balance the deaths in the population. Such population, in the absence of migration, ultimately stops growing and becomes a stationary population.

Sterility. The sterility or infecundity is known as the lack of capacity of a man, a woman or a couple to participate in reproduction (i.e., production of a live child). A woman with primary sterility may not be able to have any children till a specific period after marriage. Sometimes, secondary sterility arises after one or more children are born. Sterility may be permanent or temporary.

Stillbirth. The delivery of a fetus is called stillbirth if the fetus is of at least 20 weeks of pregnancy and dies before or during the delivery. The death is indicated by the fact that after delivery the fetus does not breathe or show any other evidence of life (e.g., beating of the heart, pulsation of the umbilical cord, or definite movement of voluntary muscles). The minimum period of pregnancy considered in this regard may vary among various studies/reports (e.g., between 20 and 28 weeks). Hence, one should be careful about considered period of pregnancy while making comparison between studies.

12.2.7. Morbidity/Mortality-related Terms

Complete expectation of life. Complete expectation of life, also called the expectation of life at birth (i.e., at age zero), is the average age at death (or the average longevity) of a person belonging to a given birth cohort. It may be defined as the ratio of the total number of person-years lived by all the members of a birth cohort to the size of that cohort.

Death/mortality. The death of a person is permanent disappearance of all evidence of life at any time after his/her live birth. Obviously, the fetal deaths are not considered as deaths. Mortality is nothing but death. It is a major component of population change. However, as it affects all age groups, it does not disrupt the composition of the population significantly.

Epidemic. The spread of an infectious disease capable of infecting a large number of persons within a relatively short time interval is called an epidemic. For example, cholera and viral fever may turn to be epidemics, unless appropriate public health measures are taken.

Epidemic model. A mathematical model developed for describing any of the various aspects of an epidemic, like expected duration, rate of spread or rate of removal, is called an epidemic model.

Generation life table. A life table based on the mortality rate experienced by a particular birth cohort (e.g., all persons born in a calendar year) may be called a generation life table.

Infant mortality. The mortality of a live-born child before he/she reaches the first birthday is called infant mortality. In other words, it is the magnitude of mortality among those aged less than one year. It is one of the best health indicators for a community and many international comparisons of the prevailing health scenario are made using this index.

Life table. A life table is a table devised for describing the mortality experience of a hypothetical cohort as it gradually decreases in size until all its members die. It has seven columns and all the seven columns are obtained through the corresponding life table functions originating from a set of probabilities of death within each interval of age. They are mathematically related and, hence, can be derived if the value of one of them is known. Such a life table that deals with intervals of one year is often referred to as "Complete Life Table", whereas that obtained using age intervals of more than 1 year is called "Abridged Life Table".

Morbidity statistics. Details with respect to the number, frequency, duration, magnitude, severity, etc., of morbid conditions are called morbidity statistics. Here it is implied that different terms such as morbid condition, the diagnostic basis, severity, etc., are well defined and uniformly followed in compiling the different statistics. Otherwise, such statistics have little relevance. However, these definitions might vary from place to place or study to study and often contradictory reports on the same morbid condition are due to the differences in the definitions.

Morbidity. A specific condition of a disease, illness, sickness or ill health in a person, due to any cause is known as morbidity. Three aspects of morbidity, namely, frequency, duration and severity are commonly measured using appropriate indices in terms of morbidity rates and ratios.

Mortality differential. Like fertility, mortality is also known to vary between various categories of a population. Such mortality variation between different groups is called differential mortality. To study this, specific death rates are used.

Perinatal mortality. The word 'peri' means around and 'natal' means birth. So perinatal refers to the time around birth. Mortality during the time of birth – just before and a few days after birth — is called perinatal mortality. It mainly includes stillbirths and neonatal deaths up to seven days of life. It is so because, in general, the causes of death of fetuses during the last few weeks of pregnancy and of live-born infants during the first few days of life after birth may often result from similar underlying factors.

Person-years lived. It is the sum of the years lived by all the persons of a hypothetical cohort during their life time. For instance, if the individuals in a cohort of 7 persons lived for 0, 11, 87, 19, 40, 0 and 48 years, respectively, the person years lived by the cohort is: $0 + 11 + 87 + 19 + 40 + 0 + 48 = 205$ years. It is included as one of the columns in a life table.

Survival rate. The proportion of persons in a specified group (e.g., age, sex group) alive at the beginning of an age (or an age interval) who survive till the end of that age (or age interval) is defined as the survival rate.

Survival ratio. The proportion of survivors in a cohort from one age (or age-group) to another or next age (or age group) according to the mortality of the life table is defined as a survival ratio:

$$\text{Survival ratio} = \frac{L_{X+1}}{L_X}$$

Where, L_X in a life table is the number of years lived by the life-table cohort between the ages x and x + 1.

Obviously, the expected number of surviving persons at an age (or age-group) can be obtained by multiplying the survival ratio by the number of people in the cohort at the earlier age (or age-group).

Survivors at a given age. The survivors at a given age, say X, are defined as the number of persons in the original cohort surviving till age X. This is obtained by multiplying the radix of the original cohort by the probability of survival till age X.

12.2.8. Migration-related Terms

Emigration. The process of persons moving out of one country to another, involving a change in the residence at least for one year, is called emigration. It does not involve the movement of temporary visitors.

Exodus. It generally means a sudden emigration of persons in very large numbers (or mass migration), mainly caused by some emergency or catastrophe. For example, in case of flood and/or other disasters, people move in large numbers.

Immigration. The process of entering of individuals into one country from another with the intention of taking up esidence for at least one year there is called immigration. It does not involve the movement of temporary visitors.

In-migration. Within a country, the process of entering of individuals in one administrative unit (e.g., district) from another administrative unit with the intention of permanently residing there is known as in-migration. In other words, it relates to internal migration, within a country. It is different from immigration that relates to international migration.

International migration. The process of migration from one country to another country with an intention to reside there permanently is called international migration. Both immigration and emigration constitute international migration.

Marital migration. As a result of marriage, traditionally, female partners move to their spouses' house. In some societies, after marriage, male partners may move to their spouses' house. Such type of movement, as a result of marriage, is called marital migration.

Migration. A geographical mobility across specified geographical units, generally involving a change of residence from the place of departure to the place of arrival, is known as migration. It may be either international migration (migration between two countries) or internal migration (migration within a country).

Net migration. It is the net balance of the emigration and immigration for a country or a region, for a given period. US and other developed countries might register a negative net migration, implying that the emigrants are outnumbered by the immigrants. Similarly, developing countries might show a positive net migration, as many qualified and unemployed people might emigrate to other countries in search of employment, etc.

Out-migration. Out-migration is defined as the process of individuals going out of one administrative unit of a country to another administrative unit within the same country with the intention of residing there. It relates to external migration, within a country. It is to be distinguished from emigration that relates to international migration.

Return migration. Coming back of migrated individuals to their place of origin, after they have been away for a considerably long time (e.g., one year or so), is known as return migration.

12.2.9. Miscellaneous Terms

Graduation of data. It is a technique designed to obtain a smooth series of values from a given irregular series of observed values. It may be carried out using either graphical or mathematical methods. It is also known as smoothing of data. This process, as is obvious, alters the values in a series. However, the obtained smoothed series shows greater regularity and throws up the underlying law governing the behaviour of the observed data.

Simulation study. Simulation is an imitation of some real thing or a process in which certain characteristic or behaviour of a selected system is represented and it helps to gain insight into the functioning of the selected system. In demography, a simulation study is a study to evaluate how a selected population would behave if the characteristics or parameters of another population are adopted in the selected population. Simulation can also be for some other point of time in the same selected population.

Transition matrix. The change of a person moving from one state of condition to another is called transition and the associated probability is called the transition probability. A matrix showing the probabilities of moving from one condition to another in a population is called the transition matrix. The transition probabilities are computed using the prevailing rates of the movement from one stage to another in the population. This concept can also be applied in clinical medicine, such as the transition probabilities of a patient on treatment to a condition. The patient may get cured, develop complications, get discharged against medical advice or die, etc.

Trend. It is a component of a time series representing its long-range movement; involving possible fluctuations. It may generally be determined by graphical analytical methods like the method of moving averages. Since most of the demographic data are available in the form of time series, long-range movements or trends therein may be of interest, e.g., trend of population growth, trend of migration or fertility/mortality trend.

Urbanization. Urban area is an area with an increased density of population and man-made structures (such as buildings, etc.) in comparison to its surrounding areas. As per the Registrar General of India[5] (1991), urban areas are defined as follows:

(a) All places with a municipality, corporation, cantonment board, notified town area committee or other such places.
(b) All places that satisfy the criteria: (i) a minimum population of five thousand, (ii) at least 75% of the male working population engaged in non-agricultural pursuits, and (iii) density of population at least 400 per sq. km.
(c) Besides, the major project colonies, areas of industrial development, railway colonies and important tourist destinations are also treated as urban, though they might not fulfill above criteria strictly.

Urbanization is a phenomenon in which the proportion of the population living in urban areas tends to increase with time. It is an important aspect of study of internal migration.

12.3. Basic Indices of Vital Events

Crude rate. In a specified period (usually one calendar year), crude rate of a demographic event in a population is defined as the ratio of the number of such events in the population during the considered period, to the population corresponding to the middle of that period. As such, this rate of a demographic event is computed for an entire population, without regard to any specific characteristics of that population. It measures the prevailing proportion of the concerned events in the total population. It may be computed, irrespective of the vital event to which it refers, as follows:

$$\text{Crude rate} = \frac{\text{Number of events occurred among the population of a given geographic area during a given period}}{\text{Mid-period total population of the given geographic area during the same period}} * 1000$$

Specific rate. A rate defined in relation to one or more characteristics of a population is known as specific rate. Any relevant characteristic of the population (e.g., age, sex, occupation, education, marital status, birth order and parity), may be the basis for a specific rate. For example, the rate obtained for a specific age group in respect of any event (e.g., marriage, fertility, migration, divorce, death) is called age-specific rate. A specific rate can be calculated as follows:

$$\text{specific rate} = \frac{\text{number of events which occurred among a specific group of the population of a given geographic area during a given period}}{\text{Mid-period population of the specified group in the given geographic area during the same period}} * 1000$$

Annual rate. All demographic indices are usually computed as annual rates, which are computed for a period of one year. Even the rates that are calculated for periods different from a year may often be converted to an annual rate through multiplication by an appropriate factor under certain assumptions.

Decennial rate. Sometimes a rate per annum is required to be computed based on a ten-year period such as decennial census data in India. Though we consider the events and population for the ten-year period, to make a comparable index with an annual rate, we divide the total events that occurred in a ten-year period by ten. In other words, decennial rate is an annual rate based on ten year data on events and the population. It may be computed as follows:

$$\text{Decennial rate} = \frac{\text{number of vital events which occurred among the population of a given geographic area during the period of ten years}}{\text{Population estimated at the middle of the ten years}} * \frac{1}{10} * 1000$$

Quinquennial rate. If the annual rate is based on 5 year data instead of ten, it is called a quinquennial rate. It is computed as follows:

$$\text{Quinquennial rate} = \frac{\text{number of vital events which occurred among the population of a given geographic area during the period of five years}}{\text{Population estimated at the middle of the five years}} * \frac{1}{5} * 1000$$

Both decennial and quinquennial rates are useful in studying long term trends.

Monthly rate. Sometimes, like decennial/quinquennial rates, monthly rates may also be required in situations like symptomatic morbidity studies. In this case, to make the rate comparable with the annual rate, the total events that occurred in a month must be multiplied by twelve. This multiplier may be more accurate in the form of the following fraction:

$$\frac{365}{\text{number of days in the considered month}}$$

Weekly rate. The weekly rates may be preferred to study the seasonal variation of diseases. This rate can be computed as follows:

$$\text{Weekly rate} = \frac{\text{number of vital events which occurred in one week}}{\text{Total mid-year estimated population}} * 1000$$

Standardization. A crude rate related to any vital event may not be comparable between two or more populations because of differences in the population characteristics with respect to some potential characteristic (like age composition) that might influence the event under consideration. A procedure of adjusting the crude rates to eliminate from them the effect of differences in age-composition of populations is called standardization. In this procedure, a standardized summary measure may be derived for each of the populations being compared, keeping in view the age composition of a standard population. This exercise in relation to age-composition of the population helps in removing the effect of any variations in the age-structure of study populations. Generally, the age distribution of another population (not under study) is considered as a standard population. Standardized rates are comparable among study populations, as the effect of age compositions on the event is removed.

There are two methods of standardization - direct and indirect. These methods are described in detail in Chapter 8.

12.4. Indices of Marriage

Age-specific marriage rate. Once the marriage rate is computed for specified age-groups, it is called age-specific marriage or nuptiality rate. It is usually computed by considering the number of married persons and the number of marriageable persons in the desired age group in a year.

Average age at marriage. The average ag at marriage can be computed separately for men and women. It is an indicator of nuptiality. For women, one has to consider age at marriage of all women that marry in a year in a specific region and find the average of all such ages. It is called the average age at marriage of women during that year in the considered region. Like wise, it can be calculated for men. The lower age at marriage among women is likely to result into higher fertility especially in absence of contraceptive adoption. Third round of NFHS[4] (2005-2006) indicated that women and men aged 20-49 years had the median age at marriage as 17.2 years and 23.4 years respectively.

Crude marriage rate. Crude marriage rate is the number of marriages (n) in a population during a period (usually a calendar year), expressed as number per 1000 population. The population (N) is taken corresponding to the middle of the period. In other words, it is computed as [{n/ N} *1000]. For example, in a village of 3000 population (as on July first) if 12 marriages take place in a year, the crude marriage rate works out to be 12 per 3000 or 4 per 1000 during that year. Though marriage involves a man and a woman and so two persons are getting married, it is counted as one. One should also be clear about inclusion/ exclusion of remarriages while calculating this rate. As per objective, one may or may not include remarriages in the calculation.

Marriage rate. It may be defined as the number of marriages in a given period (usually a calendar year) in the considered region per thousand *midyear marriageable population* of that region. The marriageable age usually depends on prevailing policy of that region. In countries like India, marriages in some of the states take place even before prescribed age at marriage (18 years for females and 21 years for males). As per the 3rd round of National Family Health Survey (2005-2006), more than half of women are married before the legal minimum age of 18.

12.5. Indices of Abortion/Stillbirth/Fetal Deaths

Abortion rate. This is generally defined as the estimated number of abortions per thousand women of age 15-49 years in a given year in a specified region. Sometimes, women of age group 15-44 years only are be considered. Further, to be more accurate, denominator may consist of only total number of pregnancies in the considered year.

Abortion ratio. Abortion ratio is defined as the estimated number of abortions per thousand live births in a given year in a specified region. Abortion rate refers to the population of women, while abortion ratio refers to live births. This distinction between the two should be understood to avoid inappropriate comparisons and also misusing them interchangeably.

Fetal death rate. The ratio of the number of fetal deaths (i.e., a total of abortions and stillbirths) in a given year in a specified region to the total number of pregnancies in the same year in that region is defined as fetal death rate. Sometimes this is considered as synonym of stillbirth rate. Therefore, one should be clear about the definitions to avoid errors in understanding, interpreting, comparing across studies/places as well as public health implications.

Fetal death ratio. Instead of all pregnancies in the denominator of a fetal death rate, if we consider all live births it is called fetal death ratio. Sometimes this is considered as a synonym of stillbirth ratio. Therefore, one should be clear about considered definitions to avoid errors in understanding, interpretation, comparison as well as public health implications.

Stillbirth rate. The proportion of the number of stillbirths per thousand total births (i.e., stillbirths and live births) in a given year in a specified region is defined as stillbirth rate. While comparing stillbirth rates among different studies, we should be alert to the pregnancy gestations used to define stillbirths in each study.

Stillbirth ratio. The ratio of the number of stillbirths per thousand live births in a given year in a specified region is defined as stillbirth ratio. As in comparison of stillbirth rates, comparison of stillbirth ratios across studies requires similar consideration of gestations for defining stillbirths.

12.6. Indices of Fertility

Sex ratio. The sex ratio is defined as the number of females per 1000 males in a population. In other words:

$$\text{Sex ratio} = \frac{F}{M} * 1000$$

Where, F is the number of females recorded in the population and M is the number of males recorded in the same population.

As per report of 3rd round of NFHS[4] (2005-2006), the sex ratio in India among the population aged 0-6 years is 918 girls per 1000 boys. This is lower than sex ratio of 927 girls per 1000 boys as per the 2001 Indian census. Hence, it remains a matter of concern for the policy planners.

Child-woman ratio. Child women ratio is defined as the ratio of the number of children up to four years of age per thousand women of childbearing age in a population. It is a crude measure of fertility.

Crude birth rate. The crude birth rate is defined as the ratio of the total number of births in a population during a given period (usually a calendar year) to the mid period (year) population. It means:

$$\text{Annual crude birth rate} = \frac{\substack{\text{number of live births which occurred among the population} \\ \text{of a given geographic area during a given year}}}{\substack{\text{Mid-year total population of the given geographic} \\ \text{area during the same year}}} * 1000$$

If the crude birth rate is 30, it implies that on an average, there are 30 births per 1000 population in that year.

Though the crude birth rate appears to be simple and conveys the general magnitude of fertility in the community, it should be noted that like any crude rate, CBR is affected by several factors such as age-sex structure of the population and distribution of married women in the reproductive period. Further, persons not involved in births are included in the computation of the crude birth rate. Because of these, it cannot be used for comparison of two or more populations, but can be used for the same population over a period of time.

General fertility rate (GFR). This is an improvement in the crude birth rate. Instead of taking all population in the denominator, we consider only those at risk of giving birth, i.e., women in the reproductive age group. Thus, the ratio of all live births registered during a year to the mid-year population of women of childbearing age (usually taken as 15 years to 44 years) is defined as GFR. In other words:

$$GFR = \frac{\text{number of live births in one year}}{\text{mid-year number of women in age group 15-44 years}} * 1000$$

In usual practice, all live births to all women of reproductive age are considered regardless of marital status. Further, sometimes childbearing age is considered as 15-49 years.

It should be noted that births to women aged less than 15 years and also to women aged more than 44/49 years should also be part of numerator.

For example, if there are 300 live births in a village with a female population of 3500 in the age-group 15-44 years during a year, the general fertility rate works out to be 86 per 1000 women. It implies that for every 1000 women aged 15-44 years, there were on the average 86 births during the year in the village.

GFR no doubt, is more acceptable than CBR as it considers only the persons at risk of giving birth. It is also easy to compute and interpret. But still it is a crude estimate as the denominator includes all women in 15-44 years including unmarried, divorced, widowed, sterile, etc. It is not helpful in comparing 2 or more populations, as it is dependent on the age-composition of women between 15 and 44/49 years.

General marital fertility rate (GMFR). Instead of all women aged 15-44 years, if we consider only married women in the denominator of GFR, it is called General Marital Fertility rate (GMFR). Accordingly, GMFR is defined as the total number of live births in a given year, per 1000 mid-year population of married women aged 15 years to 44 years in a given region. In other words:

$$GMFR = \frac{\text{number of live births in one year to married women aged 15-44 years}}{\text{mid year number of married women in age group 15-44 years}} * 1000$$

Sometimes, married women's age is considered as 15-49 years.

Age-specific fertility rate (ASFR). If fertility rate is computed for a specific age or age-group, it is called age-specific fertility rate (ASFR). It means:

$$ASFR = \frac{\begin{array}{c}\text{number of live births which occured to mothers of a specifed age group}\\ \text{of the population of a given geographic area during a given year}\end{array}}{\begin{array}{c}\text{Mid-year female population of the specified age group in the given}\\ \text{geographic area during the same year}\end{array}} * 1000$$

Generally ASFR rises from zero at age 15 years to a peak in the early or mid twenties (depending upon the marriage pattern) and thereafter declines gradually again to zero at about 45 years. Generally, specific rates for 5-year age-groups are calculated to have more stable estimates.

Total fertility rate (TFR). Total fertility rate (TFR) is an age-adjusted measure of fertility, which takes into account the age distribution of women within the childbearing period. This is the sum of the age-specific birth rates of women observed in a given year over their complete reproductive period. This is the average number of children that would be born alive to a woman during her lifetime, who would be subjected to ASFR of a given year. In other words, this is the number of children born per woman in a cohort of women by the end of their childbearing period (i.e., 44 or 49 years of age). Thus,

TFR= (sum of all ASFR)*(width of each age group)/1000

In other words, TFR per thousand women may be worked out as:

$$TFR = \left(\sum_{15}^{44} \frac{B_x}{P_x^f} \right) * 1000$$

Where, B_x is the number of births registered during the year to mothers aged x and P_x is the mid-year population of women of the same age.

Sometimes, married women's age is considered up to 49 years of age. TFR indicates the number of children which a woman would bear during her life time, if she were to bear children throughout her life at the prevailing age-specific fertility rates and does not die before completion of reproductive span.

According to the report of 3rd round of NFHS (2005-2006), the current TFR in India is 2.7 children per woman. Though it is still well above the replacement level, it has reached replacement level (2.1) in urban areas while in rural areas it is still about 3.0.

Standardization of birth rate. In general, the procedure of adjustment of the crude rate to eliminate from it the effect of differences in age-composition of populations is called standardization. Thus, birth rates adjusted for age are called standardized birth rates.

Direct method of standardization of fertility. Usually, crude bi th rate depends on the age structure of the population as well as on the levels of fertility. For comparison of the fertility performance of different study populations, the crude rates have to be adjusted to eliminate the effect of the possible differences in the age-composition of study populations. A 'standard population' with a given age structure (say P_X^s) is considered in this regard. For example, for comparison of fertility between Uttar Pradesh (A) and Kerala (B), age structure of India may be more appropriate to be considered as a standard population.

If age specific birth rates for the population (e.g., A) under study are available, these rates (m_X^A) are applied to the corresponding age groups of the standard population for standardization. Standardized fertility rate is calculated as:

$$\frac{P_X^S \, m_x^A}{P_X^S}$$

Such a method of standardization is called the direct method of standardization of fertility. In the same way, standardized fertility rate for Kerala may also be calculated. These standardized rates are useful to study the differences in the fertility experiences of two states. Using a similar approach, one may even assess differences in the fertility experiences of the same state/ community at two different periods of time.

Indirect method of standardization of birth rate. Sometimes, the age specific birth rates for the states may not be available; only their age structures might be available. In such circumstances, indirect standardization is a technique that may be employed for the adjustment of crude birth rate by applying the age-specific birth rates of a standard population separately to the given age-structure of each of the study populations. In other words:

Standardized birth rate = CBR of the given population* $\dfrac{\text{CBR of the standard population}}{\begin{array}{c}\text{CBR obtained by applying the specific birth rates of the}\\ \text{standard population to the given population}\end{array}}$

Like direct standardized rates, these standardized rates are also useful to study the differences in the fertility experiences of two states. Using a similar approach, one may even assess differences in the fertility experiences of the same state/ community at two different periods of time.

12.7. Indices of Mortality

Age-specific mortality rate. The mortality rates computed for specific ages or age-groups are called age-specific mortality rates. If D_i is the number of deaths registered during a year in the ith age–group and P_i is the mid-year population in the same age-group, then the age-specific mortality rate for the ith age-group, is calculated as:

$$\frac{D_i}{P_i} \times 1000$$

According to the report of 3rd round of NFHS (2005-2006), more than one in 13 die before reaching age five (i.e., 74.3 deaths per 1000 under-five children) and the rate remains higher in rural areas (82.0) compared to that in urban areas (51.7), as in the case of IMR.

Cause specific death rate. Mortality rates may further be reported in terms of the cause of death. In general, as a number of diseases may be the cause of death, a combined classification of illness is frequently used as cause of death. Most of the cause specific death rates are computed on total population. Accordingly, the number of deaths due to a specific cause (per 100,000 population) in a given year is called the cause-specific mortality rate (CSMR). It means:

$$\text{Anual cause-of-death rate} = \frac{\substack{\text{number of deaths from a specified cause which occurred among the} \\ \text{population of a given geographic area during a given year}}}{\substack{\text{Mid-period total population of the given} \\ \text{geographic area during the same year}}} * 100,000$$

These rates are useful in understanding the major causes of death in the study population.

Crude death rate. The ratio of the number of deaths occurring during a given period (usually a calendar year) to the number exposed to the risk of dying at the middle of the period is defined as crude death rate (CDR):

$$\text{Crude Death Rate} = \frac{\substack{\text{number of deaths which occurred among the population of a} \\ \text{given geographic area during a given year}}}{\substack{\text{Mid-period total population of the given} \\ \text{geographic area during the same year}}} * 1000$$

If a town has a CDR of 20, it means that there were 20 deaths on the average per 1000 population in the town, during the year.

Perinatal mortality rate. More conventionally, for a given year and considered region, the perinatal mortality rate is defined as follows:

$$\text{Perinatal mortality rate} = \frac{\substack{\text{late foetal deaths (28 weeks of gestation or more)} \\ + \text{deaths of live births under one week}}}{\text{live births } + \text{late foetal deaths}} * 1000$$

In view of its components, obviously, level of perinatal mortality may reflect the quality of antenatal care and delivery facilities.

As per the report of 3rd round of NFHS (2005-2006) in India, perinatal mortality rate is 49 deaths per 1000 pregnancies that lasted 7 months or more. It is comparatively higher in rural areas.

Neonatal mortality rate. The neonatal mortality refers to death of live-born children before attaining four weeks of age. Accordingly, neonatal mortality rate is defined as the number of deaths of live-born infants dying before attaining four weeks per thousand live births in a specified area during one year. It means:

$$\text{Neonatal mortality rate} = \frac{\substack{\text{No. of deaths of live-born infants within four weeks} \\ \text{after birth in a year in a specified area}}}{\text{Total number of live births in a year in a specified area}}$$

Because of the very high level of mortality in the first few hours, days and weeks of life of live-born children and the differences in the causes of infant deaths at this early and later ages of infancy, the conventional infant mortality rate is broken-up into a rate covering the first four weeks and a rate for the remainder of the year. This index can be further categorized into early neonatal (deaths within 1 week of life) and late neonatal rates (after one week but before 4 weeks of life).

Neonatal mortality rate in India as per the NFHS 3rd round is 39 deaths per 1000 live births. It is seen to be higher in rural areas (42.5) than that in urban areas (28.5).

Post-neonatal mortality rate. The number of infant deaths at 28 days through one year of age during a year for 1000 live births during that year is defined as post-neonatal mortality rate. However, the formula for the post-neonatal mortality rate does not quite reflect the true probability, because denominator includes those live births also that resulted in neonatal deaths.

$$\text{Post neonatal mortality rate} = \frac{\substack{\text{number of dealth of infants of age 28 days to under 1 year which occurred} \\ \text{among the population of a given geographic area during a given year}}}{\substack{\text{number of living births which occurred among the population of the} \\ \text{given geographic area during the same year}}} * 1000$$

As is obvious, such indices are very relevant measures of community health. According to the report of 3rd round of NFHS (2005-2006), post-neonatal mortality rate in India is 18 deaths per 1000 live births. It is high in rural areas (19.7) as compared to urban areas (13).

Infant mortality rate (IMR). The ratio of the number of infant deaths (i.e., deaths under one year of age) registered in a given year in a population to the total number of live births registered in the same year in the same population multiplied by 1000 is defined as IMR. In other words:

$$\text{Annual infant mortality rate} = \frac{\substack{\text{number of dealths under one year of age which occurred among} \\ \text{the population of a given geographic area during a given year}}}{\substack{\text{number of live births which occurred among the populaton of} \\ \text{the given geographic area during the same year}}} * 1000$$

Infant mortality rate is an age-specific death rate. Usually, it is high in developing countries like India. Mortality rates of infants receive special considerations, as they are different from rates for other ages. This is a very sensitive health index of a community.

According to the report of 3rd round of NFHS (2005-2006), the IMR in India is 57 deaths per 1000 live births. It remains higher in rural area (62 deaths per 1000 births) compared to the urban areas (42 deaths per 1000 births).

Standardized mortality ratio (SMR). The SMR is defined as the ratio of the observed number of deaths (d) in a study population to the expected number of deaths ($\Sigma d_x P_x$) obtained through the application of the age-specific death rates (d_x) of a standard population to the corresponding age groups (P_x) of that study population.

Standardized death rate. Like standardized birth rate, the procedure of adjustment of the crude death rate to eliminate the influence of differences in age-composition of the populations being compared, is called standardization. Death rates thus adjusted for age are called standardized death rates. Similar to those in case of fertility, there are again two types of these rates.

Direct method of standardization of mortality. Crude death rate depends upon the age structure of the population as well as on the levels of mortality. If a comparison of the mortality performance of different populations is to be made, the crude rates have to be adjusted to eliminate the effect of the possible differences in the population structure (e.g., age composition). This is generally done by considering a 'standard population' with a given age structure (say, P_x^s). If specific death rates for the population (A) under study are available, these rates (P_x^A) are applied to the corresponding age groups of the standard population for standardization. Such a method of standardization is called the direct method of standardization of mortality in relation to age. Accordingly, standardized mortality rate becomes:

$$\sum \frac{P_x^S m_x^A}{P_x^S}$$

A similar standardization may be carried out for another population (B). These standardized rates are useful in studying the differences in the mortality experiences of two communities or even in the mortality experiences of the same community at two different periods of time.

Indirect method of standardization of mortality. Sometimes the age specific death rates for the study populations (A & B) may not be available, only their age structures might be available. In such circumstances, indirect standardization is a technique that may be employed for the adjustment of crude death rate by applying the age-specific death rates of a standard population separately to the given age-structure of each of the study populations. In other words:

$$\text{Standardized death rate} = \text{CDR of the given population} * \frac{\text{CDR of the standard population}}{\substack{\text{Obtained CDR of the given population by applying} \\ \text{the age specific deaths rates of the standard population} \\ \text{to the given population}}}$$

= [Standardized mortality ratio (SMR) in the given Population] * [CDR in the standard population]

The standardized rates calculated for areas A and B may be useful in studying the differences in the mortality experiences of two communities. In the same way, differences even in the mortality experiences of the same community at two different periods of time may be studied.

Maternal mortality rate (MMR). Death of a woman due to complications of pregnancy, child-birth (or labour) and the puerperium is called maternal mortality. This is an important cause specific mortality. Maternal mortality rate is the number of female deaths in a year due to cause of maternal mortality per 1000 live births. Accordingly,

$$\text{Maternal mortality rate} = \frac{\substack{\text{Number of female deaths due to causes of maternal mortality} \\ \text{in a given year in a population}}}{\text{Number of live births in that year in the same study population}} * 1000$$

As a matter of fact, the index as described here is a ratio. For practical convenience, the denominator – number of live births — is taken to be a proxy for the number women at risk of the numerator. Further, to have better estimate of MMR, the denominator should ideally include all deliveries and abortions. Further, sometimes, consideration of denominator as number of women in reproductive age group (e.g., 15-44; 15-49) may provide another index namely maternal mortality ratio.

According to the report of 2nd round of NFHS[6] (1998-99), in India, MMR was 540 deaths per 100,000 live births. This index has its own public health importance, especially from mother's health point of view.

Life expectancy. As a convention, life expectancy may be defined at birth or at any other age (x). If current mortality trends are to continue, the life expectancy at birth is the average number of years a newly born child would live. Accordingly,

Life expectancy at birth = e_0^o

$$= \frac{\text{Total person-years lived by the birth cohort}}{\text{The size of the birth cohort}}$$

Likewise, the average number of additional years a person aged x would live, if current mortality trends are to continue, is called expectation of life at age x. It means:

Life expectancy at age x = e_o^o

$$= \frac{\text{Total person-years lived by the cohort from age x}}{\text{The size of cohort at age x}}$$

The additional person - years

$$= \frac{\text{lived by the cohort at age x}}{\text{the size of the cohort at age x}}$$

$$= \frac{T_x}{l_x}$$

For illustration, a worked example of a complete life table is shown below as Table 12.1.

Table 12.1: Life Tables India, Males 1961-1970

Age	Number living at age x	Survival ratio	Mortality rate	Number living between ages x and x +1	Number living above age x	Expectation of life
x	l_x	p_x	q_x	L_x	T_x	e_x^o
1	2	3	4	5	6	7
0	100000	0.86500	0.13500	89175	4707539	47.1
1	86500	0.99944	0.04056	84430	4617664	53.3
2	82992	0.98744	0.01056	82440	4533234	54.6
3	81950	0.99315	0.00685	81658	4450794	54.3
4	81388	0.99422	0.00578	81149	4369136	53.7
5	80918	0.99509	0.00491	80720	4287987	53.0
6	80521	0.99577	0.00423	80351	4207267	52.3
7	80181	0.99627	0.00373	80032	4126916	51.5
8	79882	0.99659	0.00341	79746	4046884	50.7
9	79609	0.99672	0.00328	79479	3967138	49.8
10	79348	0.99698	0.00302	79229	3887659	49.0
11	79109	0.99736	0.00264	79004	3808430	48.1
12	78900	0.99755	0.00245	78803	3729426	47.3
13	78706	0.99756	0.00244	78611	3650623	46.4
14	78514	0.99739	0.00260	78411	3572012	45.5
15	78309	0.99724	0.00276	78201	3493601	44.6
16	78092	0.99722	0.00278	77984	3415400	43.7
17	77875	0.99715	0.00258	77764	3337416	42.9
18	77653	0.99703	0.00297	77538	2359652	42.0
19	77422	0.99688	0.00312	77301	3112114	41.1
20	77181	0.99686	0.00314	77060	3104813	40.2
21	76938	0.99676	0.00324	76813	3027753	39.4
22	76689	0.99667	0.00333	76561	2950940	38.5
23	76433	0.99627	0.00373	76065	2874379	37.6
24	76148	0.99566	0.00434	75983	2798314	36.7
25	75818	0.99507	0.00493	75632	2722331	35.9
26	75445	0.99462	0.00538	75242	2646699	35.1
27	75039	0.99414	0.00586	74820	2571457	34.3
28	74599	0.99364	0.00639	74463	2496637	33.5
29	74125	0.99311	0.00689	73871	2422274	32.7
30	73615	0.99307	0.00693	73360	2378403	31.9

31	73105	0.99225	0.00775	72822	2275043	31.1
32	72538	0.99149	0.00851	72230	2202221	30.4
33	71921	0.99080	0.00920	71591	2129991	29.6
34	71260	0.99017	0.00983	70910	2058400	28.9
35	70559	0.98949	0.01051	70189	1987490	28.2
36	69818	0.98874	0.01126	69425	1987301	27.5
37	69032	0.98812	0.01188	68622	1847876	26.8
38	68212	0.98755	0.01245	67787	1779254	26.1
39	67362	0.98705	0.01295	66926	1711467	25.4
40	66490	0.98673	0.01327	66049	1644541	24.7
41	65607	0.98635	0.01365	65159	1578492	24.1
42	64711	0.98572	0.01428	64249	1513333	23.3
43	63787	0.98485	0.01515	63304	1449084	22.7
44	62821	0.98373	0.01627	62310	1385780	22.1
45	61799	0.98276	0.01724	61266	1323470	21.4
46	60733	0.98196	0.01804	60185	1262204	20.8
47	59637	0.98093	0.01907	59068	1202049	20.2
48	58500	0.97968	0.02032	57905	1142951	19.5
49	57311	0.97820	0.02180	56682	1085046	18.9
50	56062	0.97682	0.02318	55413	1028364	18.3
51	54763	0.97560	0.02440	54095	972951	17.8
52	53426	0.97422	0.02578	52737	918856	17.2
53	52049	0.97270	0.02730	51338	866119	16.6
54	50627	0.97103	0.02897	49894	814781	16.1
55	49161	0.97001	0.02999	48424	764887	15.6
56	47687	0.96908	0.03092	46950	716463	15.0
57	46212	0.96720	0.03280	45455	669513	14.5
58	44697	0.96437	0.03563	43901	624058	14.0
59	43105	0.96059	0.03741	42255	580157	13.5
60	41406	0.95684	0.04316	40512	537902	13.0
61	39618	0.95374	0.04626	38703	497390	12.6
62	37786	0.95062	0.04938	36853	454687	12.1
63	35920	0.94748	0.05252	34977	421834	11.7
64	34034	0.94432	0.05568	33087	386857	11.4
65	32139	0.34079	0.05921	31188	353770	11.0
66	30236	0.93728	0.06272	29288	322582	10.7
67	28340	0.93437	0.06563	27410	293294	10.3
68	26480	0.93205	0.06795	25580	265884	10.0
69	24680	0.93030	0.06970	23821	240304	9.7
70	22960	0.92879	0.07121	22142	216483	9.4
71	21325	0.92690	0.07310	20546	194341	9.1
72	19766	0.92467	0.07533	19022	173795	8.8
73	18277	0.92212	0.07788	17566	154773	8.5
74	16854	0.91924	0.08076	16174	137207	8.1
75	15494	0.91658	0.08342	14848	121033	7.8
76	14201	0.91416	0.08584	13593	106185	7.5
77	12983	0.91142	0.08858	12408	92592	7.1
78	11832	0.90835	0.09165	11290	80184	6.8
79	10747	0.90497	0.09503	10237	68894	6.4
80	9726	0.90182	0.09818	9249	58657	6.0
81	8771	0.89890	0.10110	8328	49408	5.6
82	7884	0.89566	0.10434	7473	41080	5.2
83	7062	0.89212	0.10788	6682	33607	4.8
84	6300	0.88826	0.11174	5948	26925	4.3
85+	5597	—	—	—	20977	3.7

Source: Life Tables, 1961-70 Census of India, 1971 Census, Registrar General, INDIA

The expectation of life at birth of the population of a region/country generally indicates their current health status. The life expectancy is one of the most frequently used indices for comparisons between populations. However, as is obvious, changing mortality trends may change life expectancy of a population.

12.8. Indices of Population Growth

Crude rate of increase. Crude rate of increase in a population size of a region in a year is the difference between crude birth rate and crude death rate in that region in the same year. Obviously, net migration is assumed to be zero while calculating this index. If crude rate of increase is 12, it means that for every 1000 population, 12 new members are getting added per annum.

Gross reproduction rate (GRR). It is same as Total Fertility Rate, restricted to only female births. It conveys the average number of daughters that a woman would have at the end of her reproductive span. Since the total fertility rate (TFR) measures the total number of children a cohort of women can have, the GRR becomes a special case of the TFR. To be more specific, given the TFR for a region in a year, GRR can be obtained by simply multiplying the TFR by the proportion of female births to total births in that year. It cannot be compared between populations with differing sex ratios at birth. Another limitation of GRR is that it does not consider mortality.

Growth rate. The rate, expressed as a percentage of the base population, at which a population increases (or decreases) in a given year is called growth rate. There are different ways of calculating the growth rate such as exponential rate, geometric rate, etc.

Net reproduction rate (NRR). As described earlier, with a considered age-specific fertility rate in a year, GRR is the average number of female live children that would be born to a woman during her lifetime. But all daughters born to women do not survive to reach reproductive span of life. So an adjustment for mortality in GRR gives a new reproduction rate called Net Reproduction Rate (NRR). Accordingly,

$$\text{Net reproduction rate} = F * \sum_{15}^{44} m_x * s_x$$

Where, F is the proportion of female births to all births; is the age-specific fertility rate at age x; and s_x is the life table survival rate at age x.

NRR has long term implications for population growth. It indicates the rate of replacement of females in the population per generation, with the current schedules of fertility and mortality. A NRR of one indicates that a woman in a population is getting replaced by one female child.

12.9. Indices of Morbidity

As reported earlier in chapter 8, there are mainly the following indices that are commonly used as measures of burden of disease.

Average duration per spell of morbidity. This may be defined as the total of the entire durations of all spells of sickness ending during a defined period divided by the number of spells ending during that period.

Average morbidity duration per person. This may be defined as the total duration of all spells of sickness that occurred wholly or partly during certain period divided by the average number of persons at risk during that period.

Average morbidity duration per sick person. This may be defined as the total of the entire durations of all spells of sickness ending during a defined period divided by the number of persons who experienced at least one spell ending during that period.

Cumulative incidence rate (CIR). This is defined as the number of newly diagnosed cases during a given period of time per 1000 non-diseased population in the beginning of the given time period. Accordingly,

$$CIR = \frac{\text{Number of persons newly contracting a disease during a given time period}}{\text{population free from disesse at the middle of the given time period}} * 1000$$

However, CIR can be calculated only if morbidity status of each of the non-diseased persons enumerated in the study is known till contracting the disease, or completely for the considered fixed period.

Fatality ratio. This may be expressed as the ratio of the number of deaths from a disease occurring during a defined period and the number of new cases of that disease recorded during the same period.

Incidence density rate (IDR). In practice, in any study, the period of follow-up of non-diseased persons for observing, whether they contract the disease or not, is same for all the study participants. Hence, instead of using CIR, IDR per 1000 person time at risk (i.e., total person time followed up till contracting a disease or end of the study) is used. Accordingly,

$$CIR = \frac{\text{Number of persons newly contracting a disease during a given time period}}{\text{Total person time followed up in the given time period}} * 1000$$

Using the concepts of prevalence and incidence rates, a number of morbidity indices can be defined.

Incidence rate (persons). This may be defined as the number of persons who experience at least one spell of sickness during a defined period per 1000 persons at risk during that period.

Incidence rate (spells). It means the average number of spells of sickness that have been observed during a defined period per 1000 non-diseased persons at risk during that period.

Notification rate. This is defined as the number of notifications of an event (e.g., mortality) during a defined period per thousand persons exposed to risk during that period.

Period prevalence (persons). It means the number of persons who are found sick at least sometime during a defined period per 1000 persons during that period.

Period prevalence (spells). It means the average number of spells of sickness reported sometime during a defined period per 1000 persons during that period.

Point prevalence (persons). This may be defined as the number of persons who are found sick at a given time per 1000 persons exposed to risk at that time.

Point prevalence (spells). This may be defined as the number of spells of sickness reported at a given time per 1000 persons at that time. A spell of sickness is a period during which a person is sick on one day or on each day of a consecutive series of days.

Prevalence. This is defined as the number of persons found with a disease (newly diagnosed as well as old cases) during a given period of time per 1000 population, who were either diseased or non-diseased in the beginning of the given time period. Here, numerator is part of the denominator. In other words:

$$Prevalence = \frac{\text{Number of persons with disease (either newly contracting a disease or old case) during a given time period}}{\text{Total population (morbid and non-morbid) at the middle of the given time period}} * 1000$$

It is one of the most important measures of burden of a disease. It is not a rate because it gives a snapshot of the picture and does not convey the speed with which an event is happening.

Proportion of time lost. This may be defined as the proportion of the total duration of all spells of sickness within a defined period that occurred wholly or partly within that period out of the total duration of exposure to risk in that period.

Secondary attack rate. This is defined as percentage of the number of new cases in a household out of the total number of persons in that household, excluding the index cases. In other words, this is a measure of the risk of persons in a household exposed to a disease (e.g., tuberculosis) present in another member (index case) in the same household. It shows the increase in contracting the disease due to familial exposure.

This chapter, as mentioned earlier, deals with only introductory aspects of medical demography. However, as described in earlier chapters for other areas of public health/ epidemiology, similar methodological approaches in further analytical work may be useful. The basic principles of biostatistics (e.g., scales of measurements of dependent/independent covariates; study design, distributions of collected data and methods used in all analysis including advance multiple variable analysis) remain the same in dealing with data analysis in this field.

A host of literature is available on this topic. Some of them are listed under 'Further Reading'.

Multiple Choice Questions

Choose the correct answers in the following multiple choice questions. The correct answers are listed on p. 345.

Q.1. **If the fatality rate of a certain disease has been observed as 30% in children and a sample consists of 500 sick children with this disease, then the expected number of survivors from the disease would be:**
a. 150
b. 500
c. 30
d. 350

Q.2. **In defining crude birth rate, the denominator is:**
a. Population between 15 and 49 years of age
b. Women population between 15 and 49 years of age
c. Mid-year population
d. Live births

Q.3. **In defining general fertility rate, denominator is:**
a. Population between 15 and 45 years of age
b. Women population between 15 and 49 years of age
c. Mid-year population
d. Live births

Q.4. **Mortality experience of daughters born to women is also taken care of in defining:**
a. Net reproduction rate
b. Gross reproduction rate
c. Total reproduction (fertility) rate
d. None of the above

Q.5. **The best indicator for the health status of any country is:**
a. Crude death rate
b. Crude birth rate
c. Infant mortality rate
d. Stillbirth rate
(For questions 6 & 7)
In a community survey of 1,00,000 population, a total of 5000 pregnancy outcomes were recorded during last one year as: (1) abortions = 600, (2) stillbirths = 400, (3) live births = 4000.

Q.6. **Crude birth rate per 1000 population will be:**
a. 50
b. 44
c. 40
d. None of the above

Q.7. If 100 infant deaths are recorded in that place in that year then the infant mortality rate will be:
  a. 25   b. 21.7
  c. 20   d. 22.7

Q.8. The sample registration scheme (SRS) is the main source of information on:
  a. Morbidity at state and national level
  b. Fertility at state and national level
  c. Mortality of state and national level
  d. Both fertility and mortality at state and national level

Q.9. In defining neonatal death rate, the numerator of the rate includes deaths of infants up to:
  a. One week of age   b. Two weeks of age
  c. Four weeks of age   d. Beyond four weeks of age

Q.10. The denominator of maternal mortality rate is:
  a. No. of married women   b. No. of total women
  c. No. of live births   d. No. of women in the reproductive age group

References

1. Registrar General, India. *Census of India, 2001 Census*. Ministry of Home Affairs, Govt. of India, Delhi.
2. Paul Demeny. *Population Policy, A Concise Summary*. Population Council, 2003, No. 173.
3. Ministry of Health and Family Welfare (MOHFW). *National Population Policy, 2000*. New Delhi: Department of Family Welfare, MOHFW; 2000.
4. International Institute for Population Sciences (IIPS) and Macro International. 2007. National Family Health Survey (NFHS-3), 2005-06: India: Volume I. Mumbai: IIPS. Website: http://www.nfhsindia.org
5. Registrar General, India. Provisional Population Totals: Workers and their Distribution. *Census of India, 1991*. Ministry of Home Affairs, Govt. of India, Delhi.
6. International Institute for Population Sciences (IIPS) and ORC Macro . 2000. National Family Health Survey (NFHS-2), 1998-99: India: Mumbai: IIPS. Website: http://www.nfhsindia.org
7. Registrar General, INDIA. Life Tables, 1961-70. *Census of India, 1971 Census*. Ministry of Home Affairs, Govt. of India, Delhi.

13 Medical Records, Hospital Statistics and International Classification of Diseases

- Importance of medical records and hospital statistics: Uses of medical records in planning health services and assessing their efficiency
- Types of statistics
- Hospital based statistical indices: Computation of admission rate, discharge rate, hospital death rate, fatality ratio, autopsy rate, average duration of stay, percentage of bed occupancy
- The international classification of diseases, injuries and causes of death (ICD)

13.1. Importance of Medical Records and Hospital Statistics

"Quod non apparent non est" is a time-honored juridicial maxim. That which does not appear in the record does not exist, at least not in the eyes of the law. In olden ays the adherents of three great religions — Jews, Christians and Muslims — were collectively referred to as the people of the Book. This might mean that everything concerning the people (probably the vital events) was recorded in some way or the other. For, we understand the life of the people in ancient days through the record books which contained details regarding the important events in their life. These events included medical events also to some extent.

Recording of an event means that the event is set down for remembrance or reference and it assumes a permanent form. Many problems can be avoided by keeping proper records. In the fields of medicine and public health also records provide much help at the hospital level, at the community level and also at the National level. The most direct way of obtaining facts and figures on the diseases from which people are suffering and the causes of death is through hospital statistics as obtained from medical records. These records together with other data collected on ad hoc basis, are the main source of information about the health of the community. Information on diseases, which accumulates in hospitals, is not only valuable for planning and assessment of the treatments for various diseases reported in the hospitals, but also in planning National Health Programmes. Eradication of diseases is possible only if the Health Departments or Agencies keep up-to-date records of the diseases. The Public Health reports of U.S.A. under prevalence of diseases say that "No health department, state or local, can effectively prevent or control diseases without the knowledge of when, where and under what conditions cases are occurring. Based on this information, the public health administrator draws plans for public health improvement. Book keeping of public health is one of the essential activities of every public health agency at every level of Government. It is very important that it not only constitutes a primary legal responsibility of health agencies, but also provides the foundation upon which all the public health programmes are planned constructed and implemented. A sound programme of maternal and child health, communicable disease control, environmental health or even the laboratory services is not possible without these valuable records.

Generally, medical records contain information about the admission of the patient and history, which states the patient's present complaint, family history and behavioural factors such as smoking, alcohol use, drug abuse, diet and other factors which might be related to the present disease. The physician after a thorough medical check-up arrives at the diagnosis of the disease. The nurse keeps a bedside record which contains the body temperature, pulse rate and respiration. All these, analyzed quantitatively and qualitatively, help the physician to suggest the best possible treatment modality (ies) to cure the disease of the patient. A physician can do something to cure the disease of a patient. But in a wider perspective, he may not be able to say whether the disease is to be tackled at the community level and whether anything can be done against it without the help of a group of medical personnel. And this group of medical persons can do something against it only if they get information about the nature of the disease, history of the patients regarding the disease, the circumstances which led the patient to contact the disease and the prevalence and incidence of the particular disease. Medical records fulfill these requirements.

For example, if a health report says that cholera has spread to many countries in Asia, killing thousands of people and WHO warns that there is a threat of further spread of the disease to many other countries, this information (accumulated and analyzed from the medical records in different countries) would allow the country to take immediate steps to prevent the disease from spreading or at least minimizing the number of cases of the disease. If another report says that cholera deaths in India have declined steeply from a few thousands to a few hundreds, and smallpox has been eradicated, this information reflects the progress of the public health in India. Such information derived from the medical records is very important in public health planning.

13.1.1. Planning Health Services

One of the major goals of the Indian health sector, since the submission of the Bhore Committee report[1] in 1946, has been to achieve the planned development of a comprehensive and an equitable nation-wide network of health services. To effectively plan and deliver health services in the country, well-recorded and well-maintained hospital statistics are very important. These are the major sources of morbidity statistics. In other words, hospital statistics are the major components of the statistics required for planning, administration and evaluation of health services.

Efficient hospital statistics enable health authorities to evaluate the relationship between demand and supply, i.e., the number of various categories seeking treatment in hospitals and the number and types of hospitals and beds available. The recognition, as quickly as possible, of any lack of balance between the two will save patients and their relatives from unnecessary strain by placing them without delay in hospital beds appropriate to the treatment of their special diseases, and will save the public authorities from unnecessary expenditure caused by an inadequate occupancy policy. In fact, health statistics kept in the hospitals and public health departments are the main key for the National Health Programmes. If they are properly recorded, analyzed and interpreted, they are the eyes and ears of the public health administrator for planning public health programmes. They suggest solutions for many demographic problems and also suggest methods for eradicating many diseases. They bring out many facts which might have been kept in dark due to ignorance and lack of availability of information. Facts and figures conveyed by medical records, serve as background information in planning and improving the hospital services.

13.1.2. Assessing Efficiency of Health Services

At another level, medical statistics are the best measures for assessing the efficiency of a hospital and its medical staff and for the effectiveness of medical care. They provide a basis for the improvement in medical care of the patients. The quality and quantity of the work in a hospital can be interpreted from these medical records and, in turn, further steps may be taken for improving the quality of medical facilities in the hospitals. Hospital statistics includes not only the details of the patients and patient related laboratory tests, it also includes the facilities in the hospital such as utilization of equipment, laboratories, personnel, doctors, nurses, paramedical staff, finances, etc.. This will facilitate in planning maximum use of hospital beds, to adjust the allotted finances and personnel to the maximum possible benefits to the patients and to assess the future needs and requirements,

Medical records containing laboratory and clinical reports and dietary records help the hospitals in the best utilization of allotted l aboratory equipment and thus by maintaining the standards of care of patients at minimum possible cost. It helps in planning regional services and facilities, in reviewing hospital budgeting and in evaluating applications for National Health grants for research, training and equipment. It gives information about the personnel engaged in the hospital work and helps to plan the needs of the hospital staff, to prepare hospital budgets and to detect technical staff shortages or surpluses. At the community level, medical records which contain statistics relating to patients from admission to discharge, are useful in adjusting allocation of beds and staff by type of service and identify community health problems. Also, it helps to control operation rates, to plan operating staff and facilities and to distribute the surgical services and facilities according to the number and type of cases.

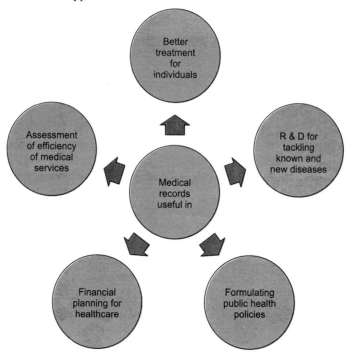

Fig. 13.1: Uses of medical records

In short, medical records are essential for the efficient working of the hospitals and health centers and progress in public health, both at the community level and at the National level can be achieved by keeping up-to-date accurate and complete medical records systematically.

13.2. Types of Hospital Statistics

Hospital morbidity statistics consist of the facts systematically collected and compiled in numerical form, relating to or derived from individual records of hospital stays or hospital visits containing personal characteristics of the patient and medico-administrative data on the hospitalization. Hospital statistics may be obtained by using either the hospital or the hospitalized patient as the statistical unit. If the hospital is used as the unit, important administrative information can be obtained concerning number of beds, number of admissions and discharges, data on diseases diagnosed in the hospital, data on staff, services rendered, expenditure on certain activities, etc. Such information forms the basis of the traditional type of hospital statistics and is of value for the guidance of health authorities in hospital planning and administration. Hospital morbidity statistics may relate to either in-patients or out-patients. The statistical treatment of these two types will be widely different.

The information necessary for the evaluation of hospital activities is in most cases to be found in two groups of data: one, concerned with the disease categories, related to various medico-administrative details such as sex, age, duration of stay in hospital, etc.; the other, comprising purely administrative information, i.e., data on staff, hospital premises, expenditure on certain activities, such as hospital kitchens and laundries, laboratories, mechanical equipments, etc. The amount and type of information needed by hospital and public health administrators in various countries must, to a large extent, depend on the organization of their hospital systems; and this in turn will depend on the prevailing social, economic and geographical conditions.

A typical hospital statistics as existing at the All India Institute of Medical Sciences (AIIMS), New Delhi is shown in Table 13.1.

Table 13.1: A typical monthly hospital statistics sheet

   I. **Total No. of patients discharged:**
       (a) Adults & children   (b) Newborn infants

  II. **Days of care to patients discharged:**
       (a) Adults & children   (b) Newborn infants

 III. **Average length of stay (based on days of care to patients discharged)**
       (a) Adults & children   (b) Newborn infants

  IV. **Total deaths including newborn:**
       (a) Deaths under 48 hours   (b) Deaths over 48 hours
       (c) Gross death rate in percentage   (d) Net death rate in percentage

   V. **Total No. of patient admitted:**
       (a) Adults & children   (b) Newborn infants

  VI. **Daily census of hospital patients:**
       (a) Maximum on any one day this month
       (b) Minimum on any one day this month
       (c) Total No. of patients cared for in hospital (as per daily census)
       (d) Adults & children
       (e) Newborn infants

 VII. **Daily average number of patients:**
       (a) Adults & children   (b) Newborn infants

VIII. **Average percentage of bed occupancy:**
       (a) Adults & children   (b) Newborn infants

  IX. **Birth in the hospital:**
       (a) Male babies   (b) Female babies

   X. **Type of admission (based on discharges):**
       (a) Routine   (b) Emergency   (c) M.L.C

  XI. **Department-wise information on the following items:**
       No. of admissions,   No. of discharges,   No. of days of care,
       Average length of stay,   Total deaths,   Deaths under 48 hours,
       Deaths over 48 hours,   Deaths gross on %ge ,   Net deaths in %ge

13.3. Hospital Based Statistical Indices

A number of summary statistics about hospitalized patients are generally abstracted using data available at a hospital. Further, using this information, some of the additional statistics may be worked out at hospital level. These statistics cannot generally be used for epidemiologic purposes leading to assessment of representativeness and generalization. This is mainly because such data do not generally have a defined denominator. Further, as per study period and hospitalization frequency, the same person might be counted more than once. However, these statistics still go a long way in helping the policy planners to work towards improvement in health services.

A rate usually consists of a numerator denoting the number of events under consideration divided by a denominator which is usually the population of the area that gave rise to the events. However, the population from which hospitals receive their patients is often not known and estimates may be impossible to make. In these cases, ratios may be used in which populations at risk are not required. Examples of these are the ratio of male to female cases, or the ratio of the number of discharges from one cause to the number from all causes. Other examples are discharges in any one age group to those at all ages, hospital death ratios, ratios based on characteristics of patients or ratios concerned with duration of stay. Some of the important hospital indices usually given in hospital statistics are given below.

13.3.1. Admission Rate

Using the principle of incidence density rate, admission rate in a hospital is defined as the number of all admissions during a given time period divided by sum of the time that each bed remained vacant in that period. As a matter of fact, a bed being vacated by a patient and occupied by another patient on the same day will be contributing one vacant day in this computation. For example, in a hospital, let us presume that there are 5000 new admissions during 2008 against 100,000 vacant bed days. Admission rate in that hospital for the year 2008 will be 50 per 1000 vacant bed days $\{(5000/100,000) \times 1000\}$.

13.3.2. Discharge Rate

Again, using the principle of incidence density rate, discharge rate is defined as the number of discharged (including deaths) patients during a time period divided by sum of the time that each bed remained occupied during the same period. As a matter of fact, a bed being vacated by a patient and occupied by another patient on the same day will be contributing one occupied day in this computation. For example, in a hospital, let us presume that there are 5000 discharges during 2008 against 25,000 occupied bed days. Discharge rate in that hospital for the year 2008 will be 200 per 1000 occupied bed days $\{(5000/25,000) \times 1000\}$.

13.3.3. Hospital Death Rate

This is defined as a ratio of the total number of hospital deaths in a considered period to the number of discharges including deaths during the same period. For example, if there are 500 deaths in a hospital out of 5000 discharges in the hospital, hospital death rate will be 10%.

13.3.4. Fatality Ratio

The ratio of the number of deaths from a disease occurring in a hospital during a fixed period and the number of new cases of that disease admitted to that hospital during the same period is defined as fatality ratio. For instance, in a hospital during 2008, if there have been 50 deaths due to coronary heart diseases (CHD) out of a total of 500 new CHD patients admitted, fatality ratio related to CHD will be 10 deaths per 100 new CHD patients.

13.3.5. Autopsy Rate

This is defined as the total number of hospital autopsies divided by all hospital deaths during any given period. As an example, in a hospital, out of 500 deaths during 2008, autopsies could be carried out only in 100. Accordingly, autopsy rate is 20%.

13.3.6. Average Duration of Stay

This index uses the information related to only discharged patients. This may be defined as total duration of stay of discharged patients divided by the number of discharged patients during a considered period. In a hospital during 2008, for example, 25,000 days of total stay has been recorded on 5000 discharged patients. Accordingly, average duration of stay is 5 days.

13.3.7. Percentage of Bed Occupancy

Using the principle of point prevalence, as an average daily census during any given period of time, percentage of bed occupancy is defined as the actual patient-days divided by the maximum bed-days based on available number of beds. In other words, if the number of beds remains the same throughout the year in a hospital, percentage of bed occupancy is simply the average of daily reported percentage of bed occupancy. This is an estimate of the efficiency with which beds are used. However, this index might be sensitive in relation to many aspects. For example, in a popular hospital, this may be 100% because of the fact that demand even exceeds the availability.

13.4. The International Classification of Diseases, Injuries and Causes of Death (ICD)

Classification is fundamental to the quantitative study of any phenomenon. It is recognized as the basis of systematic statistical analysis of diseases for their description and scientific generalizations and, therefore, is an essential element in statistical methodology. Uniform definitions of diseases and systems of classification are a pre-requisite for achieving this purpose and, hence, in the study of illnesses and cause of death, a standard classification of diseases and injuries and cause of death is essential.

A statistical classification is different from a nomenclature. A medical nomenclature is a list or a catalogue of approved terms for describing and recording clinical and pathological observations, which would be extensive for more accuracy. The complete specificity of a nomenclature may prevent it from serving satisfactorily as a statistical classification. When we speak of statistics, we speak of the behaviour of the group and not of the individuals separately. The purpose of statistical compilation of diseases is primarily to furnish quantitative data that will answer questions about group of cases. A statistical classification of diseases must be confined to a limited number of major categories which will encompass the entire range of morbid conditions classified in subgroups according to their occurrence and importance.

The development of the International Statistical Classification of diseases has a long history of intensive work dating back to the beginning of the 18th century. During the First International Statistical Congress at Brussels in 1853, a request was made to William Farr of England and Mare Diespine of Geneva, to prepare a uniform classification of causes of death applicable to all countries. Their list, which was adopted at the next Congress in Paris, contained 139 rubrics. The list was subsequently revised in 1874, 1880 and 1886. In 1891, the International Statistical Institute, the successor to the Congress, appointed a committee with Jacques Bertillon of Paris as Chairman, to revise the classification. Bertillon's classification represented a synthesis of English, German and Swiss classifications and contained 161 titles. The French Government convened in 1900 the First International Conference for the Revision of the International Statistical Classification of Causes of Death and adopted a classification consisting of 169 groups, together with an abridged classification of thirty-five groups. The desirability of decennial revisions was recognized. Substantial contributions were made by Jacques Bertillon, who continued to be the guiding force in the revisions of 1900, 1909 and 1920. Further revisions took place in 1929, 1938, 1948 and 1955 and 1965. Since 1948 the responsibility for the revision of the International Classification has been entrusted to the World Health Organization (WHO).

ICD provides codes to classify diseases and a wide variety of signs, symptoms, abnormal findings, complaints, social circumstances and external causes of injury or disease. Every health condition can be assigned to a unique category and given a code. This system is designed to promote international comparability in the collection, processing, classification and presentation of these statistics. The ICD is revised periodically and the current one is its tenth edition.

In the International Classification of diseases, two volumes have been prepared by the WHO. Volume 1 gives the classification according to the codes serially arranged. Standardized codes have been assigned to the different diseases and injuries. Volume 2 of the International Classification of diseases gives the alphabetical index to the Tabular list of Vol. 1.

ICD-10 was endorsed by the Forty-third World Health Assembly in May 1990 and came into use in WHO Member States with effect from 1994. The World Health Assembly adopted in 1967 the WHO Nomenclature Regulations that stipulate use of ICD in its most current revision for mortality and morbidity statistics by all Member States. The ICD is the international standard diagnostic classification for all general epidemiological, many health management purposes and clinical uses. These include the analysis of the general health situation of population groups and monitoring of the incidence and prevalence of diseases and other health problems in relation to other variables such as the characteristics and circumstances of the individuals affected, reimbursement, resource allocation, quality and guidelines etc. It is used to classify diseases and other health problems recorded on many types of health and vital records including death certificates and health records. In addition to enabling the storage and retrieval of diagnostic information for clinical, epidemiological and quality purposes, these records also provide the basis for the compilation of national mortality and morbidity statistics by WHO Member States.

Statistical Classification of Diseases and Related Health Problems of the 10th Revision Version for 2007 of ICD[2] is given in Table 13.2. This table gives the list of Chapters (main categories), Blocks (sub-categories) and titles of the diseases and conditions.

Alphabets and the numbers shown under 'Blocks' indicate the number of sub-categories of the main disease given under each Chapter (main group). For example, the number of sub-categories under "certain infectious and parasitic diseases" is A00 to B99 = A01 to A99 + B00 to B99. For example, A00 to A09 are codes for intestinal infectious diseases; A15-A19 for tuberculosis, etc., and C00-C14 for malignant neoplasms in lip, oral cavity and pharynx, C15-C26 for malignant neoplasms in digestive organs and so on.

Detailed codes for specific diseases like oncological problems are also brought out separately by the WHO. International Classification of Diseases – Oncology (ICD – O) is one such system[3]. ICD-10 codes help to know only the anatomical site of cancer. But the same anatomical site can have different types of tumors, depending on the morphological patterns of the tumour cells. ICD-O codes help to capture this additional information. The ICD-O codes are of 6 digits, the first 4 indicate the cell type, the 5th one indicates the behavior (benign, in situ, malignant, metastatic, etc.) and the 6th indicates the cells differentiation pattern (well differentiated, moderately differentiated, poorly differentiated, anaplastic, etc.). For example, small cell carcinoma of the lung is coded as 8043/3, intermediate cell carcinoma of lung is coded as 8044/3 and non-small cell carcinoma of lung is coded as 8046/3. All these 3 types of carcinomas are assigned to the same anatomical site – lung, coded in ICD 10 as C34. The data from different cancer registries, coded according to ICD-O classification has not only been very helpful in knowing the time trends in the incidences of different cancers in different regions of the world, but also facilitate comparisons among different regions.

Table 13.2: List of chapters (main categories), blocks (sub-categories) and title of diseases and conditions

Chapter	Blocks	Title
I	A00-B99	Certain infectious and parasitic diseases
II	C00-D48	Neoplasms
III	D50-D89	Diseases of the blood and blood-forming organs and certain disorders involving the immune mechanism
IV	E00-E90	Endocrine, nutritional and metabolic diseases
V	F00-F99	Mental and behavioural disorders
VI	G00-G99	Diseases of the nervous system
VII	H00-H59	Diseases of the eye and adnexa
VIII	H60-H95	Diseases of the ear and mastoid process
IX	I00-I99	Diseases of the circulatory system
X	J00-J99	Diseases of the respiratory system
XI	K00-K93	Diseases of the digestive system
XII	L00-L99	Diseases of the skin and subcutaneous tissue
XIII	M00-M99	Diseases of the musculoskeletal system and connective tissue
XIV	N00-N99	Diseases of the genitourinary system
XV	O00-O99	Pregnancy, childbirth and the puerperium
XVI	P00-P96	Certain conditions originating in the perinatal period
XVII	Q00-Q99	Congenital malformations, deformations and chromosomal abnormalities
XVIII	R00-R99	Symptoms, signs and abnormal clinical and laboratory findings, not elsewhere classified
XIX	S00-T98	Injury, poisoning and certain other consequences of external causes
XX	V01-Y98	External causes of morbidity and mortality
XXI	Z00-Z99	Factors influencing health status and contact with health services
XXII	U00-U99	Codes for special purposes

Multiple Choice Questions

Choose the correct answers in the following multiple choice questions. The correct answers are listed on p. 345.

Q.1. Admission rate in a hospital is calculated using the principle of:
a. Cumulative incidence
b. Incidence density
c. Point prevalence
d. Period prevalence

Q.2. If average duration of stay in a hospital goes up, then admission rate will comparatively be:
a. Same
b. High
c. Low
d. Either high or low

Q.3. A hospital index that depends on principle of point prevalence is:
a. Admission rate
b. Discharge rate
c. Death rate
d. Percentage of bed occupancy

Q.4. The number of volumes in the *International Classification of Diseases* is:
a. One
b. Two
c. Three
d. Four

Q.5. **The major health survey in India is:**
    a. NFHS (national family health survey)   b. Census
    c. SRS (sample registration scheme)   d. Civil registration system

Q.6. **The Registrar General of India is responsible for:**
    a. Census   b. Medical research
    c. National family health survey   d. Medical education

Q.7. **If total number of days of stay of patients in a hospital during the years 2007 and 2008 is same but the number of discharges is double in 2008 as compared that in 2007, the average duration of stay in 2008 will be:**
    a. Same   b. High
    c. Low   d. Either high or low

Q.8. **If total number of CHD patients admitted in a hospital during the year 2008 is twice that in 1998, the case fatality rate of 2008 as compared to that of 1998 will be:**
    a. Same   b. High
    c. Low   d. Nothing can be said conclusively

Q.9. **The following, except one, are related to hospital statistics:**
    a. Admission rate   b. Migration rate
    c. Discharge rate   d. Average duration of stay

Q.10. **In defining fatality ratio for CHD in a hospital during a certain period, the denominator will be:**
    a. Deaths due to all diseases
    b. All cases in that hospital
    c. Deaths due to CHD from that hospital
    d. All CHD cases admitted in that hospital during the period

References

1. Government of India. *Report of the Health Survey and Development Committee*, Vol. II (Chairman: Bhore). Delhi: Manager of Publications; 1946.
2. WHO. *International Statistical Classification of Diseases and Related Health Problems*, ICD, version, 10th revision; 2007.
3. Fritz April, Percy Constance, Jack Andrew, Shanmugaratnam Kanagaratnam, Sobin Leslie, Max Parkin D, Whelan Sharon, eds. *International Classification of Diseases for Oncology, ICD-O*. 3rd ed. Geneva: WHO; 2000.

14 | Computers and Statistical Software for Data Analysis

- Introduction
- Some common differences in the statistical software: Continuity correction in a 2x2 Chi-square test, test for equality of variances while applying Student's t test and ANOVA, creation of design variables, confidence intervals, storage of data values in the memory, missing values
- Common statistical software: Epi Info, SYSTAT, statistical package for social scientists (SPSS), statistical analysis system (SAS), Stata, BioMeDical package (BMDP)

14.1. Introduction

The introduction of personal computers has really changed the practical application of analytical techniques in research. From the age of punched card system and manual calculators we have progressed gradually to the present system of personal computers. Many statistical techniques, which were earlier thought to be cumbersome and tedious are now common and are easily applied with the help of personal computers and statistical programs. This change has been largely beneficial to the medical research community and has also helped Biostatistics and Bio-statisticians in getting due recognition. The earlier practice of a statistician drawing a set of dummy tables, a computer programmer developing a suitable program, running this program on a mainframe computer to produce a bulky output and passing this to the statistician for appropriate interpretation, etc., is outdated. Instead, nowadays, a statistician himself along with the investigator sits before a personal computer and with appropriate software analyzes the data in an interactive manner before culling out the best from the available data. Such an approach was not possible earlier. Though there are several advantages of the use of computers in statistical analyses, there are certain disadvantages too. Dependence on computers should be made a boon and not a bane. Altman[1] (1991) has listed several advantages and disadvantages of using a computer in statistical analyses.

As Hofacker[2] (1983) has put it, the advent of computers and software enabled access to statistical analysis techniques much faster than the understanding of the analysis techniques themselves. It should be understood that the use of computers in itself does not guarantee correct and valid results. Computers only help in doing the analysis fast and with accuracy. Proper understanding of the techniques is a must before application of such techniques on any data set. Unfortunately, the easy availability of computers and statistical packages led to an erroneous impression and belief among many non-statisticians that they have acquired professional statistical expertise. Lack of proper understanding of application of the analytical techniques by such persons can further aggravate the existing problem of misuse of statistics and statistical errors (see Chapter 15) in medical/health literature.

Even among many statisticians, mainly beginners, who do not have an appropriate understanding of the application of advanced analytical techniques, there appears to be a tendency to perform such procedures by simply running suitable software without the ability of proper interpretation of the results. The intricacies of various options and assumptions, etc., require a thorough understanding, without which the best out of the data cannot be brought out. At times, such attempts might also give misleading results. In view of this, it should be remembered that a computer can never be a substitute for a competent statistician.

14.2. Some Common Differences in the Statistical Software

There are a number of computer programs available for statistical analyses. Some are free and can be downloaded from the respective sources on the web, while some are to be purchased. Again, certain programs are of general purpose, while some are for specific needs such as sample size estimation, analysis of sample surveys, statistical process control, drawing graphs, etc. It is very difficult to generalize that a particular program or software is universally better than the rest. Each software or program has its own advantages and disadvantages. It is for the user to understand these in the context of his/her working environment and abilities, and decide accordingly. A thorough knowledge of at least one software program is essential these days for any practicing biostatistician. Most of the programs have similar approach in executing different commands, but the syntax or the grammar of specific commands may vary. Whatever the package or program one may use, the users must be aware how various techniques are implemented and their limitations, etc., while using any computer program for statistical analyses. Some of these are listed below.

14.2.1. Continuity Correction in a 2 × 2 Chi-square Test

Certain programs incorporate the Yate's continuity correction in a 2 × 2 chi-square automatically and some offer it as an option, while some programs do not implement it at all. While the logic or reasoning behind this is beyond the scope of this book, one should be alive to this issue and how it is implemented in the software being used as the significance of the results depend on that. Similarly, when analyzing matched binary data, implementation of continuity correction for Mc-Nemar chi-square test is also different in different software.

14.2.2. Test for Equality of Variances while applying Student's t Test and ANOVA

While testing the equality of two means, some programs show the results of the test for equality of the two variances, so that the analyst is alerted if the two variances are unequal. If significant difference is indicated, data may need to be appropriately transformed or dealt with a modified t test with unequal variances or with an appropriate non-parametric test. Some programs do not show the test of equality of variances and it entirely rests on the analyst to take the blame or credit. Same situation is also applicable for the application of analysis of variance.

14.2.3. Creation of Design Variables

While fitting regression models, often one has to create design variables for an indicator variable to estimate the effect in each exposure category, compared to a baseline category. Most of the programs create the design variables automatically if the variable under consideration is designated as an indicator variable. While this avoids considerable effort by the statistical analyst, it should be borne in mind that the method of creating design variables varies from program to program. Some programs automatically take the category with the smallest code as the baseline and proceed to next category with the next higher code, etc. Certain programs take the category with the largest code as the baseline and design variables are created keeping that as the comparison category. Accordingly, the category-specific estimates and related interpretations vary. Optional feature for choosing a baseline category as to the least or largest code is also available in some specific programs. Therefore, the analyst should be aware of the features implemented in the software that he/she is using.

14.2.4. Confidence Intervals

There are a variety of ways to estimate the standard error and confidence intervals for an Odds Ratio or Relative Risk, etc. It is important for the statistical analyst to know this, because the confidence intervals may vary according to the method and the significance level also may change at times.

14.2.5. Storage of Data Values in the Memory

When a data item consists of decimal values, one should be careful as to how the software stores it as a default. For example, a value of 8.45 may be stored as 8.44999999 or a value of 0.49 may be stored as 0.49000001 in the memory. While the numerical difference between the actual and its stored value is negligible, it matters a lot when one has to categorize the study subjects using these specific values as a cut-off. For example, if for a variable, a value of less than 8.45 is to be taken as a normal value and greater than or equal to 8.45 as abnormal, a person having a value exactly as 8.45 has to be categorized as abnormal. But if the program stores the value as 8.44999999, he/she will be categorized in the other way. So a user of computer programs for statistical analyses has to be aware of such problems.

14.2.6. Missing Values

It is important for the users to know how the missing values for any variable are treated by the software program. Certain programs treat missing values for numeric variables as the smallest values, while certain other programs treat these as the largest values. Further, most commands in any software program ignore missing values by default. Certain commands, however, may use missing values in a way that will surprise the users. Take for example age measured as completed years and we are interested in generating a new variable with age categorized as < 45 and ≥ 45 years. If age is not recorded for certain cases/subjects, the missing values get included in < 45 or ≥ 45 in the generated variable, depending on the way the missing values are treated in the program/software. Therefore, it is essential to be aware of this to avoid spurious or erroneous results.

14.3. Common Statistical Software

14.3.1. Epi Info

This software was developed by the Centre for Disease Control (CDC), Atlanta as a public domain software package for public health practitioners and researchers. The program and documentation can be freely copied, distributed and translated. Originally launched as a DOS version in 1984, Epi Info Windows version was released in the year 2000. The main advantage of Epi Info is that it can be used as a Word Processor, as a database and also as an analysis program. Epidemiologists, public health and medical professionals can develop a questionnaire or form, enter and analyze data quickly with the help of Epi Info™ and a personal computer. Statistical analysis, tables, graphs, and maps are produced with simple commands such as READ, FREQ, LIST, TABLES, GRAPH, and MAP.

Epi Info™ for Windows retains many features of the earlier Epi Info™ for DOS, while offering Windows ease of use strengths, such as point-and-click commands, graphics, fonts, and printing. It is also compatible with Microsoft Access, SQL and ODBC databases, Visual Basic and World Wide Web browsers and HTML. Epi Report is a tool that allows the user to combine analysis output, enter data and edit any data contained in Access or SQL Server and present it in a professional format. The generated reports can be saved as HTML files for easy distribution or web publishing. Double entry of data can be carried out using Data Compare. Data can be protected, encrypted and compressed using Epi Lock. Data files of different types can be imported into Epi Info and analyzed.

Analysis program is used to manage, print and analyze data. It has a *command choice* window (left-hand aspect of screen), *output* window (top), and *command log* window (bottom). Simple clicking on the commands in the *command* window performs the various operations. This brings up dialogue boxes, which help construct commands that appear in the *command log* window. READ command is generally the first command to open a file at the beginning of any analysis session. Output to the commands given can be directed to an output file by the ROUTEOUT command.

Epi Map displays geographic maps with data from Epi Info™. NutStat, a nutrition anthropometry program calculates percentiles and z-scores using reference values. A recent version of Epi Info (Version 3.5) was released in May 2008.

The program and documentation can be downloaded from *www.cdc.gov/epiinfo*. For a guided tour of Epi Info, *www.cdc.gov/epiinfo* can be visited.

14.3.2. SYSTAT

SYSTAT is another popular, general-purpose statistical software. It was first developed by Leland Wilkinson in the late 1970's, at the University of Illinois, Chicago. SYSTAT was acquired by SPSS, which in turn sold it to Cranes Software, Bangalore, India. SYSTAT is easy to learn with its intuitive Windows interface and flexible command language. A beginner can work with its user-friendly and simple menu-dialogs, while an experienced user can use its intuitive command language. Comprehensive dialogs can help to locate advanced options.

Creation of command files is easy. The functions executed using the menus and dialog selections are tracked by the command log. One can simply save the command log script to re-run the analysis. Over 500 examples of command files are available so that one can carry out similar analysis on his/her data sets.

It incorporates robust algorithms, so that one can obtain meaningful results even with extreme data. Bootstrapping and simulation are easy with SYSTAT's powerful random number generator. We can generate random samples from a variety of univariate and multivariate, discrete and continuous distributions.

SYSTAT offers a large number of options for scientific and technical graphs. One very useful feature of SYSTAT is that it offers publication quality graphics. A variety of online help is available.

The latest version is version 12. More information on SYSTAT can be found at URL *http://www.systat.com*.

14.3.3. Statistical Package for Social Scientists (SPSS)

SPSS was first developed for mainframe computers in 1968 at the Stanford University. It was the first statistical software to be introduced on the personal computers during the mid 80s. Today, it is one of the most widely available and powerful statistical software packages used by social scientists. SPSS products are modular in nature and include SPSS Professional Statistics, SPSS Advanced Statistics, SPSS Tables, SPSS Trends, SPSS Categories, SPSS CHAID, SPSS LISREL 7, SPSS Developer's Kit, SPSS Exact Tests, Teleform, and MapInfo. It covers a broad range of statistical procedures that allow to summarize data, perform statistical tests of significance, examine relationships among variables such as correlation and multiple regression, and graphs. SPSS can take data from almost any type of file, including Excel, dBASE, Lotus, and SAS.

SPSS Windows is by far the most used and is extremely user-friendly. It provides a user interface that makes statistical analysis more intuitive for all levels of users. Simple menus and dialog box selections make it possible to perform complex analyses without typing a single line of command syntax. Through the syntax editor, it is also possible to write down the commands or to paste those selected through the dialog boxes in order to keep a record of the job. Moreover, the built-in SPSS Data Editor offers a simple and efficient spreadsheet-like utility for entering data and browsing the working data file. In addition, high-resolution, presentation-quality charts and plots can be created and edited. Using the SPSS Viewer, one can handle the output with greater flexibility.

The latest version is SPSS Statistics 17.0. More on this software can be seen at URL *http://www.spss.com.*

14.3.4. Statistical Analysis System (SAS)

SAS began as a statistical analysis system in the late 1960's, growing out of a project in the Department of Experimental Statistics at the North Carolina State University. Later, the SAS Institute was founded in 1976. SAS System has expanded to become an evolving system for complete data management and analysis since that time. It contains products for management of large databases and modules for advanced statistical analyses. A geographic information system is also available in the system. Perhaps, it is one of the most comprehensive statistical software available.

A variety of simulation studies are possible with SAS, as random numbers can be generated for many different distributions. Ease of data management is the strength of SAS as we can subset, merge and rearrange databases. User written functions can be integrated into the system. Many applications can be accomplished using simple point and click operations.

SAS is generally considered as an industry standard statistical software package. The demand for professionals SAS programmers is considerably greater than for those with skills in other statistical packages. Familiarity with SAS itself is an essential qualification for many positions in pharmaceutical industries as can be noted from many vacancy notifications. SAS vendors in each region conduct different training programs from time to time for the benefit of SAS users.

Some useful URLs are *http://www.sas.com/,* which is the main URL for SAS and also *http://is.rice.edu/~radam/prog.html*, which contains some user-developed tips on using SAS.

14.3.5. Stata

Stata is a powerful and easy to use statistical program, which can be used by both beginners and professionals. Stata uses online commands, which can be entered one at a time. Alternatively, one can use the dropdown menu to execute the required analysis. Beginners generally prefer such a mode. Experienced users can enter many commands at a time through a Stata program called Stata 'do file'.

Data management capabilities of Stata may not be as extensive as those of SAS, but it has many powerful yet simple data management commands that allow us to perform complex manipulations of the data with ease. Data files from one software to another can be easily converted with the Stat/Transfer utility. Tasks that involve working with multiple data files may be cumbersome with Stata as it primarily works with one data file at a time.

Most of the statistical analyses can be easily performed on Stata. Very good regression diagnostic tools, which are simple to use, are perhaps the greatest strengths of Stata. Another important feature Stata has is a very nice array of robust methods that are very easy to use, including robust regression, regression with robust standard errors. Many other estimation commands also include robust standard errors. Survey data can also be easily analyzed for different types of regression analyses.

Apart from the standard features, one can easily download programs developed by other users for any specific Stata application. High quality graphs for publication can be created using Stata commands and they are very helpful for supplementing statistical analysis.

There is a Stata Journal, published quarterly (www.stata-journal.com). *The Stata Technical Bulletin* after ten years of publication evolved into the *Stata Journal*. It contains articles on data analysis, teaching methods, and effective use of Stata's language. The journal also publishes reviewed papers together with short notes and comments, regular columns, book reviews, and other material of interest to researchers applying statistics in a variety of disciplines. In addition, StataCorp has a variety of resources to help learn Stata. Prospective users can enroll in short courses and web-based NetCourses. Friendly and knowledgeable staff is available to answer questions and resolve problems, free of charge, for registered users of Stata. Additionally, an active Stata community provides a wealth of resources, including books, tutorials, third-party short courses, and users group meetings.

Latest version of Stata is version 10. Visit URL: *http://www.stata.com/* for more information.

14.3.6. BioMeDical Package (BMDP)

BMDP was developed at the Health Sciences Computing Facility, School of Medicine, University of California, Berkeley in 1961 and was first implemented in FORTRAN for the IBM 7090 mainframe computer. It is a comprehensive library of statistical routines from simple data description to advanced multivariate analysis. BMDP comes with an extensive documentation, which itself can be a learning resource for many statisticians. For every analysis module, a model instructions file is available, so that one can carry out similar analysis on his/her data sets easily. The documentation of BMDP is one of the best, so much so, even a beginner statistician will be able to understand and interpret the results easily. The program modules are known to be based on the most competitve algorithms available and the different modules have been rigorously field-tested.

The earlier versions were less user friendly, as one needed to create a command file and execute it to get the required analysis done. Current version is BMDP 2007, which has a dialog interface to generate BMDP Command Language. Through this easy-to-use interface, even beginners would be able carry out data analysis with simple point and click and fill-in-the-blank interactions. Pop-up windows and dialog boxes will prompt the user until the analysis is complete.

The BMDP package contains over 40 interrelated statistical modules and all of them share common instructions and convenience features to save time and effort. The BMDP instructions are English-based, free-formatted and may be abbreviated to facilitate data input. All instructions are logically grouped into sentences and paragraphs. The same basic BMDP instructions can be used to perform several types of analyses with only minimal instruction changes. Paragraphs that describe the data remain the same for all programs. Only those paragraphs that describe statistical procedures need to be changed to initiate new analyses with other programs.

Though BMDP is less user friendly, users with fairly good statistics background or professional statisticians find it an extremely good statistical software.

A reference URL for BMDP is *http://www.statsol.ie/*

Multiple Choice Questions

Choose the correct answers in the following multiple choice questions. The correct answers are listed on p. 345.

Q.1. The following software, except one, are statistical software:
    a. SPSS   b. SAS
    c. Microsoft   d. SYSTAT

Q.2. The expansion of SPSS is:
    a. Statistical Package for Social Sciences   b. Statistical Package for Social Scientists
    c. Science Package for Social Sciences   d. Standard Package for Social Scientists

Q.3. **The expansion of SAS is:**
  a. Statistical Analysis Systems
  b. Statistical Application Systems
  c. Statistical Application Studies
  d. Standard Analysis Systems

Q.4. **Statistical analysis of data can be done if the data is entered, except in:**
  a. MS-Excel
  b. SPSS
  c. SAS
  d. MS-Word

Q.5. **The statistical software Epi info was developed by:**
  a. WHO
  b. UNICEF
  c. Centre for Disease Control, Atlanta
  d. ICMR

Q.6. **All the following, except one, are connected with computers and statistical software:**
  a. PC
  b. Doors
  c. Programs
  d. Windows

Q.7. **In the analysis of data the results obtained in the computer using a statistical software is generally known as:**
  a. Windows
  b. Output
  c. Input
  d. CD

Q.8. **For a computerized analysis of any data, which one the following is not suitable for the data entry?**
  a. Word
  b. excel
  c. SAS
  d. SPSS

Q.9. **For analysis of data using statistical software, the data can be stored in the following devices, except:**
  a. Hard drive
  b. CD
  c. Pen drive
  d. MS Word

Q.10. **Computer software means:**
  a. Computer memory
  b. Package containing program(s) for analysis
  c. Data input
  d. Output

References

1. Altman DG. *Practical Statistics for Medical Research*. London: Chapman and Hall; 1991.
2. Hofacker C.F. Abuse of statistical packages: the case of the general linear model. *Am. J. Physiol*. 1983; 245: R299-302.

15 Misuse of Statistics

- Common pitfalls
- Averages
- Variation measures
- Correlation coefficients
- Chi-square tests
- Student's t-test (independent samples)
- Paired t-test in place of independent sample t-test
- One-way ANOVA in place of two-way ANOVA
- Parametric test in place of nonparametric test — independent samples
- Parametric test in place of nonparametric test — paired samples
- Parametric test in place of nonparametric test — independent samples (more than two groups)
- Graphs

There are three types of lies — lies, damn lies and statistics.

Benjamin Disraeli

This famous statement made by the former British Prime Minister Benjamin Disraeli clearly implies a disdain for the statistical interpretations. Indeed, if the statistical methods are not used properly, the result may be more dangerous than damn lies. Of course, if applied properly and appropriately, statistical methods provide potent and very helpful tools in the collection, compilation and analysis of data in scientific research. But applied inappropriately, these can lead to blunders.

Another view of statistical methods is provided by a statement by Aaron Leven Stein, who said, 'Statistics is like a bikini — what it reveals is suggestive, but what it conceals is vital'. Thus, statistics may be used to reveal important details, but it may also be misused to conceal crucial information.

We often assume results described in quantitative terms to be factual. But quantity does not always guarantee quality. Statistics for some people is like a lamp post to a drunkard – it is used more for support rather than illumination. Because of such a tendency, people are rightly skeptical of statistics, especially when used for promoting a particular cause, say, for boosting sale of a product or in predicting election results. Charts are drawn and statistical figures are given just to impress the consumers, sometimes at the cost of truth. Skepticism about statistics is reinforced when we read claims of some investigators in newspapers that coffee and chocolates are good for heart /brain/ some other body function on one day and after some days we again read that they are harmful.

Even the results of some clinical trials may be manipulated by the vested interests to enhance saleability and credibility of their products. For example, in a clinical trial, if the results show that the improvement rate with the standard treatment is 20% and that with the new treatment is 50%, we would tend to accept the claim that the new treatment is more effective than the standard treatment. But, if we know that two patients out of ten who received the standard treatment showed improvement (20%) and one patient out of two who received the new treatment showed improvement (50%), we would not accept the claims made for the new treatment. Similarly, if the majority of the patients in the standard treatment group have a severe degree of disease and if most of those in the new treatment group have disease of a mild degree, the results will not be valid. Hence, balancing the groups in terms of adequate sample size, selecting the patients by applying appropriate method of sampling and matching the patients in the two groups with respect to those factors which may affect the responses become very important for a valid comparison of the results.

Statistically Speaking

1. If somebody says that in a group of students 2% of boys are married to 50% of girls, it may sound very odd and misleading, though nothing is wrong in that statistics — there were 50 boys and 2 girls and there was one married couple among them (2% of 50 = 1 and 50% of 2 = 1).

2. A surgeon was very popular for a particular type of surgery. One morning when he went to the operation theatre with a very happy face, the patient who was to be operated was nervous and asked the surgeon, the reason for his happiness. The surgeon replied that statistically the rate of success in the operation was 10% and since all the nine patients he had operated upon earlier had died, he was sure that this operation, being the tenth, would be successful. But, unfortunately that patient also died.

3. A villager wanted to cross a river and he asked the person standing near the river, what was the depth of the river. That person replied, on an average the depth was 3 feet. The villager started crossing the river confidently, but the poor fellow got drowned after taking a few steps. The information about the depth was correct; the problem lay in the details — at some places, the depth was 10 feet and at other places it was only half a foot, making the overall average three feet. The villager would have been safe if he had compared his height with the maximum depth of the river.

15.1. Common Pitfalls

One common problem is generalization of results obtained from non-probability sampling (quota sampling), which may lead to misleading results. We know that in quota sampling there is no randomness at all and the sample is selected purely based on some criteria of number and category. In market research and sometimes in predicting election results, this type of sampling is adopted giving completely misleading results many a time.

In clinical research, while making generalization of results obtained from the sample for the population, there is a contradiction between statistical significance and clinical significance. Introduction of any new pharmacotherapy always follows large scale randomized clinical trials that report the results of quantitative comparisons between a new treatment and the standard treatment or with placebo. Statisticians are interested to quote the statistical significance in terms of the popular 'p' value, but the clinicians are interested in knowing whether the difference is clinically significant or not. When the sample size is very large, even a small difference in the value, say of blood pressure, may be statistically significant, but may not be a clinically important difference for the clinician.

Statistical significance depends exclusively on a judgment based on probabilities of how likely a difference between groups was due to chance alone. All tests of statistical significance are based on considerations of a theoretical sampling distribution, all possible values the statistic can take and the probability of obtaining any possible value by chance alone. Those values that occur less than 5% of the time by chance alone are counted as especially unlikely and, in fact, are judged as not likely to be due to chance at all. Rather, they are interpreted as resulting from a systematic difference between groups. It is always better to show both statistical and clinical significance. But, sometimes, it may not be practicable due to certain unavoidable reasons. Apart from quoting the popular 'p' value the corresponding confidence intervals, effect size and possibly the number needed to treat (number of patients who need to be treated in order to produce one additional good outcome or to avoid one additional bad outcome) should also be stated for revealing the complete picture of the results.

Another common mistake is committed by combining results obtained from studies having different designs. Apart from the possible conflicting results from these studies, the designs of these studies may not be uniform and standardized. Appropriate meta-analysis methods should be applied for combining the results from various studies and caution should be exercised while interpreting the results obtained from studies having different designs.

Scope of arriving at misleading conclusions is substantial in another important aspect of statistical analysis: establishing the cause and effect relationship. Care should be taken in establishing that the risk factor under study is indeed the cause of the disease. For example, eating too much food without any exercise may be the cause of obesity, but it may not be the causative factor or may not be the only causative factor for diabetes or heart disease. Before making the interpretation, other possible factors like age, heredity, smoking habit and use of alcohol, etc., should also be investigated by applying appropriate statistical analysis, without which the results could be misleading. In medical diagnosis based on quantitative parameters such as blood pressure and blood glucose levels, the cut off values based on which a person may be considered as having the disease and putting him under treatment are very important. If the cut off values are not statistically identified, normal persons may be given treatment unnecessarily and the persons with the disease may not receive the treatment, which may lead to complications in some of them and also to ethical and legal problems.

All these examples clearly show what statistics can reveal and what it can conceal, or whether statistics is used or misused, or whether statistics is a boon or a bane. It is definitely a bane if the methods are misused or are not properly and appropriately applied. It is in the hands of the statisticians to make use of the tools properly after understanding the conditions and appropriateness of the methods to be used. Biostatisticians have to play a positive role together with the medical researchers, clinicians, epidemiologists and medical and public health administrators in making the application of statistical methods a boon. Applied with care, these methods can yield unambiguous results and interpretations and thus benefit millions of patients afflicted by various diseases and health conditions.

Given below are some examples of possible misuse/wrong application of statistical methods for the empirical data with the corresponding correct/better method of analysis.

15.2. Averages

15.2.1: The following are the number of malaria cases reported in a town from 1998 to 2007:

Year:	1998	1999	2000	2001	2002	2003	2004	2005	2006	2007
No. of cases:	200,	120,	350,	100,	90,	110,	130,	270,	3000,	200

Compute the average number of malaria cases reported in that town over a period of 10 years from 1998 to 2007.

Wrong average

Arithmetic mean = 457 (affected by the extreme value of 3000 in one year)

Correct average

Median = (130+200)/2 = **165**

(Arrange the values in ascending order. Median is the average of the two middle values (5th & 6th values) in the ten values arranged in ascending order. Fifth value is 130 & 6th value is 200).

15.2.2: An epidemiologist wanted to conduct a study on the prevalence of diabetes and hypertension in a village. As a part of this study he obtained information on income of the 100 villagers living in that village.

He found that income of 98 villagers (labourers) was Rs. 500/- each and that of two landlords was Rs.30, 000/- each. He wanted to compute the mean income in that village.

Wrong method

Arithmetic mean (A.M.)

$$A.M. = \frac{(98 \times 500 + 2 \times 30000)}{100} = \frac{Rs. \, 1,09,000}{100} = Rs. \, 1090$$

It may be noted that the arithmetic average of income (Rs. 1090) in that village cannot be considered as representative income in that village since income of 98 persons was only Rs.500 and the A.M. was inflated because of the high income of the two landlords.

Correct method

In such a case of extreme values in the sample, the best average will be either the median or the mode (the value which is repeated most often among all the values).

In this example, Median = **Rs 500** and Mode = Rs. 500 (value repeated 98 times in the data)

15.2.3: One researcher (a podiatrist — specialist in diabetic foot problems) wanted to instruct the shoemaker to make shoes for the patients affected by diabetic foot deformities. He had only limited funds. To keep expenditure within the available funds, he told the shoe maker to take the measurements of all the patients and make shoes for them based on the arithmetic average of the measurements. But, only very few patients could make use of the shoes made by the shoemaker since they didn't fit their feet leading to wastage of money.

The podiatrist consulted a statistician on this problem. The statistician told him that the wastage could have been avoided if the podiatrist had instructed the shoemaker to make shoes based not on the arithmetic average of measurements but according to the modal value of the measurements. The foot measurement corresponding to this maximum number is the mode average.

Data

Foot measurement size	No. of patients
5	11
6	18
7	27
8	35
9	5
10	3
11	1

Wrong method

A.M. = 7.18

Correct method

Mode = **8** (corresponding to the maximum number of patients (35).

15.2.4: Titre values of hormones (in ng/ml) of 6 patients are given below:

1/10, 1/10, 1/40, 1/20, 1/80 and 1/80

Compute the average titre value from this sample.

Wrong method

A.M. = (10+10+40+20+80+80+) / 6 = 1/40

Correct method

Since these observations show a geometric progression (multiples of 2), arithmetic mean (A.M.) will not be a good average to use. Geometric average will be the most appropriate average in such cases.

G.M. = Antilog of {(log10+log10+log40+log20+log80+log80)/6}
       = **28.2**

15.2.5: In testing the speed, per hour, of a particular brand of cars the following data were obtained:

Car No.	1	2	3	4	5
Speed (km per hour)	40	35	45	50	60

Method which may be OK

Average speed of the car: A.M. = 46 km

Better method (accurate)

When we require the average value of rates Harmonic mean would be a better average

Harmonic mean $\quad = 1/\{(1/x_1)+(1/x_2)+(1/x_3)+\ldots\ldots\}$

$\qquad = 5/\{(1/40)+(1/35)+(1/45)+(1/50)+(1/60)\}$

$\qquad = 5/(0.025+0.0286+0.0222+0.02+0.0167)$

$\qquad = \mathbf{44.5\ km}$

15.3. Variation Measures

15.3.1: Suppose we have to find out which variable has more variation in a given population. Mean, standard deviation and the coefficient of variation are the usual indicators of variation in the values of parameters. Consider the following data where the two variables (birth weight & systolic blood pressure (SBP) are recorded (in different units of measurements, g and mm Hg, respectively):

Variable	Mean	SD	CV
Birth weight (g)	2592.0	354.90	13.69%
SBP (mm Hg)	135.6	19.84	14.63%

Wrong method

If the conclusion regarding variation is drawn from the SD values, the interpretation would be that variation in birth weight is more than that in SBP. This conclusion is wrong since the units of measurement of the two variables are different and, hence, variation should not be compared based on SD values

Correct method

Conclusion should be drawn from the CV (coefficient of variation) values.

CV is defined as the SD expressed as a percentage of the arithmetic mean. Unlike mean and SD, CV does not have any units. It is expressed as percentage.

Coefficient of variation, $CV = \frac{\sigma}{\bar{X}} \times 100$; where s is the estimated SD.

In the example CV of birth weights = (354.90 ÷ 2592) × 100 = **13.69%**

CV of SBP $\qquad\qquad\qquad = (19.84 \div 135.6) \times 100 = \mathbf{14.63\%.}$

Correct interpretation would be that the variation in both birth weight and SBP is almost the same (slightly more in SBP).

15.3.2: Suppose we have to find out which variable has more variation in the following data where the two populations (children & adults) are heterogeneous with respect to the variable weight:

Variable	Mean	SD	CV
Weight of children (kg)	20.7	4.20	20.3%
Weight of adults (kg)	62.5	10.5	16.8%

Wrong method

If the conclusion is drawn from the SD values, the interpretation would be that the variation in weight of adults is more than that in children. But, since the two populations (children & adults) are heterogeneous with respect to weight, conclusion should not be drawn on the basis of SD values.

Correct method

Conclusion should be drawn from CV (coefficient of variation) values.

CV of weight in children = $(4.2 \div 20.7) \times 100$ = **20.3%**

CV of weight in adults = $(10.5 \div 62.5) \times 100$ = **16.8%.**

Correct interpretation would be that the variation in weight of children is slightly more than that in adults.

15.4. Correlation Coefficient

15.4.1: Age (years) and cholesterol (mg%) values of 6 men are listed below. Calculate the appropriate correlation coefficient (ρ).

Age:	25	80	65	90	60	75	Mean = 65.8	SD = 22.7
Cholesterol:	180	450	220	250	200	500	Mean = 300.0	SD = 138.4

Wrong method

Pearson's product moment correlation coefficient = 0.529

(p-value = 0.281 — more than 0.05 — not statistically significant)

Since the distribution of values of both the variables is not normal and the sample size is very small, use of Pearson's product moment correlation coefficient will not be appropriate. In such a situation, use of Spearman rank correlation coefficient (nonparametric) will be more appropriate.

Correct method

Spearman rank correlation coefficient = 0.771

(p-value = 0.072-slightly more than 0.05 – statistically-borderline significant)

15.4.2: Weight (kg) and cholesterol (mg%) values of 10 men are listed below. Calculate the appropriate correlation coefficient (ρ).

Cholesterol	Weight
123.7	43.5
121.2	51.8
125.5	63.4
119.2	52.9
117.5	57.1
116.6	53.6
118.0	58.7
115.6	43.7
290.3	74.5
374.9	80.6

Variable	Mean	SD
Cholesterol	162.25	92.02
Weight	57.98	12.07

Wrong method

Pearson's product moment correlation coefficient = 0.863

(p-value = 0.001 — statistically very highly significant)

Since the distribution of cholesterol values is not normal and the sample size is very small, use of Pearson's product moment correlation coefficient will not be appropriate. In such a situation, use of Spearman rank correlation coefficient (nonparametric) will be more appropriate.

Correct method

Spearman rank correlation coefficient = 0.552

(p-value ± 0.098 — s ightly more than 0.05 — statistically not significant, but may be considered as borderline significant)

15.5. Chi-square Tests

15.5.1: The following data pertains to smoking habit in lung cancer patients and in comparative normal subjects. Test whether lung cancer is associated with smoking habit.

		Lung cancer		
		Yes	No	Total
Smoking	Yes	8	6	14
	No	2	14	16
	Total	10	20	30

Wrong method

On applying chi-square test the p-value obtained was = 0.0097.

Correct method

Since the sample size is very small in both the normal and cancer groups, a more appropriate analysis would be use of chi-square test with Yate's correction factor. On applying chi-square test with Yate's correction factor, the p-value obtained was = 0.0278.

A better analysis when the sample size is very small would be Fisher's exact test. On applying Fisher's exact test, p-value obtained was = 0.0187

15.5.2: The following data gives the results of treatment by two drugs (A-standard drug and B-new drug) for the relief of pain in patients having some ear problem. Compare the efficacy of the drugs in pain relief. Research hypothesis is that the new drug is more effective than the standard drug.

		Pain relief		
		Yes	No	Total
Treatment	A	2	10	12
	B	8	5	13
	Total	10	15	25

Wrong method

On applying chi-square test, the p-value obtained was = 0.022.

Correct method

Since the sample size is very small in both the treatment groups, a more appropriate analysis would be chi-square test with Yate's correction factor. On applying chi-square test with Yate's correction factor, the p-value obtained was = 0.06.

A better analysis when the sample size is very small would be Fisher's exact test. On applying Fisher's exact test, p-value obtained was = 0.041.

15.5.3: The following data gives the results of a diagnosis test by two methods A & B. Test whether the difference in results by the two tests is statistically significant or not.

		Test A		
		+ve	-ve	Total
Test B	+ve	13	7	20
	-ve	2	28	30
	Total	15	35	50

Wrong method

On applying chi-square test, the p-value obtained was <0.001 with and without the Yate's correction factor.

Correct method

However, since the samples are paired (same 50 specimens are subjected to both the tests A & B), the correct analysis would be McNemar's chi-square test. On applying McNemar's chi-square test, the p-value obtained was = 0.18.

The conclusion is that the difference in results by the two tests is statistically not significant. Both the tests give statistically comparable results.

15.5.4: The following data gives the results of a diagnosis test by two technicians A & B. Compute an appropriate agreement parameter between the results of the two technicians.

		Test A		
		+ve	-ve	Total
Test B	+ve	7	4	11 (0.22)
	-ve	9	30	39 (0.78)
	Total	16 (0.32)	34 (0.68)	50 (1.0)

Wrong method

Observed agreement (O) =

(where both A & B gave +ve results + where both A & B gave -ve results)/total specimens

$$= (7+30)/50 = 0.74$$

Correct method

However, chance element has not been considered in computing the agreement percentage. Since the results are obtained from a sample study, chance corrected proportion of agreement has to be computed. This is obtained by computing Kappa statistic:

Kappa = (O-C)/ (1-C)
O = Observed proportion of agreement
C = Proportion of chance agreement
C = $(0.22 \times 0.32) + (0.78 \times 0.68) = 0.6$
Kappa = $(0.74 - 0.60)/ (1-0.60)$
$\qquad = 0.35$

15.6. Student's t-test (Independent Samples)

15.6.1: Heights (in cm) of 15 children from public schools and 12 children from Govt. schools are given below. Test whether the difference in heights of children from the two types of schools is statistically significant.
Public school: 173, 155, 158, 150, 151, 152, 153, 159, 154, 179, 164, 172, 168, 178, 174
Govt. school: 148, 154, 152, 160, 154, 151, 158, 163, 157, 153, 155, 152

Type of School	Mean	SD
Public school	162.67	10.44
Govt. school	154.75	4.16

Wrong method

By applying Student's t-test between two independent samples, p-value obtained for comparing height between the two types of schools was = 0.021

However, Fisher's F-value for testing homogeneity of variances in the two populations was found to be 6.30 with a p-value of 0.01 indicating that the two populations were heterogeneous with respect to height. Hence, modified t-test should be applied.

Correct method

On applying modified t-test, p-value was obtained as 0.015.

Though both tests gave statistically significant difference in heights between the two groups, p-value was smaller in case of modified t-test compared to that for t-test without modification.

15.7. Analysis of Variance (Independent Samples)

15.7.1: The following data gives the cholesterol values for diabetic patients, hypertension patients and normal subjects. Test whether the differences in cholesterol values among the three groups are statistically significant or not.

	Cholesterol level	
Diabetic	Hypertension	Normal
160	252	124
190	290	128
170	265	140
200	286	152
165	300	165
	260	148
		155
		136

Group	Mean	SD
Normal (1)	143.50	14.02
Hypertension (2)	275.5	19.6
Diabetic (3)	177.0	17.18

On applying one-way ANOVA, p-value obtained was < 0.001. Since the ANOVA showed that the variation in cholesterol between groups is statistically significant, we are interested in finding the pairs of groups which are statistically significant.

Groups	Multiple comparisons** p-value	Student's t-test* p-value
1 & 2	< 0.001	< 0.001
1 & 3	0.008	0.003
2 & 3	<0.001	< 0.001

*Wrong method
The p-values obtained by applying Student's t-test for comparing pairs of groups are given in column 3.
Since there are three groups in the study, the comparison should be based on one error variation. However, in Student's t-test different error variations are used in each comparison. Hence, for a valid comparison of the variable between pairs of groups, an appropriate multiple comparison test should be used.

**Correct method
On applying Student-Newman-Keul's multiple comparison test, the p-values obtained for all the comparisons were < 0.01 (column 2).
It may be noted that the p-values obtained on applying the wrong & the correct methods are not very different. The difference could be more pronounced in certain cases.

15.8. Paired t-Test in Place of Independent Sample t-Test

15.8.1: The following data gives the systolic blood pressure (SBP) values of 10 hypertension patients before and one week after giving a drug. Test whether the reduction in SBP after treatment is statistically significant or not.

Systolic B.P	Patient Number									
	1	2	3	4	5	6	7	8	9	10
Before drug	160	150	170	130	140	170	160	160	120	140
After drug	150	140	160	140	145	150	140	150	120	120

Time	Mean	SD
BF	150.00	17.00
AF	141.50	12.91

Wrong method
On applying independent samples t-test, p-value obtained for comparing between time was 0.224

Correct method

However, since the design of the study is a paired design, paired t-test is the appropriate analysis and not independent samples t-test. Paired t-test will give lesser error variation making the comparison more valid. On applying Paired t-test p-value obtained was 0.031.

It may be noted that the decrease in SBP was statistically not significant on applying independent samples t-test; it was statistically significant on applying paired t-test.

15.9. One-way ANOVA in place of Two-way ANOVA

15.9.1: The following data gives the systolic blood pressure (SBP) values of 10 hypertension patients before and one week and two weeks after giving a drug. Test whether the reduction in SBP after treatment is statistically significant or not.

Sl.No.	Before	After 1 week	After 2 week
1.	170	165	150
2.	165	160	155
3.	180	175	165
4.	175	165	160
5.	170	165	155
6.	180	175	165
7.	175	170	165
8.	160	150	145
9.	155	150	135
10.	165	160	150

Time	Mean	SD
Before	169.50	8.32
After One week	163.50	8.84
After two weeks	154.50	9.85

Wrong method

On applying one-way ANOVA, p-value obtained for comparing between time was 0.0035.

Correct method

However, since the design of the study is randomized complete block design (block is time), two-way ANOVA is the appropriate analysis and not one-way ANOVA. Two-way ANOVA will give lesser error variation making the comparison more valid. On applying two-way ANOVA p-value obtained was found to be <0.0001.

The p-value obtained for variation between subjects was <0.0001, which is very highly significant. This was ignored while applying one-way ANOVA.

15.10. Parametric Test in Place of Nonparametric Test — Independent Samples

15.10.1: The following data gives the cholesterol values of normal subjects (1) and hypertension patients (2). Test whether the difference in cholesterol values between the two groups is statistically significant or not.

Group	Cholesterol
1	124
1	128
1	140
1	152
1	165
1	180
1	179
1	136
2	192
2	290
2	125
2	186
2	388
2	210

Group	Mean	SD
1	150.50	22.12
2	231.83	93.11

Wrong method

On applying Student's t-test, p-value obtained for the test was 0.033 and the p-value obtained for the modified t-test (due to statistically significant heterogeneity of variances in the two groups) was = 0.086.

However, since the distribution of values among the patients is not normal and the sample size is very small, Student's t-test or modified t-test will not be appropriate.

Correct method

The correct statistical test for this data would be an appropriate nonparametric test. On applying Wilcoxon's rank sum test, the p-value obtained was 0.028.

15.11. Parametric Test in Place of Nonparametric Test — Paired Samples

15.11.1: The following data gives the systolic blood pressure (SBP) values of 10 hypertension patients before and one week after giving a drug. Test whether the reduction in SBP after treatment is statistically significant or not.

Before drug	After drug
210	150
150	110
240	160
180	130
150	115
170	120
160	130
160	110
140	140
130	120

Group	Mean	SD
Before	169.00	33.48
After	128.50	17.00

Wrong method

On applying paired t-test, p-value obtained for the test was <=0.001.

However, since the distribution of values among the patients is not normal and the sample size is very small, paired t-test will not be appropriate.

Correct method

The correct statistical test for this data would be an appropriate nonparametric test. On applying Wilcoxon's signed rank test, the p-value obtained was 0.007.

15.12. Parametric Test in Place of Nonparametric Test — Independent Samples (More Than Two Groups)

15.12.1: The following data gives the sodium values of three groups of patients (Group 1: normal subjects; Group 2: mild to moderate grade patients; and Group 3: severe patients). Test whether the differences in sodium values among the three groups are statistically significant or not.

Group	Sodium(mEq/L)
1	135
1	152
1	140
1	145
2	162
2	184
2	210
2	218
2	198
2	290
3	268
3	280
3	182
3	246
3	500
3	235
3	298
3	480

Group	Mean	SD
1	143.00	7.26
2	210.33	43.79
3	311.13	115.82

Wrong method

On applying one-way ANOVA, p-value obtained for comparing between Groups was 0.012.

Since the SD values were very much different, applying the test for homogeneity of variances, 'p' value was found to be 0.022 showing that they were heterogenous. Hence, ANOVA has to be applied on log values.

Correct method

On applying ANOVA on log values, p-value obtained was 0.001.

The p-value obtained on applying ANOVA on original values was 0.012.

Groups	Multiple comparison p-value	
	on original values	*on log values*
1 & 2	0.686 ×	0.139 √
1 & 3	0.014 ×	0.001 √
2 & 3	0.121 ×	0.077 √

15.13. Graphs

15.13.1: The following data gives the infant mortality rate (IMR) in a country from 2000 to 2007. Draw an appropriate graph depicting the change in IMR from 2000 to 2007.

Wrong method

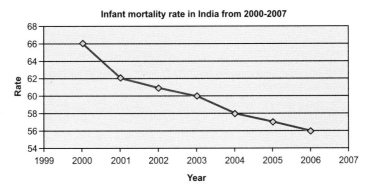

Fig. 15.1: IMR during 1999-2007

In the above given line graph (Fig. 15.1), the reading on Y-axis does not start from zero. In this graph, the reduction in IMR as depicted is steep decline, but in reality the decline is not steep.

Correct method

In an arithmetic graph paper the reading on Y-axis should start from zero. The line graph is drawn correctly in Fig. 15.2. The graph shows that there is a reduction in IMR, but it is only a small decrease.

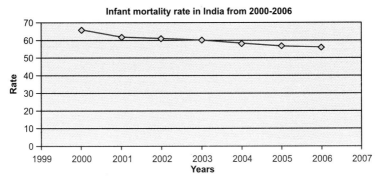

Fig. 15.2: IMR during 1999-2007

Multiple Choice Questions

Choose the correct answers in the following multiple choice questions. The correct answers are listed on p. 346.

Q. 1. **The following are the number of malaria cases reported in a town from 1998 to 2007:**

Year:	1998	1999	2000	2001	2002	2003	2004	2005	2006	2007
No. of cases:	200,	120,	350,	100,	90,	110,	130,	270,	3000,	200

For computing the average number of malaria cases reported in that town over a period of 10 years from 1998 to 2007, the correct average is:

a. Arithmetic mean   b. Mode
c. Median   d. Geometric mean

Q. 2. **Titre values of hormones (in ng/ml) of 6 patients are given below:**
1/10, 1/10, 1/40, 1/20, 1/80 and 1/80
For computing the average titre value from this sample, the best average is:
a. Arithmetic mean   b. Mode
c. Median   d. Geometric mean

Q. 3. **From the following results, to find out which variable has more variation, the best statistical parameter is:**

Variable	Mean	SD
Birth weight (g)	2592.0	354.90
SBP (mm Hg)	135.6	19.84

a. Mean   b. Standard deviation
c. Coefficient of variation   d. None of the above

Q. 4. **Age (years) and cholesterol (mg%) values of 6 men are listed below.**

Age:	25	80	65	90	60	75	Mean = 65.8	SD = 22.7
Cholesterol:	180	450	220	250	200	500	Mean = 300.0	SD = 138.4

The most appropriate correlation coefficient for this data is:
a. Pearson's correlation coefficient   b. Spearman's rank correlation coefficient
c. Coefficient of variation   d. None of the above

Q. 5. **The following data pertains to smoking habit in lung cancer patients and in comparative normal subjects.**

		Lung cancer		
		Yes	No	Total
Smoking	Yes	8	6	14
	No	2	14	16
	Total	10	20	30

To test whether lung cancer is statistically associated with smoking habit or not, the best statistical test of significance is:
a. Chi-square test without correction for continuity   b. Fisher's exact test
c. McNemar's chi-square test   d. Chi-square test for trend

Q. 6. **The following data gives the results of a diagnosis test by two methods A & B.**

		Test A		
		+ve	-ve	Total
Smoking	+ve	13	7	20
	-ve	2	28	30
	Total	15	35	50

To test whether the discordance in results by the two tests is statistically significant or not, the best statistical test of significance is:

a. Chi-square test for independent samples without continuity correction
b. Fisher's exact test
c. McNemar's chi-square test
d. Chi-square test for independent samples with continuity correction

Q. 7. **Heights (in cm) of 15 children from public schools and 12 children from Govt. schools are given below.**

Public school: 173, 155, 158, 150, 151, 152, 153, 159, 154, 179, 164, 172, 168, 178, 174
Govt. school: 148, 154, 152, 160, 154, 151, 158, 163, 157, 153, 155, 152

Type of School	Mean	SD
Public school	162.67	10.44
Govt. school	154.75	4.16

To test whether the difference in heights of children from the two types of schools is statistically significant or not, the best statistical test of significance is:

a. Paired t-test
b. Student's t-test for independent samples
c. Modified t-test
d. Analysis of variance

Q. 8. **The following data gives the systolic blood pressure (SBP) values of 10 hypertension patients before and one week after giving a drug.**

Systolic B.P	Patient Number									
	1	2	3	4	5	6	7	8	9	10
Before drug	160	150	170	130	140	170	160	160	120	140
After drug	150	140	160	140	145	150	140	150	120	120

To test whether the reduction in SBP after treatment is statistically significant or not, the best statistical test of significance is:

a. Paired t-test
b. Student's t-test for independent samples
c. Modified t-test
d. Analysis of variance

Q. 9. **To test the statistical significance of the difference in mean haemoglobin level between 50 pregnant and 100 non-pregnant women in the age group 25 to 35 years, the statistical test of significance to be used is (assuming statistical equality of variances):**

a. Paired t-test
b. Student's t-test for independent samples
c. Modified t-test
d. Analysis of variance

Q. 10. **The following data gives the results of a study on the diagnosis of diabetes and its association with regular exercise.**

		Diabetes		
		+ve	-ve	Total
Regular exercise	+ve	25	300	325
	-ve	125	550	675
	Total	150	850	1000

To test the statistical significance of the association between the occurrence of diabetes and lack of regular exercise, the appropriate statistical test of significance is:

a. Chi-square test
b. Paired t-test
c. McNemar's chi-square test
d. Analysis of variance

Answers to the MCQs along with Explanatory Hints

Chapter 1

1. c	2. c	3. b	4. a	5. a
6. d	7. b	8. c	9. d	10. b

Chapter 2

1. c	2. b	3. d	4. a	5. b
6. d	7. a	8. b	9. b	10. a

Chapter 3

1. c [Systolic blood pressure is a continuous variable.]
2. d [Because of two variables - sex & the type of disease. In each of the two gender groups, males and females, there will be multiple bars adjacent to each other for the types of diseases.]
3. c [Two variables are measurable and correlation between two measurable variables is graphically represented by scatter diagram.]
4. b [Because of the extreme value of 5000 in the year 1992.]
5. d [Because the units of measurement of height and weight are different and CV is independent of the units of measurement.]
6. d
7. b [(2/8) × 100]   8. d   9. a   10. d

Chapter 4

1. d
2. c

Mamography	Disease		
	+	–	Total
+	150	50	200
–	70	1730	1800
Total	220	1780	2000

Applying Baye's theorem P (D+/M-) = P (D+) × P (M-/D+) = $\dfrac{P\,(D+) \times P\,(M\text{-}/D+)}{\{P\,(D+) \times P(M\text{-}/D+)\} + \{P\,(D\text{-}) \times P\,(M\text{-}/D\text{-})\}}$

(Where D+ = Disease present; D- = Disease absent; M- = Mammography negative)

$$= \frac{(220/2000) \times (70/220)}{\left\{(220/2000) \times (70/220)\right\} + \left\{(1780/2000) \times (1730/1780)\right\}}$$

$$= 70/1800$$

3. c

$$\frac{12 - 14.5}{2.5} < Z > \frac{17 - 14.5}{2.5}$$

$$-1 < Z > 1 = (0.5 - 0.1587) + (0.8413 - 0.5) = 0.683$$

(From the Table of normal deviate values)
[In normal distribution Mean-1SD and Mean + 1SD will include 68.3% of the observations in the sample, i.e., the interval 12 to 17 will include 68.3% of 1000 (683) observations.]

4. b [In normal distribution mean-2SD and mean + 2SD will include about 95% of the observations in the sample, i.e., 2.5% of the observations will be lesser than the mean and 2.5% of the observations will be greater than the mean.]

5. b

$$Z = \frac{X\text{-Mean}}{SD} = \frac{140 - 160}{20} = 1$$

p = 0.84(84%)—From the Table of normal deviate values
[In normal distribution mean-1SD and mean + 1SD will include about 68% of the observations in the sample, i.e., 34% of the values will be between mean & mean -1SD. There will 50% of the observations less than the mean and 50% of the observations greater than the mean. Hence, the percentage of patients having their BP more than 140 (Mean-1SD) = 34 + 50 = 84%.]

6. d [The event is rare (3/1000) and the sample size is large (1000)]
7. d
8. c
   [p = 0.6, q = 0.4
   Required probability = nCr $p^r q^{n-r}$ = $_3C_3 \times (0.4)^0 (0.6)^3 = 0.216$]
9. d
   [p = 0.6, q = 0.4
   Required probability = nCr $p^r q^{n-r}$ = $_2C_2 \times (0.4)^0 (0.6)^2 = 0.36$]
10. b [CI= Mean ±2 × SD = 105 ± (2 × 10) = 85 & 125]

Chapter 5

1. b [More than two groups]
2. d [Because of paired samples(values before and after the administration of the drug on the same patients)]
3. d [Because of paired samples(Reponses to the question by the 2 methods were obtained from the same sample)]
4. c [Two independent samples: males & females]
5. a [For testing the statistical significance of the difference in proportion between two independent groups-Standard drug and new drug groups]
6. c [Association between two categorical variables]
7. d [Because of two independent samples - males & females]
8. b [Because of two independent samples: maternal intake of iron supplements –Good or Poor]
9. d [Two categorical variables - breast cancer status and using oral contraceptives]
10. d [Paired samples - two techniques-PCR & culture are tested on the same samples]

Chapter 6

1. c	2. c	3. c	4. b	5. a
6. c	7. d	8. c	9. b	10. c

Chapter 7

1. c	2. a	3. b	4. d	5. c
6. d	7. b	8. a	9. b	10. d

Chapter 8

1. c   2. c   3. b
4. b

		Lung cancer	
		Yes	No
Exposure	Yes	24	40
	No	96	960

Odds Ratio= (ad/bc) = $(24 \times 960)/(40 \times 96) = 6$

5. a   6. a   7. b   8. c   9. d   10. c

Chapter 9

1. d	2. c	3. c	4. c	5. c
6. d	7. b	8. c	9. c	10. c

Chapter 10

1. d
$$[n = 4 \times p \times (100\text{-}p)/L^2 = (4 \times 50 \times 50/5^2 = 400]$$
2. d
3. c
$$[L = [4 \times p \times (100\text{-}p)/n]^{1/2} = (4 \times 20 \times 80/100)^{1/2} = 8]$$
4. c
5. a $[n = (2.58)^2 \times SD^2/L^2 = (6.656 \times 10^2/6^2) = 19]$
6. b

$$n = \frac{[Z_{1-\alpha/2} \sqrt{\{2p(1-p)} + Z_{1-\beta} \sqrt{\{p_1(1-p_1) + p_2(1-p_2)\}}]^2}{(p_1 - p_2)^2}$$

where $p = (p_1 + p_2)/2 = (60 + 80/2 = 70 = 0.7)$

$$n = \frac{[1.96.\sqrt{\{2 \times 0.7 \times 0.3\}} + 0.84 \sqrt{\{0.6 \times 0.4 + 0.8 \times 0.2\}}]^2}{(0.8 - 0.6)^2} = 85$$

7. c
$$p = (p_1 + p_2)/2 = (0.7+0.5)/2 = 0.6$$

$$p = (p_1 + p_2)/2 = (0.7 + 0.5)/2 = 0.6)$$

$$n = \frac{[1.96.\sqrt{\{2 \times 0.6 \times 0.4\}} + 1.28\sqrt{\{0.7 \times 0.3 + 0.5 \times 0.5\}}]^2}{(0.7 - 0.5)^2} = 125$$

8. a

$$n = \frac{\left(SD_1^2 + SD_2^2\right)\left(Z_{1-\alpha/2} + Z_{1-\beta}\right)^2}{(M_1 - M_2)^2}$$

$$n = \frac{\left(0.5^2 + 0.7^2\right)\left(1.96 + 1.28\right)^2}{(3.0 - 2.5)^2} = 31$$

9. b

$$n = \frac{[Z_{1-\alpha/2.}\sqrt{\{2p(1-p)} + Z_{1-\beta}\sqrt{\{p_1(1-p_1) + p_2(1-p_2)\}}]^2}{(p_1 - p_2)^2}$$

where $p = (p_1 + p_2)/2 = (0.05 + 0.15)/2 = 0.1$

$$n = \frac{[1.96.\sqrt{\{2 \times 0.1 \times 0.9\}} + 1.28\sqrt{\{0.05 \times 0.95 + 0.15 \times 0.85\}}]^2}{(0.15 - 0.05)^2} = 190$$

10. c

Chapter 11

1. d   2. a   3. b
4. b [99 × 100/100) = 99%]
5. a [90 × 100/100) = 90%]
6. b [Sensitivity/(100-Specificity) = 99/10 = 9.9]
7. b [100-Sensitivity)/Specificity = 1/90 = 0.01]
8. c
9. a [20 × 100/40) = 50%]
10. c

Chapter 12

1. d [500-(500 × 30%)]   2. c   3. b   4. a   5. c
6. c [Crude birth rate = (live births × 1000/ total population) = (4000 × 1000)/100,000) = 40]
7. a [Infant mortality rate = (infant deaths/live births) × 1000 = (100/4000) × 1000 = 25]
8. d   9. c   10. c

Chapter 13

1. b   2. c   3. d   4. b   5. a
6. a   7. c   8. d   9. b   10. d

Chapter 14

1. c   2. b   3. a   4. d   5. c
6. b   7. b   8. a   9. d   10. b

Chapter 15

1. c   [Because of one extreme value - 3000 in 2006.]
2. d   [The values are in geometric progression.]
3. c   [Because of the difference in the unit of measurements of birth weight and SBP.]
4. b   [Because of small sample size and large SD compared to the mean : non-normal distribution.]
5. b   [Both of the two groups has less than 20 samples.]
6. c   [Paired samples - Both the tests A & B are done on the same subjects.]
7. c   [Because of the heterogeneity of variances in the two groups.]
8. a   [Paired samples - before and after design.]
9. b   [Two independent samples (pregnant & non-pregnant women) with equal variances.]
10. a   [Association between two independent variables - diabetes & exercise.]

Further Reading

Chapter 2

1. Ardilly P, Tillé Y. *Sampling Methods: Exercises and Solutions.* 1st ed. Springer; 2005.
2. Benedetto JJ, Ferreira PJSG. *Modern Sampling Theory.* 1st ed. Boston: Birkhäuser; 2001.
3. Chaudhuri A, Stenger H. *Survey Sampling: Theory and Methods.* 2nd ed. CRC; 2005.
4. Cochran W G. *Sampling Techniques.* 3rd ed. New Age International Pvt Ltd; 2008.
5. Groves RM, Floyd J, Fowler Jr., Couper MP, Lepkowski J M. *Survey Methodology.* 1st ed. New York: Wiley-Interscience; 2004.
6. Hektner JM, Schmidt JA, Csikszentmihalyi M. *Experience Sampling Method: Measuring the Quality of Everyday Life.* Sage Publications; 2006.
7. Kessler R, Ustun TB. *The WHO World Mental Health Surveys: Global Perspectives on the Epidemiology of Mental Disorders.* 1st ed. Cambridge University Press; 2008.
8. Korn EL, Graubard BI. *Analysis of Health Surveys.* 1st ed. New York: Wiley-Interscience; 1999.
9. Lavallée P. *Indirect Sampling (Springer Series in Statistics).* 1st ed. Springer; 2007.
10. Levy PS, Lemeshow S. *Sampling of Populations: Methods and Applications (Wiley Series in Survey Methodology).* 4th ed. New York: Wiley; 2008.
11. Lohr SL. *Sampling: Design and Analysis.* 1st ed. Duxbury Press; 1999.
12. Lynn P. *Methodology of Longitudinal Surveys.* New York: Wiley; 2009.
13. Mukhopadhyay P. *Theory and Methods of Survey Sampling.* New Delhi: Prentice-Hall of India Pvt. Ltd; 2004.
14. Paik Yung-Han, Ko Ung-Ring, Patwari Kamini Mohan, eds. WHO. *Health Research Methodology (A Guide for Training in Research Methods), 1992.* Delhi: Oxford University Press; 1993.
15. Pandey B N. *Statistical Techniques in Life Testing, Reliability, Sampling Theory.* New Delhi: Narosa Pub House; 2007.
16. Rao PSRS. *Sampling Methodologies with Applications (Texts in Statistical Science).* 1st ed. Chapman & Hall/CRC; 2000.
17. Rubin DB. *Matched Sampling for Causal Effects.* 1st ed. Cambridge University Press; 2006.
18. Sampath S. *Sampling Theory and Methods.* 2nd ed. Alpha Science International, Ltd; 2005.
19. Särndal C-E, Swensson B, Wretman J. *Model Assisted Survey Sampling.* Springer; 2003.
20. Särndal C-E, Swensson B, Wretman J. *Model Assisted Survey Sampling.* Springer; 2003.
21. Scheaffer RL, Mendenhall W, Ott RL. *Elementary Survey Sampling (with CD-ROM).* 6th ed. Duxbury Press; 2005.
22. Stephens K S. *The Handbook of Applied Acceptance Sampling: Plans, Procedures & Principles.* 1st ed. ASQ Quality Press; 2001.
23. Stephens KS. *The Handbook of Applied Acceptance Sampling: Plans, Procedures & Principles.* 1st ed. ASQ Quality Press; 2001.
24. Thompson SK. *Sampling (Wiley Series in Probability and Statistics).* 2nd ed. New York: Wiley-Interscience; 2002.
25. Thompson W. *Sampling Rare or Elusive Species: Concepts, Designs, and Techniques for Estimating Population Parameters.* 1st ed. Island Press; 2004.
26. Tillé Y. *Sampling Algorithms.* 1st ed. Springer; 2006.
27. White P. *Basic Sampling (The Basic Series).* Sanctuary; 2004.
28. Zhang C. *Fundamentals of Environmental Sampling and Analysis.* New York: Wiley-Interscience; 2007.

Chapter 3

1. Altman Douglas G. *Practical Statistics for Medical Research.* New York: Chapman & Hall/ CRC, 1991.
2. Armitage Peter, Berry Geoffrey, Matthews JNS. *Statistical Methods in Medical Research.* London: Blackwell Science. 4th ed. 2002.

3. Bourke GJ, Daly LE, Mcgilvray J. *Interpretation and Uses of Medical Statistics*. London: Blackwell Scientific Publications; 1988.
4. Campbell Michael J, Machin David, Walters Stephen J. *Medical Statistics: A Textbook for the Health Sciences*. 4th ed. New York: John Wiley, 2007.
5. Castle WM. *Statistics in Small Doses*. Edinburgh: Churchill, Livingstone; 1984.
6. Colquohoun D. *Lectures on Biostatistics – An Introduction to Statistics with Applications in Biology and Medicine*. Oxford: Clarendon Press; 1971.
7. Colton T. *Statistics in Medicine*. Boston: Little Brown & Co.; 1974.
8. Feinstein Alvin R. *Clinical Biostatistics*. New York: The C.V. Mosby & Co.; 1977.
9. Martin Bland. *An Introduction to Medical Statistics*. 3rd ed. Oxford: Oxford University Press, 2000.
10. Pagano Marcello, Gauvreau Kimberlee. *Principles of Biostatistics*. 2nd ed. Brooks / Cole; 2000.
11. Petrie Aviva. *Lecture Notes on Medical Statistics*. London: Blackwell Scientific Publications; 1978.
12. Robert R, Sokal & James Rohlf F. *Introduction to Biostatistics*. New York: W.H. Freeman; 1987.
13. Schor SS. *Fundamentals of Biostatistics*. New York: G.P. Putnam & Sons; 1968.

Chapter 4

1. Armitage P, Berry G, Matthews JNS. *Statistical Methods in Medical Research*. 4th ed. London: Blackwell Science; 2002.
2. Bourke GJ, Daly le, Mcgilvray J. *Interpretation and Uses of Medical Statistics*. London: Blackwell Scientific Publications; 1988.
3. Colquohoun D. *Lectures on Biostatistics–An Introduction to Statistics with Applications in Biology and Medicine*. Oxford: Clarendon Press; 1971.
4. Colton T. *Statistics in Medicine*. Boston: Little Brown & Co.; 1974.
5. Feinstein Alvin R. *Clinical Biostatistics*. New York: The C.V. Mosby & Co.; 1977.
6. Matthews DE, Farewell V. *Using and Undertaking Medical Statistics*. London: Karger; 1985.
7. Schor SS. *Fundamentals of Biostatistics*. New York: G.P. Putnam & Sons; 1968.

Chapter 5

1. Altman DG, Machin D, Bryant TN, Gardner MJ, eds. *Statistics with Confidence*. 2nd ed. London: BMJ Books, 2000.
2. Altman Douglas G. *Practical Statistics for Medical Research*. New York: Chapman & Hall/ CRC, 1991.
3. Armitage Peter, Berry Geoffrey, Matthews JNS. *Statistical Methods in Medical Research*. London: Blackwell Science. 4th ed. 2002.
4. Bourke GJ, Daly LE, Mcgilvray J. *Interpretation and Uses of Medical Statistics*. London: Blackwell Scientific Publications; 1988.
5. Campbell Michael J., Machin David, Walters Stephen J. *Medical Statistics: A Textbook for the Health Sciences*. 4th ed. New York: John Wiley, 2007.
6. Castle WM. *Statistics in Small Doses*. Edinburgh: Churchill, Livingstone; 1984.
7. Colquohoun D. *Lectures on Biostatistics – An Introduction to Statistics with Applications in Biology and Medicine*. Oxford: Clarendon Press; 1971.
8. Colton T. *Statistics in Medicine*. Boston: Little Brown & Co.; 1974.
9. Feinstein Alvin R. *Clinical Biostatistics*. New York: The C.V. Mosby & Co.; 1977.
10. Fleiss Joseph L., Levin Bruce, Cho Paik Myunghee. *Statistical Methods for Rates and Proportions,* 3rd ed. New York: John Wiley, 2003.
11. Martin Bland. *An Introduction to Medical Statistics*. 3rd ed. Oxford: Oxford University Press, 2000.
12. Matthews DE, Farewell V. *Using and Undertaking Medical Statistics*. London: Karger; 1985.
13. Maxwell AE. *Analysing Qualitative Data*. London: Methuen & Co. Ltd.; 1961
14. Pagano Marcello, Gauvreau Kimberlee. *Principles of Biostatistics*. 2nd ed. Brooks/Cole, 2000.
15. Petrie Aviva. *Lecture Notes on Medical Statistics*. London: Blackwell Scientific Publications; 1978.
16. Robert R, Sokal & James Rohlf F. *Introduction to Biostatistics*. New York: W.H. Freeman; 1987.
17. Schor SS. *Fundamentals of Biostatistics*. New York: G.P. Putnam & Sons; 1968.

Chapter 6

1. Armitage P, Berry G, Matthews JNS. *Statistical Methods in Medical Research.* 4th ed. London: Blackwell Science; 2002.
2. Aviva Petrie. *Lecture Notes on Medical Statistics.* Oxford: Blackwell Scientific Publications; 1978.
3. Bourke GJ, Daly LE, Mcgilvray J. *Interpretation and Uses of Medical Statistics.* London: Blackwell Scientific Publications; 1988.
4. Castle WM. *Statistics in Small Doses.* Edinburgh: Churchill, Livingstone; 1984.
5. Colquhoun D. *Lectures on Biostatistics – An Introduction to Statistics with Applications in Biology and Medicine.* Oxford: Clarendon Press; 1971.
6. Colton T. *Statistics in Medicine.* Boston: Little Brown   Co.; 1974.
7. Conover WJ (ed). *Practical Non-Parametric Statistics.* 2nd ed. New York: John Wiley; 1980.
8. Daniel Wayne W. *Biostatistics - A Foundation for Analysis in the Health Sciences.* 7th ed. New York: John Wiley & Sons; 1999.
9. Feinstein Alvin R. *Clinical Biostatistics.* New York: C.V. Mosby & Co.; 1977.
10. Martin Bland. *An Introduction to Medical Statistics.* 3rd ed. Oxford: Oxford University Press; 2000.
11. Matthews DE, Farewell V. *Using and Undertaking Medical Statistics.* London: Karger; 1985.
12. Pett MA. *Non-Parametric Statistics for Health Care Research.* London: Sage Publications; 1997.
13. Schor SS. *Fundamentals of Biostatistics.* New York: G.P. Putnam & Sons; 1968.
14. Siegel S. *Non-parametric Statistics for Behavioural Sciences.* New York: McGraw-Hill; 1956.
15. Sokal Robert R, Rohlf F. James. *Introduction to Biostatistics.* New York: W.H. Freeman; 1987.

Chapter 7

1. Afifi Abdelonem, May Susanne, Clark Virginia. *Computer Aided Multivariate Analysis.* New York: Chapman & Hall (CRC); 2003.
2. Altman DG. *Practical Statistics for Medical Research.* London: Chapman & Hall; 1991.
3. Anderson TW. *An Introduction to Multivariate Statistical Analysis.* New York: John Wiley & Sons. Inc.; 1984.
4. Armitage P, Berry G, Matthews JNS. *Statistical Methods in Medical Research.* 4th ed. London: Blackwell Science; 2002.
5. Bland M. *An Introduction to Medical Statistics.* Oxford: Oxford University Press; 2000.
6. Collett David. *Modelling Binary Data.* 2nd ed. London: Chapman & Hall; 2003.
7. Daniel Wayne W. *Biostatistics.* New York: John Wiley & Sons. Inc.; 2005.
8. Dillon WR, Goldstein Matthew. *Multivariate Analysis: Methods and Applications.* New York: John Wiley & Sons. Inc.; 1984.
9. Everett Brain S, Dunn Graham. *Applied Multivariate Data Analysis.* Oxford: Oxford University Press; 2001.
10. Flury Bernard. *A First Course in Multivariate Statistics.* New York: Springer; 1997.
11. Hosmer David W, Lemeshow Stanley. *Applied Logistic Regression.* 2nd ed. New York: John Wiley and Sons; 2000.
12. Jobson JD. *Applied Multivariate Data Analysis, Volume II: Categorical and Multivariate Methods.* New York: Springer; 1992.
13. Kendall MG. *Multivariate Analysis.* London: Griffin; 1980.
14. Lebart L, Morineau A, Warwick KM. *Multivariate Descriptive Statistical Analysis.* New York: Wiley; 1984.
15. Morrison Donald F. *Multivariate Statistical Methods.* New York: McGraw Hill; 1990.
16. Neter John, Wasserman William, Kutner Michael H. *Applied Linear Regression Models.* 2nd ed. Boston: Irwin; 1989.
17. Norusis MJ. *The SPSS Guide to Data Analysis.* Chicago: SPSS Inc.; 1991.
18. Snedecor GW, Cochran WG. *Statistical Methods.* Iowa State University Press; 1989.

Chapter 8

1. Abramson LH. *Survey Methods in Community Medicine.* London: Churchill Livingstone; 1990.
2. Barker DJP, Hall AJ. *Practical Epidemiology.* NY: Churchill Livingstone; 1991.
3. Greenberg Raymond S, Daniels Stephen RW, Flanders Dana, Eley John William, Boring III John R. *Medical Epidemiology.* New York: Lange Medical Books/McGraw Hill; 1996.
4. Hennekens Charles H, Burning Julie E. In: Sherry L Mayrent (ed.). *Epidemiology in Medicine.* Boston: Little Brown and Co.; 1987.

5. Kelsey AR, Thompson WD, Evans AS. *Methods of Observational Epidemiology*. Oxford: Oxford University Press; 1986.
6. Lilienfeld AE, Lilienfeld DE. *Foundation of Epidemiology*. Oxford: Oxford University Press; 1980.
7. MacMahon B, Pugh. *Epidemiology: Principles and Methods*. Boston: Little Brown; 1970.
8. Rothman KJ. *Modern Epidemiology*. Boston: Little Brown; 1997.

Chapter 9

1. Angell M. The ethics of clinical research in the third world. *N Engl J Med*. 1997; 337(12):847.
2. Byron, Kenward Michael G. *Design and Analysis of Cross-over Trials*. 2nd ed. New York: Chapman Hall/ CRC; 2003.
3. Cook Thomas D, DeMets David L. *Introduction to Statistical Methods for Clinical Trials*. New York: Chapman & Hall/ CRC; 2008.
4. Fleiss JL. *Statistical Methods for Rates and Proportions*. New York: John Wiley & Sons; 1981.
5. Frieman JA, Chalmers TC, Smith H, Kubler RR. The importance of beta, the type II error and sample size in design and interpretation of the randomized control trial: survey of "negative" trials. *N Eng J Med*. 1978; 299: 690-694.
6. Kleinbaum DG, Kupper LL, Muller KE. *Applied Regression Analysis and other Multivariable Methods*. Boston: PWS-KENT Publishing Company; 1988.
7. Last John M. *A Dictionary of Epidemiology*. 2nd ed. New York: Oxford University Press; 1988.
8. Lee ET. *Statistical Method for Survival Data Analysis*. Belmont, California: Lifetime Learning Publications; 1980.
9. Lemshow SL, Hosmer DW, Klar JN, Lwanga KS. *Adequacy of Sample Size in Health Studies*. New York: John Wiley & Sons; 1990.
10. Lilford RF, Jackson J. Equipoise and the ethics of randomization. *J R Soc Med*. 1995; 88(10):552-559.
11. Machin D, Campbell MJ. *Statistical Tables for the Design of Clinical Trials*. Oxford: Blackwell Scientific Publications; 1987.
12. Moher David, Dulberg Corinne S, Wells George A. Statistical power, sample size, and their reporting in randomized controlled trials. *JAMA*. 1994; 272:122-124.
13. Retherford RD, Choe MK. *Statistical Models for Causal Analysis*. New York: John Wiley & Sons, Inc.; 1993
14. Rothman KJ, Michels KB. The continuing unethical use of placebo controls. *N Engl J Med*.1994; 331(6):394-398.

Chapter 10

1. Blackwelder WC. Equivalence trials. In: *Encyclopedia of Biostatistics*. New York: John Wiley and Sons, Inc; 1997.
2. Donner A. Approaches to sample size estimation in the design of clinical trials-a review. *Statistics in Medicine*, 1984; 3:199-214.
3. Gould AL. Sample size for event rate equivalence trials using prior information. *Statistics in Medicine*.1993; 12: 2009-2023.
4. Julious S A. Tutorial in biostatistics, sample size for clinical trials with normal data. *Statistics in Medicine*. 2004; 23:1921-1986.
5. Lee KL. Sample size and interim analysis issues for dose selection. *American Heart Journal*. 2000; 139 (4): S161-S165.
6. Lwanga SK, Lemeshow S. Sample size determination in health studies. *A Practical Manual*. Geneva: World Health Organization; 1991.
7. Proschan MA, Liu Q, Hunsberger S. Practical midcourse sample size modification in clinical trials. *Controlled Clinical Trials*. 2003; 24:4-15.
8. Rosenberger WF, Lachin JM. *Randomization in Clinical Trials, Theory and Practice*. New York: John Wiley & Sons; 2002.
9. Whitehead J. Sample size for phase II and phase III clinical trials: an integrated approach. *Statistics in Medicine*.1986; 5:459-464.

Chapter 11

1. Altman Douglas G. *Practical Statistics for Medical Research*. New York: Chapman & Hall/ CRC; 1991.
2. Armitage Peter, Berry Geoffrey, Matthews JNS. *Statistical Methods in Medical Research*. 4th ed. London: Blackwell Science; 2002.

3. Feinstein Alvin R. *Clinical Biostatistics.* New York: The C.V. Mosby & Co.; 1977.
4. Martin Bland. *An Introduction to Medical Statistics.* 3rd ed. Oxford: Oxford University Press; 2000.
5. Sox HC, Blatt MA, Higgins MC, Marton KI. *Medical Decision Making.* Stoneham, Massachusetts: Butterworth-Heinemann; 1988.

Chapter 12

1. Beard RE. Some aspects of theories of mortality, cause of death analysis, forecasting and stochastic process. In: Brass W (ed.). *Biological Aspects of Demography.* London: Taylor and Francis Ltd.
2. Bogue DJ. *Principles of Demography.* New York: John Wiley and Sons Inc.; 1969.
3. Chiang CL. *Introduction to the Stochastic Processes in Biostatistics.* New York: John Wiley and Sons Inc.; 1968.
4. Johnson RC Elandt, Johnson Norman L. *Survival Models and Data Analysis.* New York: John Wiley and Sons Inc.; 1980.
5. Land KC, Rogers A. *Multidimensional Mathematical Demography.* New York: Academic Press; 1982.
6. Last John M. *A Dictionary of Epidemiology.* 2nd ed. Oxford: Oxford University Press; 1988.
7. Lwanga SK, Tye Cho-Yook. *Teaching Health Statistics: Twenty Lesson and Seminar Outlines.* Geneva: World Health Organization; 1986.
8. Ministry of Health and Family Welfare (MOHFW). *Family Welfare Programme in India Year Book: 1990-91.* New Delhi: Department of Family Welfare, MOHFW; 1992.
9. Ministry of Health and Family Welfare (MOHFW). *National Health Policy, 2002.* New Delhi: MOHFW; 2002.
10. Ministry of Health and Family Welare (MOHFW). *Reproductive and Child Health Programme: Schemes for Implementation.* New Delhi: Department of Family Welfare, MOHFW; 1997.
11. Pathak KB, Ram F. *Teaching of Demographic Analysis.* New Delhi: Himalayan Publishing House; 1992.
12. UN Asian Development Institute, Bangkok, Thailand. *A Glossary of Some Terms of Demography.* New Delhi: Hans Raj Gupta & Sons; 1980.
13. United Nation. *Indirect Techniques for Demographic Estimation. ManualX, Population Studies* No. 81, ST/ ESA/ SER. A/ 81; New York.

Chapter 13

1. Last John M. *A Dictionary of Epidemiology.* 2nd ed. Oxford: Oxford University Press; 1988.
2. Lwanga SK, Tye Cho-Yook. *Teaching Health Statistics: Twenty Lesson and Seminar Outlines.* Geneva: World Health Organization; 1986.
3. Sunder Rao PSS, Richard J. *An Introduction to Biostatistics: A Manual for Students in Health Sciences.* 3rd ed. New Delhi: Prentice Hall of India Private Limited; 1996.

Chapter 14

Most of the statistical software have their own manuals which will be very handy for a beginner. In addition, help files are also part of the software, so that context based help can easily be accessed. Further, some books dealing with the usage, obtaining the output and the interpretation of results, etc., for the beginners are available; some of these are listed below.

1. Acock Alan C. *A Gentle Introduction to Stata.* 2nd ed. Boca Raton, Florida: CRC Press; 2008.
2. Bissett Brian D. *Automated Data Analysis Using Excel.* Boca Raton, Florida: Chapman & Hall/ CRC; 2007.
3. Der Geoff, Everitt Brian S. *A Handbook of Statistical Analyses using SAS.* 3rd ed. New York: Chapman & Hall/ CRC; 2008.
4. Der Geoff, Everitt Brian S. *Statistical Analysis of Medical Data Using SAS.* New York: Chapman & Hall/CRC; 2005.
5. Foster Jeremy J. *Data Analysis Using SPSS for Windows*: New Ed. Version 8-10. London: Sage Publication.
6. Griffith Arthur. *SPSS for Dummies.* New York: John Wiley; 2007.
7. Gupta Sunil, Edmonds Curt. *Sharpening Your SAS Skills.* New York: Chapman & Hall/CRC; 2005.
8. Juul Svend. *An Introduction to Stata for Health Researchers.* 2nd Ed. Boca Raton, Florida: CRC Press; 2008.
9. Kohler Ulrich, Kreuter Frauke. *Data Analysis Using Stata.* Boca Raton, Florida: Chapman & Hall/CRC; 2005.
10. Landau Sabine, Everitt Brian S. *A Handbook of Statistical Analyses using SPSS.* Boca Raton, Florida: Chapman & Hall/ CRC; 2003.

11. Marasinghe Mervyn G, Kennedy William J. *SAS for Data Analysis*. New York: Springer; 2008.

12. Rabe-Hesketh Sophia, Everitt Brian S. *A Handbook of Statistical Analyses using Stata*. 4th ed. New York: Chapman & Hall/ CRC; 2006.

13. Spencer Neil H. *SAS Programming: The One-Day Course*. New York: Chapman & Hall/CRC; 2003.

Chapter 15

1. Altman DG, Bland JM. Absence of evidence is not evidence of absence. *BMJ*. 1995; 4-85.

2. Altman DG. Statistics in medical journals: development in the 1980s. *Statistics in Medicine*. 1991; 10:1897-1913.

3. Badgley RF. An assessment of research methods reported in 103 scientific articles in two Canadian medical journals. *Canadian Medical Association Journal*. 1961; 85: 246-250.

4. Browner W, Newman T. Are all significant P values created equal? The analogy between diagnostic test and clinical research. *JAMA*. 1987; 257:2459-2463.

5. Carven RP. The case against statistical significance testing. *Harvard Educ Rev*. 1978; 48:378-399.

6. Cruess DF. Review of use of statistics in the *American Journal of Tropical Medicine and Hygiene* for January-December 1988. *American Journal of Tropical Medicine and Hygiene*. 1989; 41:619-626.

7. Cullagh MC, Nehder JA. The most common form of misinterpretation involved in compraisis. *Statistics in Medicine*. 1993; 12:1459-1469.

8. Elwood JM. *Causal Relationship in Medicine: A Practical System for Critical Appraisal*. Oxford: Oxford University Press; 1988.

9. Felson DT, Cupples LA, Meenan RF. Misuse of statistical methods in *Arthritis and Rheumatism* 1882 versus 1967-68. *Arthritis and Rheumatism*. 1984; 27:1018-1022.

10. Gigerenzer G. Mindless statistics. *J Socio Economics*. 2004; 33:587-606.

11. Glantz SA. Biostatistics: how to detect, correct and prevent errors in the medical literature. *Circulation*. 1980; 61:1-7.

12. Gonzales VA, Ottenbacher KJ. Measures of central tendency in rehabilitation research: what do they mean? *Am J Physical Medicine & Rehab*. 2001; 80(2):141-146.

13. Goodman NW, Hughes AO. Statistical awareness of research workers in British anaesthesia. *British Journal of Anaethesia*. 1992; 68:321-324.

14. Gorey KM, Trevisan M. Secular trends in the United States black/white hypertension prevalence ratio: potential impact of diminishing response rates. *Am J Epidemiol*. 1998; 147:95-99.

15. Hamitton GW, Williams DL, Kennedy JW. Misuse of statistics - correlation coefficient (r) - Thy head is treacherous. *The Journal of Nuclear Medicine*. 1978; 19: 8:974.

16. Hill AB. *A Short Textbook of Medical Statistics*. London: The English Language Book Society; 1977: 261.

17. James E. De. Muth. *Basic Statistics and Pharmaceutical Statistical Application*. 2nd ed. New York: Chapman and Hall / C.R.C. Taylor Francis Group; 2006.

18. James RB. Understanding P-value misuse. *Statistics in Medicine*. 1989; 8:1413-1417.

19. Janso TC. The value of a p-valueless paper. Misinterpretation and misuse of the kappa statistic. *Am J Epidemiol*. 2004; 126(2):161-169.

20. Landies JR, Koch GG. Misinterpretation and misuse of kappa statistics. *American Journal of Epidemiology*. 1987; 4:2191-2205.

21. Ludwing EG, Collette JC. Some misuse of health statistics. *JAMA*. 1971; 216:493-499.

22. Nagele P. Misuse of standard error of the mean (SEM) when reporting variability of a sample. A critical evaluation of four anesthesia journals. *American Journal of Anesthesia*. 2003; 90: 4514-4516.

23. Siegrist M. Communicating low risk magnitudes: incidence rates expressed as frequency versus rates expressed as probability. *Risk Anal*. 1997; 17:507-510.

24. Silber JH, Rosenbaum PR. A spurious correlation between hospital mortality and complication rates: the importance of severity adjustment. *Med Care*. 1997; 35(10 Suppl):OS77-OS92.

25. Steven N, Goodman G. Toward evidence-based medical statistic 1: the P value fallacy. *Annals of Internal Medicine*. 1999; 130,12:995-1004.

26. Stimson GV, Hickman M, Turnbull PJ. Statistics on misuse of drugs have been misused. *BMJ*. 1998; 317: 1388.

27. Wulff HR, Andersen B, Brandenhoff P, Guttler F. What do doctors know about statistics? *Stat Med*. 1987; 6:3-10.

Appendices 1-7: Statistical Tables

Appendix 1 - Random Numbers*

Row No.	1 - 5	6 - 10	11 - 15	16 - 20	21 - 25	26 - 30	31 - 35	36 - 40	41 - 45	46 – 50
1	71556	27674	40671	20661	42145	00612	90036	80532	65995	59492
2	13210	31996	30331	67516	53475	06948	09342	78837	20361	75857
3	38596	70650	14781	43138	43989	25548	62121	15639	31958	93631
4	27508	97412	03351	49833	09059	46011	79390	64628	30911	53341
5	77922	95566	77623	94712	51454	78495	06197	83264	27944	41911
6	95947	43157	68869	44577	89844	70670	16417	86811	66520	67268
7	20392	99828	69987	26479	01183	90479	35816	45011	34315	28992
8	90041	83005	84857	50301	32228	36633	01910	89559	22486	43676
9	54299	49454	36604	70276	89288	82544	24803	99954	36471	9906
10	75630	65134	42358	03585	54293	33643	02760	53568	33094	31396
11	84125	29568	99986	05557	89177	82771	55954	83585	05366	79379
12	33057	26645	88237	10842	56495	62091	63063	64580	16467	12196
13	78771	20627	78701	32277	40868	72282	52441	01132	37399	5738
14	54927	71725	30118	23503	00859	58676	92248	03635	51602	27737
15	29073	04244	50314	19576	54884	85195	20510	67260	31945	69670
16	98769	42805	76933	84640	30408	47601	29307	89905	63818	29770
17	45237	32536	47290	53572	61679	48277	80404	42950	23093	95560
18	58857	80929	23102	09170	07392	93055	91786	64314	31209	25978
19	02484	59611	88605	11515	33120	06929	24751	68747	21324	50462
20	28552	50943	14619	52572	97286	05178	40917	13172	18764	12005
21	10165	86115	57305	54003	85559	31872	97033	78682	48693	60081
22	13689	63612	61164	41847	54088	44718	28942	70046	28245	41422
23	46483	15930	32669	70430	91231	36328	83968	38198	68456	24512
24	00317	80892	16740	10290	04937	43147	00541	36555	99156	84978
25	67961	88584	20028	28934	74155	90668	63506	36359	34013	06029
26	60400	65198	17735	79271	74452	84535	19210	75288	03737	79479
27	65351	92168	64028	24095	94952	24719	40461	33642	60175	94680
28	04236	80323	57683	43160	97442	29068	85085	74308	85634	92757
29	89450	01499	59335	19099	19683	72461	43981	04393	46878	47364

*Generated by Microsoft Excel, 2007

(Continued)

Appendix 1 - Random Numbers* (Contd.)

Row No.	Column No.									
	1 - 5	*6 - 10*	*11 - 15*	*16 - 20*	*21 - 25*	*26 - 30*	*31 - 35*	*36 - 40*	*41 - 45*	*46 – 50*
30	91134	48294	43268	23852	81118	38528	8263	33998	41741	74222
31	01405	42835	81587	23021	67260	66425	83034	38261	66256	50765
32	40962	85808	4284	90058	30742	19503	72711	54355	49463	41311
33	79393	87840	33195	64185	09184	90794	20215	89556	89107	76808
34	94346	46303	81206	20695	07237	66246	01211	00623	86535	44184
35	51819	92239	22477	98993	84251	29518	57266	27708	24201	93784
36	00391	77211	28559	14699	15132	96729	55628	84660	10622	16346
37	71216	95709	08750	07888	86565	96358	14275	51240	82631	98471
38	06023	92279	54490	05634	13984	92479	95953	57303	30791	01729
39	27241	73450	76669	18470	08146	51711	75252	29343	95616	24350
40	17728	24524	09700	24002	30008	44324	47517	90992	06289	11235
41	98564	46145	59890	16289	07736	55627	13242	55065	56532	37231
42	50358	49731	05902	67955	14245	53953	35082	54795	58959	36840
43	61583	21321	85366	44371	13536	58426	10122	09410	45886	69408
44	09152	96029	14656	32977	15991	25099	24390	80951	15903	32951
45	93305	25399	65518	92687	23047	83482	94060	36024	16823	38476
46	71501	07028	98374	75224	84861	99359	53893	65352	12440	42185
47	28914	41410	33915	25920	31298	83271	68784	37369	69171	43065
48	52287	76710	72366	57364	34662	02100	27255	77415	31424	16887
49	52091	40980	27944	29641	22578	80619	85650	57181	14332	92727
50	81314	43603	24326	31035	30403	00673	48218	07402	72664	31718
51	80756	87672	04161	75023	84175	40165	32574	62639	34059	30908
52	55507	52164	60245	76989	39488	32642	68396	85683	57742	05431
53	18836	54714	76842	35017	02790	70806	62877	59802	27318	28867
54	86174	77461	54476	29191	56674	44084	00437	98323	89991	96714
55	09077	94096	46066	90450	79243	16347	44112	21464	89836	12560
56	05916	23537	20685	57599	90776	01571	03453	29908	74207	54753
57	47881	24782	70943	16278	79460	56945	98537	43604	77126	99901
58	99866	64163	37918	52832	20160	07875	90894	43050	40125	85635
59	78605	86508	78871	02893	91062	53971	34900	02543	37706	70012
60	35905	74575	9361	54719	43157	13231	06544	89702	65267	11871
61	47814	46549	13658	43399	13413	02997	54580	19495	35237	83704
62	80573	84659	14404	31073	54184	68122	12484	23193	88957	65771
63	10120	71328	79552	97483	56718	96118	23954	58147	93371	71644
64	76825	30499	72757	17586	19659	56110	10125	19675	95091	46704
65	61883	93764	37636	46801	52756	77178	03458	81915	04242	89278

*Generated by Microsoft Excel, 2007

(Continued)

Appendix 1 - Random Numbers* (Contd.)

Row No.	Column No.									
	1 - 5	*6 - 10*	*11 - 15*	*16 - 20*	*21 - 25*	*26 - 30*	*31 - 35*	*36 - 40*	*41 - 45*	*46 – 50*
66	31448	44963	72375	06216	30000	47647	24347	84546	13344	82134
67	19578	32720	41139	94927	09952	91218	07155	27777	15509	99622
68	45601	48194	31426	89223	94345	99905	59493	99509	34542	66822
69	81218	94200	66969	82874	00306	12187	15627	65020	69298	15514
70	10741	51837	88761	63435	89054	45735	06294	27065	67484	16866
71	92795	29457	49976	90825	55261	59672	26593	52104	17435	92659
72	30490	46130	42387	99107	41094	78661	85245	81994	19936	89359
73	21393	09606	94369	91622	21538	63022	41496	80064	62457	20705
74	49451	38575	85534	94947	22197	42164	68316	43552	68052	41062
75	14052	01167	44530	77212	89762	77560	66078	22250	64156	10088
76	82934	43405	67368	30540	00595	03810	71641	75626	39440	35598
77	94459	10387	78879	85869	30222	67499	20630	23676	98841	05357
78	09340	23635	88098	41939	75057	64837	02553	63342	01465	69193
79	59738	22035	24311	80668	82983	40422	46843	78979	95460	08485
80	06671	33049	29845	54104	99398	13385	90543	52186	35742	72064
81	93519	08374	77246	06372	95431	16995	77616	12781	29498	78655
82	15871	96921	90266	73868	32642	51978	75992	10299	30496	81067
83	14564	27679	75094	58634	90555	77271	32081	88691	66026	01050
84	87979	55804	62364	36893	82100	70900	67202	26637	29723	33925
85	41117	57887	18655	20550	05334	21325	32684	92975	39759	54207
86	65160	37113	32952	96307	74353	38095	80141	55657	64765	71814
87	71518	54831	00373	69644	61562	55994	47652	41474	83304	04093
88	12770	37917	06423	22930	88736	49697	76298	32280	82072	64893
89	86224	09775	40203	64135	34143	07530	37666	57664	00244	02303
90	04064	47312	29521	49181	25171	81024	91982	07137	30525	33477
91	55807	18216	76566	63661	17144	48197	90840	87341	84244	39992
92	86129	10705	79711	66703	93515	80211	81600	77470	45596	27225
93	42265	19912	56036	4668	29161	05270	8314	68046	75850	25745
94	62435	49762	54977	79377	52028	96828	32961	75545	71544	01770
95	49198	35101	49501	45646	88281	11585	17933	34200	25028	00914
96	97792	04992	78781	48766	39651	45291	63383	81079	54187	34020
97	81741	10489	52366	58126	94853	70053	69501	01243	13844	79587
98	76508	49889	57067	88942	98869	71452	27064	18344	53991	67195
99	50796	04356	07458	53801	69380	15894	84729	93664	13568	32895
100	96529	80239	77523	35705	16898	63794	40411	57021	59770	51686

*Generated by Microsoft Excel, 2007

Appendix 2 — Area* under the Standard Normal Curve

A: Left tail area (- ∞ to Z)
C: Right tail area (Z to ∞)

B: O to Z
D: Two tailed area (-Z to +Z)

Z	A	B	C	D	Z	A	B	C	D
0.00	0.5000	0.0000	0.5000	0.0000	0.40	0.6554	0.1554	0.3446	0.3108
0.01	0.5040	0.0040	0.4960	0.0080	0.41	0.6591	0.1591	0.3409	0.3182
0.02	0.5080	0.0080	0.4920	0.0160	0.42	0.6628	0.1628	0.3372	0.3255
0.03	0.5120	0.0120	0.4880	0.0239	0.43	0.6664	0.1664	0.3336	0.3328
0.04	0.5160	0.0160	0.4840	0.0319	0.44	0.6700	0.1700	0.3300	0.3401
0.05	0.5199	0.0199	0.4801	0.0399	0.45	0.6736	0.1736	0.3264	0.3473
0.06	0.5239	0.0239	0.4761	0.0478	0.46	0.6772	0.1772	0.3228	0.3545
0.07	0.5279	0.0279	0.4721	0.0558	0.47	0.6808	0.1808	0.3192	0.3616
0.08	0.5319	0.0319	0.4681	0.0638	0.48	0.6844	0.1844	0.3156	0.3688
0.09	0.5359	0.0359	0.4641	0.0717	0.49	0.6879	0.1879	0.3121	0.3759
0.10	0.5398	0.0398	0.4602	0.0797	0.50	0.6915	0.1915	0.3085	0.3829
0.11	0.5438	0.0438	0.4562	0.0876	0.51	0.6950	0.1950	0.3050	0.3899
0.12	0.5478	0.0478	0.4522	0.0956	0.52	0.6985	0.1985	0.3015	0.3969
0.13	0.5517	0.0517	0.4483	0.1034	0.53	0.7019	0.2019	0.2981	0.4039
0.14	0.5557	0.0557	0.4443	0.1113	0.54	0.7054	0.2054	0.2946	0.4108
0.15	0.5596	0.0596	0.4404	0.1192	0.55	0.7088	0.2088	0.2912	0.4177
0.16	0.5636	0.0636	0.4364	0.1271	0.56	0.7157	0.2157	0.2843	0.4245
0.17	0.5675	0.0675	0.4325	0.1350	0.57	0.7157	0.2157	0.2843	0.4313
0.18	0.5714	0.0714	0.4286	0.1428	0.58	0.7190	0.2190	0.2810	0.4381
0.19	0.5793	0.0793	0.4207	0.1507	0.59	0.7224	0.2224	0.2776	0.4448
0.20	0.5793	0.0793	0.4207	0.1585	0.60	0.7257	0.2257	0.2743	0.4515
0.21	0.5832	0.0832	0.4168	0.1663	0.61	0.7291	0.2291	0.2709	0.4581
0.22	0.5871	0.0871	0.4129	0.1741	0.62	0.7324	0.2324	0.2676	0.4647
0.23	0.5910	0.0910	0.4090	0.1819	0.63	0.7357	0.2357	0.2643	0.4713
0.24	0.5948	0.0948	0.4052	0.1897	0.64	0.7389	0.2389	0.2611	0.4778
0.25	0.5987	0.0987	0.4013	0.1974	0.65	0.7422	0.2422	0.2578	0.4843
0.26	0.6026	0.1026	0.3974	0.2051	0.66	0.7454	0.2454	0.2546	0.4907
0.27	0.6064	0.1064	0.3936	0.2128	0.67	0.7486	0.2486	0.2514	0.4971
0.28	0.6103	0.1103	0.3897	0.2205	0.68	0.7517	0.2517	0.2483	0.5035
0.29	0.6141	0.1141	0.3859	0.2282	0.69	0.7549	0.2549	0.2451	0.5098
0.30	0.6179	0.1179	0.3821	0.2358	0.70	0.7580	0.2580	0.2420	0.5161
0.31	0.6217	0.1217	0.3783	0.2434	0.71	0.7611	0.2611	0.2389	0.5223
0.32	0.6255	0.1255	0.3745	0.2510	0.72	0.7642	0.2642	0.2358	0.5285
0.33	0.6293	0.1293	0.3707	0.2586	0.73	0.7673	0.2673	0.2327	0.5346
0.34	0.6331	0.1331	0.3669	0.2661	0.74	0.7703	0.2703	0.2297	0.5407
0.35	0.6368	0.1368	0.3632	0.2737	0.75	0.7734	0.2734	0.2266	0.5467
0.36	0.6406	0.1406	0.3594	0.2812	0.76	0.7764	0.2764	0.2236	0.5527

(Continued)

Appendix 2 — Area* under the Standard Normal Curve (Contd.)

Z	A	B	C	D	Z	A	B	C	D
0.37	0.6443	0.1443	0.3557	0.2886	0.77	0.7794	0.2794	0.2206	0.5587
0.38	0.6480	0.1480	0.3520	0.2961	0.78	0.7823	0.2823	0.2177	0.5646
0.39	0.6517	0.1517	0.3483	0.3035	0.79	0.7852	0.2852	0.2148	0.5705
0.80	0.7881	0.2881	0.2119	0.5763	1.24	0.8925	0.3925	0.1075	0.785
0.81	0.7910	0.2910	0.2090	0.5821	1.25	0.8944	0.3944	0.1056	0.7887
0.82	0.7939	0.2939	0.2061	0.5878	1.26	0.8962	0.3962	0.1038	0.7923
0.83	0.7967	0.2967	0.2033	0.5935	1.27	0.8980	0.3980	0.1020	0.7959
0.84	0.7995	0.2995	0.2005	0.5991	1.28	0.8997	0.3997	0.1003	0.7995
0.85	0.8023	0.3023	0.1977	0.6047	1.29	0.9015	0.4015	0.0985	0.8029
0.86	0.8051	0.3051	0.1949	0.6102	1.30	0.9032	0.4032	0.0968	0.8064
0.87	0.8078	0.3078	0.1922	0.6157	1.31	0.9049	0.4049	0.0951	0.8098
0.88	0.8106	0.3106	0.1894	0.6211	1.32	0.9066	0.4066	0.0934	0.8132
0.89	0.8133	0.3133	0.1867	0.6265	1.33	0.9082	0.4082	0.0918	0.8165
0.90	0.8159	0.3159	0.1841	0.6319	1.34	0.9099	0.4099	0.0901	0.8198
0.91	0.8186	0.3186	0.1814	0.6372	1.35	0.9115	0.4115	0.0885	0.8230
0.92	0.8212	0.3212	0.1788	0.6424	1.36	0.9131	0.4131	0.0869	0.8262
0.93	0.8238	0.3238	0.1762	0.6476	1.37	0.9147	0.4147	0.0869	0.8293
0.94	0.8264	0.3264	0.1736	0.6528	1.38	0.9162	0.4162	0.0838	0.8324
0.95	0.8289	0.3289	0.1711	0.6579	1.39	0.9177	0.4177	0.0823	0.8355
0.96	0.8315	0.3315	0.1685	0.6629	1.40	0.9192	0.4192	0.0808	0.8385
0.97	0.8340	0.3340	0.1660	0.6680	1.41	0.9207	0.4207	0.0793	0.8415
0.98	0.8365	0.3365	0.1635	0.6729	1.42	0.9222	0.4222	0.0778	0.8444
0.99	0.8389	0.3389	0.1611	0.6778	1.43	0.9236	0.4236	0.0764	0.8473
1.00	0.8413	0.3413	0.1587	0.6827	1.44	0.9251	0.4251	0.0749	0.8501
1.01	0.8438	0.3438	0.1562	0.6875	1.45	0.9265	0.4265	0.0735	0.8529
1.02	0.8461	0.3461	0.1539	0.6923	1.46	0.9279	0.4279	0.0721	0.8557
1.03	0.8485	0.3485	0.1515	0.6970	1.47	0.9292	0.4292	0.0708	0.8584
1.04	0.8508	0.3508	0.1492	0.7017	1.48	0.9306	0.4306	0.0694	0.8611
1.05	0.8531	0.3531	0.1469	0.7063	1.49	0.9319	0.4319	0.0681	0.8638
1.06	0.8554	0.3554	0.1446	0.7109	1.50	0.9332	0.4332	0.0668	0.8664
1.07	0.8577	0.3577	0.1423	0.7154	1.51	0.9345	0.4345	0.0655	0.8690
1.08	0.8599	0.3599	0.1401	0.7199	1.52	0.9357	0.4357	0.0643	0.8715
1.09	0.8621	0.3621	0.1379	0.7243	1.53	0.9370	0.4370	0.063	0.8740
1.10	0.8643	0.3643	0.1357	0.7287	1.54	0.9382	0.4382	0.0618	0.8764
1.11	0.8665	0.3665	0.1335	0.7330	1.55	0.9394	0.4394	0.0606	0.8789
1.12	0.8686	0.3686	0.1314	0.7373	1.56	0.9406	0.4406	0.0594	0.8812
1.13	0.8708	0.3708	0.1292	0.7415	1.57	0.9418	0.4418	0.0582	0.8836
1.14	0.8729	0.3729	0.1271	0.7457	1.58	0.9429	0.4429	0.0571	0.8859
1.15	0.8749	0.3749	0.1251	0.7499	1.59	0.9441	0.4441	0.0559	0.8882

(Continued)

Appendix 2 — Area* under the Standard Normal Curve (Contd.)

Z	A	B	C	D	Z	A	B	C	D
1.16	0.8770	0.3770	0.1230	0.7540	1.60	0.9452	0.4452	0.0548	0.8904
1.17	0.8790	0.3790	0.1210	0.7580	1.61	0.9463	0.4463	0.0537	0.8926
1.18	0.8810	0.3810	0.1190	0.7620	1.62	0.9474	0.4474	0.0526	0.8948
1.19	0.8830	0.3830	0.1170	0.7660	1.63	0.9484	0.4484	0.5160	0.8969
1.20	0.8849	0.3849	0.1151	0.7699	1.64	0.9495	0.4495	0.0505	0.8990
1.21	0.8869	0.3869	0.1131	0.7737	1.65	0.9505	0.4505	0.0495	0.9011
1.22	0.8888	0.3888	0.1112	0.7775	1.66	0.9515	0.4515	0.0485	0.9031
1.23	0.8907	0.3907	0.1093	0.7813	1.67	0.9525	0.4525	0.0475	0.9051
1.68	0.9535	0.4535	0.0465	0.9070	2.12	0.9830	0.4830	0.0170	0.9660
1.69	0.9545	0.4545	0.0455	0.9090	2.13	0.9834	0.4834	0.0166	0.9668
1.70	0.9554	0.4554	0.0446	0.9109	2.14	0.9838	0.4838	0.0162	0.9676
1.71	0.9564	0.4564	0.0436	0.9127	2.15	0.9842	0.4842	0.0158	0.9684
1.72	0.9573	0.4573	0.0427	0.9146	2.16	0.9846	0.4846	0.0154	0.9692
1.73	0.9582	0.4582	0.0418	0.9164	2.17	0.9850	0.4850	0.0150	0.9700
1.74	0.9591	0.4591	0.0409	0.9181	2.18	0.9854	0.4854	0.0146	0.9707
1.75	0.9599	0.4599	0.0401	0.9199	2.19	0.9857	0.4857	0.0143	0.9715
1.76	0.9680	0.4608	0.0392	0.9216	2.20	0.9861	0.4861	0.0139	0.9722
1.77	0.9616	0.4616	0.0384	0.9233	2.21	0.9864	0.4864	0.0136	0.9729
1.78	0.9625	0.4625	0.0375	0.9249	2.22	0.9868	0.4868	0.0132	0.9736
1.79	0.9633	0.4633	0.0367	0.9265	2.23	0.9871	0.4871	0.0129	0.9743
1.80	0.9641	0.4641	0.0359	0.9281	2.24	0.9875	0.4875	0.0125	0.9749
1.81	0.9649	0.4649	0.0351	0.9297	2.25	0.9878	0.4878	0.0122	0.9756
1.82	0.9656	0.4656	0.0344	0.9312	2.26	0.9881	0.4881	0.0119	0.9762
1.83	0.9664	0.4664	0.0336	0.9328	2.27	0.9884	0.4884	0.0116	0.9768
1.84	0.9678	0.4678	0.0322	0.9357	2.28	0.9887	0.4887	0.0113	0.9774
1.85	0.9678	0.4678	0.0322	0.9357	2.29	0.9890	0.4890	0.0110	0.9780
1.86	0.9686	0.4686	0.0314	0.9371	2.30	0.9893	0.4893	0.0107	0.9786
1.87	0.9693	0.4693	0.0307	0.9385	2.31	0.9896	0.4896	0.0104	0.9791
1.88	0.9699	0.4699	0.0301	0.9399	2.32	0.9898	0.4898	0.0102	0.9797
1.89	0.9706	0.4706	0.0294	0.9412	2.33	0.9901	0.4901	0.0099	0.9802
1.90	0.9713	0.4713	0.0287	0.9426	2.34	0.9904	0.4904	0.0096	0.9807
1.91	0.9713	0.4713	0.0287	0.9426	2.35	0.9906	0.4906	0.0094	0.9812
1.92	0.9726	0.4726	0.0274	0.9451	2.36	0.9909	0.4909	0.0091	0.9817
1.93	0.9732	0.4732	0.0268	0.9464	2.37	0.9911	0.4911	0.0089	0.9822
1.94	0.9738	0.4738	0.0262	0.9476	2.38	0.9913	0.4913	0.0087	0.9827
1.95	0.9744	0.4744	0.0256	0.9488	2.39	0.9916	0.4916	0.0084	0.9832
1.96	0.9750	0.4750	0.0250	0.9500	2.40	0.9918	0.4918	0.0082	0.9836
1.97	0.9756	0.4756	0.0244	0.9512	2.41	0.9920	0.492	0.0080	0.9840
1.98	0.9761	0.4761	0.0239	0.9523	2.42	0.9922	0.4922	0.0078	0.9845
1.99	0.9767	0.4767	0.0233	0.9534	2.43	0.9925	0.4925	0.0075	0.9849

(Continued)

Appendix 2 — Area* under the Standard Normal Curve (Contd.)

Z	A	B	C	D	Z	A	B	C	D
2.00	0.9772	0.4772	0.0228	0.9545	2.44	0.9927	0.4927	0.0073	0.9853
2.01	0.9778	0.4778	0.0222	0.9556	2.45	0.9929	0.4929	0.0071	0.9857
2.02	0.9783	0.4783	0.0217	0.9566	2.46	0.9931	0.4931	0.0069	0.9861
2.03	0.9788	0.4788	0.0212	0.9576	2.47	0.9932	0.4932	0.0068	0.9865
2.04	0.9793	0.4793	0.0207	0.9586	2.48	0.9934	0.4934	0.0066	0.9869
2.05	0.9798	0.4798	0.0202	0.9596	2.49	0.9936	0.4936	0.0064	0.9869
2.06	0.9803	0.4803	0.0197	0.9606	2.50	0.9938	0.4938	0.0062	0.9876
2.07	0.9808	0.4808	0.0192	0.9615	2.51	0.9940	0.4940	0.0060	0.9879
2.08	0.9812	0.4812	0.0188	0.9625	2.52	0.9941	0.4941	0.0059	0.9883
2.09	0.9817	0.4817	0.0183	0.9634	2.53	0.9943	0.4943	0.0057	0.9886
2.10	0.9821	0.4821	0.0179	0.9643	2.54	0.9945	0.4945	0.0055	0.9889
2.11	0.9826	0.4826	0.0174	0.9651	2.55	0.9946	0.4946	0.0054	0.9892
2.56	0.9948	0.4948	0.0052	0.9895	3.00	0.9987	0.4987	0.0013	0.9973
2.57	0.9949	0.4949	0.0051	0.9898	3.01	0.9987	0.4987	0.0013	0.9974
2.58	0.9951	0.4951	0.0049	0.9901	3.02	0.9987	0.4987	0.0013	0.9975
2.59	0.9952	0.4952	0.0048	0.9904	3.03	0.9988	0.4988	0.0012	0.9976
2.60	0.9953	0.4953	0.0047	0.9907	3.04	0.9988	0.4988	0.0012	0.9976
2.61	0.9955	0.4955	0.0045	0.9909	3.05	0.9989	0.4989	0.0011	0.9977
2.62	0.9956	0.4956	0.0044	0.9912	3.06	0.9989	0.4989	0.0011	0.9978
2.63	0.9957	0.4957	0.0043	0.9915	3.07	0.9989	0.4989	0.0011	0.9979
2.64	0.9959	0.4959	0.0041	0.9917	3.08	0.9990	0.4990	0.0010	0.9979
2.65	0.9960	0.4960	0.0040	0.9920	3.09	0.9990	0.4990	0.0010	0.9980
2.66	0.9961	0.4961	0.0039	0.9922	3.10	0.9990	0.4990	0.0010	0.9981
2.67	0.9962	0.4962	0.0038	0.9924	3.11	0.9991	0.4991	0.0009	0.9981
2.68	0.9963	0.4963	0.0037	0.9926	3.12	0.9991	0.4991	0.0009	0.9982
2.69	0.9964	0.4964	0.0036	0.9929	3.13	0.9991	0.4991	0.0009	0.9983
2.70	0.9965	0.4965	0.0035	0.9931	3.14	0.9992	0.4992	0.0008	0.9983
2.71	0.9966	0.4966	0.0034	0.9933	3.15	0.9992	0.4992	0.0008	0.9984
2.72	0.9967	0.4967	0.0033	0.9935	3.16	0.9992	0.4922	0.0008	0.9984
2.73	0.9968	0.4968	0.0032	0.9937	3.17	0.9992	0.4992	0.0008	0.9985
2.74	0.9969	0.4969	0.0031	0.9939	3.18	0.9993	0.4993	0.0007	0.9985
2.75	0.9970	0.4970	0.0030	0.9940	31.9	0.9993	0.4993	0.0007	0.9986
2.76	0.9971	0.4971	0.0029	0.9942	3.20	0.9993	0.4993	0.0007	0.9986
2.77	0.9972	0.4972	0.0028	0.9944	3.21	0.9993	0.4993	0.0007	0.9987
2.78	0.9973	0.4973	0.0027	0.9946	3.22	0.9994	0.4994	0.0006	0.9987
2.79	0.9974	0.4974	0.0026	0.9947	3.23	0.9994	0.4994	0.0006	0.9988
2.80	0.9974	0.4974	0.0026	0.9949	3.24	0.9994	0.4994	0.0006	0.9988
2.81	0.9975	0.4975	0.0025	0.9950	3.25	0.9994	0.4994	0.0006	0.9988
2.82	0.9976	0.4976	0.0024	0.9952	3.26	0.9994	0.4994	0.0006	0.9988
2.83	0.9977	0.4977	0.0023	0.9953	3.27	0.9995	0.4995	0.0005	0.9989

(Continued)

Appendix 2 — Area* under the Standard Normal Curve (Contd.)

Z	A	B	C	D	Z	A	B	C	D
2.84	0.9977	0.4977	0.0022	0.9955	3.28	0.9995	0.4995	0.0005	0.9990
2.85	0.9978	0.4978	0.0022	0.9956	3.29	0.9995	0.4995	0.0006	0.9990
2.86	0.9979	0.4979	0.0021	0.9958	3.30	0.9995	0.4995	0.0005	0.9990
2.87	0.9979	0.4979	0.0021	0.9959	3.31	0.9995	0.4995	0.0005	0.9991
2.88	0.9980	0.4980	0.0020	0.9960	3.32	0.9995	0.4995	0.0005	0.9991
2.89	0.9981	0.4981	0.0019	0.9961	3.33	0.9996	0.4996	0.0004	0.9991
2.90	0.9981	0.4981	0.0019	0.9963	3.34	0.9996	0.4996	0.0004	0.9992
2.91	0.9982	0.4982	0.0018	0.9964	3.35	0.9996	0.4996	0.0004	0.9992
2.92	0.9982	0.4982	0.0018	0.9965	3.36	0.9996	0.4996	0.0004	0.9992
2.93	0.9983	0.4983	0.0017	0.9966	3.37	0.9996	0.4996	0.0004	0.9992
2.94	0.9984	0.4984	0.0016	0.9967	3.38	0.9996	0.4996	0.0004	0.9993
2.95	0.9984	0.4984	0.0016	0.9968	3.39	0.9997	0.4997	0.0003	0.9993
2.96	0.9985	0.4985	0.0015	0.9969	3.40	0.9997	0.4997	0.0003	0.9994
2.97	0.9985	0.4985	0.0015	0.9970	3.41	0.9997	0.4997	0.0003	0.9994
2.98	0.9986	0.4986	0.0014	0.9971	3.42	0.9997	0.4997	0.0003	0.9994
2.99	0.9986	0.4986	0.0014	0.9972	3.43	0.9997	0.4997	0.0003	0.9994
3.44	0.9997	0.4994	0.0003	0.9994	3.67	0.9999	0.4999	0.0001	0.9998
3.45	0.9997	0.4997	0.0003	0.9994	3.68	0.9999	0.4999	0.0001	0.9998
3.46	0.9997	0.4997	0.0003	0.9995	3.69	0.9999	0.4999	0.0001	0.9998
3.47	0.9997	0.4997	0.0003	0.9995	3.70	0.9999	0.4999	0.0001	0.9998
3.48	0.9997	0.4997	0.0003	0.9995	3.71	0.9999	0.4999	0.0001	0.9998
3.49	0.9998	0.4998	0.0002	0.9995	3.72	0.9999	0.4999	0.0001	0.9998
3.50	0.9998	0.4998	0.0002	0.9995	3.73	0.9999	0.4999	0.0001	0.9998
3.51	0.9998	0.4998	0.0002	0.9996	3.74	0.9999	0.4999	0.0001	0.9998
3.52	0.9998	0.4998	0.0002	0.9996	3.75	0.9999	0.4999	0.0001	0.9998
3.53	0.9998	0.4998	0.0002	0.9996	3.76	0.9999	0.4999	0.0001	0.9998
3.54	0.9998	0.4998	0.0002	0.9996	3.77	0.9999	0.4999	0.0001	0.9998
3.55	0.9998	0.4998	0.0002	0.9996	3.78	0.9999	0.4999	0.0001	0.9998
3.56	0.9998	0.4998	0.0002	0.9996	3.79	0.9999	0.4999	0.0001	0.9998
3.57	0.9998	0.4998	0.0002	0.9996	3.80	0.9999	0.4999	0.0001	0.9999
3.58	0.9998	0.4998	0.0002	0.9995	3.81	0.9999	0.4999	0.0001	0.9999
3.59	0.9998	0.4998	0.0002	0.9997	3.82	0.9999	0.4999	0.0001	0.9999
3.60	0.9998	0.4998	0.0002	0.9997	3.83	0.9999	0.4999	0.0001	0.9999
3.61	0.9998	0.4998	0.0002	0.9997	3.84	0.9999	0.4999	0.0001	0.9999
3.62	0.9999	0.4999	0.0001	0.9997	3.85	0.9999	0.4999	0.0001	0.9999
3.63	0.9999	0.4999	0.0001	0.9997	3.86	0.9999	0.4999	0.0001	0.9999
3.64	0.9999	0.4999	0.0001	0.9997	3.87	0.9999	0.4999	0.0001	0.9999
3.65	0.9999	0.4999	0.0001	0.9997	3.88	0.9999	0.4999	0.0001	0.9999
3.66	0.9999	0.4999	0.0001	0.9997	3.89	0.9999	0.4999	0.0001	0.9999

*Generated by Stata, Version–9.1

Appendix 3 — Values of F at 1% Significance Level*

N2	N1 1	2	3	4	5	6	7	8	9	10	11	12
1	4052.18	4999.50	5403.35	5624.58	5763.65	5858.99	5928.36	5981.07	6022.47	6055.85	6083.32	6106.32
2	98.50	99.00	99.17	99.25	99.30	99.33	99.36	99.37	99.39	99.40	99.41	99.42
3	34.12	30.82	29.46	28.71	28.24	27.91	27.67	27.49	27.35	27.23	27.13	27.05
4	21.20	18.00	16.69	15.98	15.52	15.21	14.98	14.80	14.66	14.55	14.45	14.37
5	16.26	13.27	12.06	11.39	10.97	10.67	10.46	10.29	10.16	10.05	9.96	9.89
6	13.75	10.92	9.78	9.15	8.75	8.47	8.26	8.10	7.98	7.87	7.79	7.72
7	12.25	9.55	8.45	7.85	7.46	7.19	6.99	6.84	6.72	6.62	6.54	6.47
8	11.26	8.65	7.59	7.01	6.63	6.37	6.18	6.03	5.91	5.81	5.73	5.67
9	10.56	8.02	6.99	6.42	6.06	5.80	5.61	5.47	5.35	5.26	5.18	5.11
10	10.04	7.56	6.55	5.99	5.64	5.39	5.20	5.06	4.94	4.85	4.77	4.71
11	9.65	7.21	6.22	5.67	5.32	5.07	4.89	4.74	4.63	4.54	4.46	4.40
12	9.33	6.93	5.95	5.41	5.06	4.82	4.64	4.50	4.39	4.30	4.22	4.16
13	9.07	6.70	5.74	5.21	4.86	4.62	4.44	4.30	4.19	4.10	4.02	3.96
14	8.86	6.51	5.56	5.04	4.69	4.46	4.28	4.14	4.03	3.94	3.86	3.80
15	8.68	6.36	5.42	4.89	4.56	4.32	4.14	4.00	3.89	3.80	3.73	3.67
16	8.53	6.23	5.29	4.77	4.44	4.20	4.03	3.89	3.78	3.69	3.62	3.55
17	8.40	6.11	5.19	4.67	4.34	4.10	3.93	3.79	3.68	3.59	3.52	3.46
18	8.29	6.01	5.09	4.58	4.25	4.01	3.84	3.71	3.60	3.51	3.43	3.37
19	8.18	5.93	5.01	4.50	4.17	3.94	3.77	3.63	3.52	3.43	3.36	3.30
20	8.10	5.85	4.94	4.43	4.10	3.87	3.70	3.56	3.46	3.37	3.29	3.23
21	8.02	5.78	4.87	4.37	4.04	3.81	3.64	3.51	3.40	3.31	3.24	3.17
22	7.95	5.72	4.82	4.31	3.99	3.76	3.59	3.45	3.35	3.26	3.18	3.12
23	7.88	5.66	4.76	4.26	3.94	3.71	3.54	3.41	3.30	3.21	3.14	3.07
24	7.82	5.61	4.72	4.22	3.90	3.67	3.50	3.36	3.26	3.17	3.09	3.03
25	7.77	5.57	4.68	4.18	3.85	3.63	3.46	3.32	3.22	3.13	3.06	2.99
26	7.72	5.53	4.64	4.14	3.82	3.59	3.42	3.29	3.18	3.09	3.02	2.96
27	7.68	5.49	4.60	4.11	3.78	3.56	3.39	3.26	3.15	3.06	2.99	2.93
28	7.64	5.45	4.57	4.07	3.75	3.53	3.36	3.23	3.12	3.03	2.96	2.90
29	7.60	5.42	4.54	4.04	3.73	3.50	3.33	3.20	3.09	3.00	2.93	2.87
30	7.56	5.39	4.51	4.02	3.70	3.47	3.30	3.17	3.07	2.98	2.91	2.84
40	7.31	5.18	4.31	3.83	3.51	3.29	3.12	2.99	2.89	2.80	2.73	2.66
50	7.17	5.06	4.20	3.72	3.41	3.19	3.02	2.89	2.78	2.70	2.63	2.56
60	7.08	4.98	4.13	3.65	3.34	3.12	2.95	2.82	2.72	2.63	2.56	2.50
70	7.01	4.92	4.07	3.60	3.29	3.07	2.91	2.78	2.67	2.59	2.51	2.45
80	6.96	4.88	4.04	3.56	3.26	3.04	2.87	2.74	2.64	2.55	2.48	2.42
90	6.93	4.85	4.01	3.53	3.23	3.01	2.84	2.72	2.61	2.52	2.45	2.39
100	6.90	4.82	3.98	3.51	3.21	2.99	2.82	2.69	2.59	2.50	2.43	2.37
120	6.85	4.79	3.95	3.48	3.17	2.96	2.79	2.66	2.56	2.47	2.40	2.34
150	6.81	4.75	3.91	3.45	3.14	2.92	2.76	2.63	2.53	2.44	2.37	2.31
200	6.76	4.71	3.88	3.41	3.11	2.89	2.73	2.60	2.50	2.41	2.34	2.27
300	6.72	4.68	3.85	3.38	3.08	2.86	2.70	2.57	2.47	2.38	2.31	2.24
400	6.70	4.66	3.83	3.37	3.06	2.85	2.68	2.56	2.45	2.37	2.29	2.23
500	6.69	4.65	3.82	3.36	3.05	2.84	2.68	2.55	2.44	2.36	2.28	2.22
∞	6.64	4.61	3.79	3.32	3.02	2.81	2.64	2.51	2.41	2.32	2.25	2.19

N1 and N2 are degrees of freedom of the numerator and denominator respectively

*Generated by Stata, Version–9.1

Appendix 3 — Values of F at 5% Significance Level*

N2	N1											
	1	*2*	*3*	*4*	*5*	*6*	*7*	*8*	*9*	*10*	*11*	*12*
1	161.45	199.50	215.71	224.58	230.16	233.98	236.77	238.88	240.54	241.88	242.98	243.91
2	18.51	19.00	19.16	19.25	19.30	19.33	19.35	19.37	19.38	19.40	19.40	19.41
3	10.13	9.55	9.28	9.12	9.01	8.94	8.89	8.85	8.81	8.79	8.76	8.74
4	7.71	6.94	6.59	6.39	6.26	6.16	6.09	6.04	6.00	5.96	5.94	5.91
5	6.61	5.79	5.41	5.19	5.05	4.95	4.88	4.82	4.77	4.74	4.70	4.68
6	5.99	5.14	4.76	4.53	4.39	4.28	4.21	4.15	4.10	4.06	4.03	4.00
7	5.59	4.74	4.35	4.12	3.97	3.87	3.79	3.73	3.68	3.64	3.60	3.57
8	5.32	4.46	4.07	3.84	3.69	3.58	3.50	3.44	3.39	3.35	3.31	3.28
9	5.12	4.26	3.86	3.63	3.48	3.37	3.29	3.23	3.18	3.14	3.10	3.07
10	4.96	4.10	3.71	3.48	3.33	3.22	3.14	3.07	3.02	2.98	2.94	2.91
11	4.84	3.98	3.59	3.36	3.20	3.09	3.01	2.95	2.90	2.85	2.82	2.79
12	4.75	3.89	3.49	3.26	3.11	3.00	2.9	2.85	2.80	2.75	2.72	2.69
13	4.67	3.81	3.41	3.18	3.03	2.92	2.83	2.77	2.71	2.67	2.63	2.60
14	4.60	3.74	3.34	3.11	2.96	2.85	2.76	2.70	2.65	2.60	2.57	2.53
15	4.54	3.68	3.29	3.06	2.90	2.79	2.71	2.64	2.59	2.54	2.51	2.48
16	4.49	3.63	3.24	3.01	2.85	2.74	2.66	2.59	2.54	2.49	2.46	2.42
17	4.45	3.59	3.20	2.96	2.81	2.70	2.61	2.55	2.49	2.45	2.41	2.38
18	4.41	3.55	3.16	2.93	2.77	2.66	2.58	2.51	2.46	2.41	2.37	2.34
19	4.38	3.52	3.13	2.90	2.74	2.63	2.54	2.48	2.42	2.38	2.34	2.31
20	4.35	3.49	3.10	2.87	2.71	2.60	2.51	2.45	2.39	2.35	2.31	2.28
21	4.32	3.47	3.07	2.84	2.68	2.57	2.49	2.42	2.37	2.32	2.28	2.25
22	4.30	3.44	3.05	2.82	2.66	2.55	2.46	2.40	2.34	2.30	2.26	2.23
23	4.28	3.42	3.03	2.80	2.64	2.53	2.44	2.37	2.32	2.27	2.24	2.20
24	4.26	3.40	3.01	2.78	2.62	2.51	2.42	2.36	2.30	2.25	2.22	2.18
25	4.24	3.39	2.99	2.76	2.60	2.49	2.40	2.34	2.28	2.24	2.20	2.16
26	4.23	3.37	2.98	2.74	2.59	2.47	2.39	2.32	2.27	2.22	2.18	2.15
27	4.21	3.35	2.96	2.73	2.57	2.46	2.37	2.31	2.25	2.20	2.17	2.13
28	4.20	3.34	2.95	2.71	2.56	2.45	2.36	2.29	2.24	2.19	2.15	2.12
29	4.18	3.33	2.93	2.70	2.55	2.43	2.35	2.28	2.22	2.18	2.14	2.10
30	4.17	3.32	2.92	2.69	2.53	2.42	2.33	2.27	2.21	2.16	2.13	2.09
40	4.08	3.23	2.84	2.61	2.45	2.34	2.25	2.18	2.12	2.08	2.04	2.00
50	4.03	3.18	2.79	2.56	2.40	2.29	2.20	2.13	2.07	2.03	1.99	1.95
60	4.00	3.15	2.76	2.53	2.37	2.25	2.17	2.10	2.04	1.99	1.95	1.92
70	3.98	3.13	2.74	2.50	2.35	2.23	2.14	2.07	2.02	1.97	1.93	1.89
80	3.96	3.11	2.72	2.49	2.33	2.21	2.13	2.06	2.00	1.95	1.91	1.88
90	3.95	3.10	2.71	2.47	2.32	2.20	2.11	2.04	1.99	1.94	1.90	1.86
100	3.94	3.09	2.70	2.46	2.31	2.19	2.10	2.03	1.97	1.93	1.89	1.85
120	3.92	3.07	2.68	2.45	2.29	2.18	2.09	2.02	1.96	1.91	1.87	1.83
150	3.90	3.06	2.66	2.43	2.27	2.16	2.07	2.00	1.94	1.89	1.85	1.82
200	3.89	3.04	2.65	2.42	2.26	2.14	2.06	1.98	1.93	1.88	1.84	1.80
300	3.87	3.03	2.63	2.40	2.24	2.13	2.04	1.97	1.91	1.86	1.82	1.78
400	3.86	3.02	2.63	2.39	2.24	2.12	2.03	1.96	1.90	1.85	1.81	1.78
500	3.86	3.01	2.62	2.39	2.23	2.12	2.03	1.96	1.90	1.85	1.81	1.77
∞	3.84	3.00	2.61	2.37	2.22	2.10	2.01	1.94	1.88	1.83	1.79	1.75

N1 and N2 are degrees of freedom of the numerator and denominator respectively

*Generated by Stata, Version–9.1

Appendix 3 — Values of F at 10% Significance Level*

N2	N1											
	1	2	3	4	5	6	7	8	9	10	11	12
1	39.86	49.50	53.59	55.83	57.24	58.20	58.91	59.44	59.86	60.19	60.47	60.71
2	8.53	9.00	9.16	9.24	9.29	9.33	9.35	9.37	9.38	9.39	9.40	9.41
3	5.54	5.46	5.39	5.34	5.31	5.28	5.27	5.25	5.24	5.23	5.22	5.22
4	4.54	4.32	4.19	4.11	4.05	4.01	3.98	3.95	3.94	3.92	3.91	3.90
5	4.06	3.78	3.62	3.52	3.45	3.40	3.37	3.34	3.32	3.30	3.28	3.27
6	3.78	3.46	3.29	3.18	3.11	3.05	3.01	2.98	2.96	2.94	2.92	2.90
7	3.59	3.26	3.07	2.96	2.88	2.83	2.78	2.75	2.72	2.70	2.68	2.67
8	3.46	3.11	2.92	2.81	2.73	2.67	2.62	2.59	2.56	2.54	2.52	2.50
9	3.36	3.01	2.81	2.69	2.61	2.55	2.51	2.47	2.44	2.42	2.40	2.38
10	3.29	2.92	2.73	2.61	2.52	2.46	2.41	2.38	2.35	2.32	2.30	2.28
11	3.23	2.86	2.66	2.54	2.45	2.39	2.34	2.30	2.27	2.25	2.23	2.21
12	3.18	2.81	2.61	2.48	2.39	2.33	2.28	2.24	2.21	2.19	2.17	2.15
13	3.14	2.76	2.56	2.43	2.35	2.28	2.23	2.20	2.16	2.14	2.12	2.10
14	3.10	2.73	2.52	2.39	2.31	2.24	2.19	2.15	2.12	2.10	2.07	2.05
15	3.07	2.70	2.49	2.36	2.27	2.21	2.16	2.12	2.09	2.06	2.04	2.02
16	3.05	2.67	2.46	2.33	2.24	2.18	2.13	2.09	2.06	2.03	2.01	1.99
17	3.03	2.64	2.44	2.31	2.22	2.15	2.10	2.06	2.03	2.00	1.98	1.96
18	3.01	2.62	2.42	2.29	2.20	2.13	2.08	2.04	2.00	1.98	1.95	1.93
19	2.99	2.61	2.40	2.27	2.18	2.11	2.06	2.02	1.98	1.96	1.93	1.91
20	2.97	2.59	2.38	2.25	2.16	2.09	2.04	2.00	1.96	1.94	1.91	1.89
21	2.96	2.57	2.36	2.23	2.14	2.08	2.02	1.98	1.95	1.92	1.90	1.87
22	2.95	2.56	2.35	2.22	2.13	2.06	2.01	1.97	1.93	1.90	1.88	1.86
23	2.94	2.55	2.34	2.21	2.11	2.05	1.99	1.95	1.92	1.89	1.87	1.84
24	2.93	2.54	2.33	2.19	2.10	2.04	1.98	1.94	1.91	1.88	1.85	1.83
25	2.92	2.53	2.32	2.18	2.09	2.02	1.97	1.93	1.89	1.87	1.84	1.82
26	2.91	2.52	2.31	2.17	2.08	2.01	1.96	1.92	1.88	1.86	1.83	1.81
27	2.90	2.51	2.30	2.17	2.07	2.00	1.95	1.91	1.87	1.85	1.82	1.80
28	2.89	2.50	2.29	2.16	2.06	2.00	1.94	1.90	1.87	1.84	1.81	1.79
29	2.89	2.50	2.28	2.15	2.06	1.99	1.93	1.89	1.86	1.83	1.80	1.78
30	2.88	2.49	2.28	2.14	2.05	1.98	1.93	1.88	1.85	1.82	1.79	1.77
40	2.84	2.44	2.23	2.09	2.00	1.93	1.87	1.83	1.79	1.76	1.74	1.71
50	2.81	2.41	2.20	2.06	1.97	1.90	1.84	1.80	1.76	1.73	1.70	1.68
60	2.79	2.39	2.18	2.04	1.95	1.87	1.82	1.77	1.74	1.71	1.68	1.66
70	2.78	2.38	2.16	2.03	1.93	1.86	1.80	1.76	1.72	1.69	1.66	1.64
80	2.77	2.37	2.15	2.02	1.92	1.85	1.79	1.75	1.71	1.68	1.65	1.63
90	2.76	2.36	2.15	2.01	1.91	1.84	1.78	1.74	1.70	1.67	1.64	1.62
100	2.76	2.36	2.14	2.00	1.91	1.83	1.78	1.73	1.69	1.66	1.64	1.61
120	2.75	2.35	2.13	1.99	1.90	1.82	1.77	1.72	1.68	1.65	1.63	1.60
150	2.74	2.34	2.12	1.98	1.89	1.81	1.76	1.71	1.67	1.64	1.61	1.59
200	2.73	2.33	2.11	1.97	1.88	1.80	1.75	1.70	1.66	1.63	1.60	1.58
300	2.72	2.32	2.10	1.96	1.87	1.79	1.74	1.69	1.65	1.62	1.59	1.57
400	2.72	2.32	2.10	1.96	1.86	1.79	1.73	1.69	1.65	1.61	1.59	1.56
500	2.72	2.31	2.09	1.96	1.86	1.79	1.73	1.68	1.64	1.61	1.58	1.56
∞	2.71	2.30	2.08	1.95	1.85	1.78	1.72	1.67	1.63	1.60	1.57	1.55

N1 and N2 are degrees of freedom of the numerator and denominator respectively

*Generated by Stata, Version–9.1

Appendix 4 — Table of t-Distribution* (Two-tailed Probability)

Degrees of freedom (DF)	0.001	0.01	0.02	0.03	0.04	0.05	0.10	0.20	0.30	0.40	0.50	0.60	0.70	0.80	0.90
1	636.6192	63.6567	31.8205	21.2049	15.8945	12.7062	6.3138	3.0777	1.9626	1.3764	1	0.7265	0.5095	0.3249	0.1584
2	31.5991	9.9248	6.9646	5.6428	4.8487	4.3027	2.9200	1.8856	1.3862	1.0607	0.8165	0.6172	0.4447	0.2887	0.1421
3	12.924	5.8409	4.5407	3.8960	3.4819	3.1824	2.3534	1.6377	1.2498	0.9785	0.7649	0.5844	0.4242	0.2767	0.1366
4	8.6103	4.6041	3.7469	3.2976	2.9985	2.7764	2.1318	1.5332	1.1896	0.9410	0.7407	0.5686	0.4142	0.2707	0.1338
5	6.8688	4.0321	3.3649	3.0029	2.7565	2.5706	2.0150	1.4759	1.1558	0.9195	0.7267	0.5594	0.4082	0.2672	0.1322
6	5.9588	3.7074	3.1427	2.8289	2.6122	2.4469	1.9432	1.4398	1.1342	0.9057	0.7176	0.5534	0.4043	0.2648	0.1311
7	5.4079	3.4995	2.9980	2.7146	2.5168	2.3646	1.8946	1.4149	1.1192	0.8960	0.7111	0.5491	0.4015	0.2632	0.1303
8	5.0413	3.3554	2.8965	2.6338	2.4490	2.3060	1.8595	1.3968	1.1081	0.8889	0.7064	0.5459	0.3995	0.2619	0.1297
9	4.7809	3.2498	2.8214	2.5738	2.3984	2.2622	1.8331	1.3830	1.0997	0.8834	0.7027	0.5435	0.3979	0.2610	0.1293
10	4.5869	3.1693	2.7638	2.5275	2.3593	2.2281	1.8125	1.3722	1.0931	0.8791	0.6998	0.5415	0.3966	0.2602	0.1289
11	4.4370	3.1058	2.7181	2.4907	2.3281	2.2010	1.7959	1.3634	1.0877	0.8755	0.6974	0.5399	0.3956	0.2596	0.1286
12	4.3178	3.0545	2.6810	2.4607	2.3027	2.1788	1.7823	1.3562	1.0832	0.8726	0.6955	0.5386	0.3947	0.2590	0.1283
13	4.2208	3.0123	2.6503	2.4358	2.2816	2.1604	1.7709	1.3502	1.0795	0.8702	0.6938	0.5375	0.3940	0.2586	0.1281
14	4.1405	2.9768	2.6245	2.4149	2.2638	2.1448	1.7613	1.3450	1.0763	0.8681	0.6924	0.5366	0.3933	0.2582	0.1280
15	4.0728	2.9467	2.6025	2.3970	2.2485	2.1314	1.7531	1.3406	1.0735	0.8662	0.6912	0.5357	0.3928	0.2579	0.1278
16	4.0150	2.9208	2.5835	2.3815	2.2354	2.1199	1.7459	1.3368	1.0711	0.8647	0.6901	0.5350	0.3923	0.2576	0.1277
17	3.9651	2.8982	2.5669	2.3681	2.2238	2.1098	1.7396	1.3334	1.0690	0.8633	0.6892	0.5344	0.3919	0.2573	0.1276
18	3.9216	2.8784	2.5524	2.3562	2.2137	2.1009	1.7341	1.3304	1.0672	0.8620	0.6884	0.5338	0.3915	0.2571	0.1274
19	3.8834	2.8609	2.5395	2.3456	2.2047	2.0930	1.7291	1.3277	1.0655	0.8610	0.6876	0.5333	0.3912	0.2569	0.1274
20	3.8495	2.8453	2.5280	2.3362	2.1967	2.0860	1.7247	1.3253	1.0640	0.8600	0.6870	0.5329	0.3909	0.2567	0.1273
25	3.7251	2.7874	2.4851	2.3011	2.1666	2.0595	1.7081	1.3163	1.0584	0.8562	0.6844	0.5312	0.3898	0.2561	0.1269
30	3.6460	2.7500	2.4573	2.2783	2.1470	2.0423	1.6973	1.3104	1.0547	0.8538	0.6828	0.5300	0.3890	0.2556	0.1267
35	3.5911	2.7238	2.4377	2.2622	2.1332	2.0301	1.6896	1.3062	1.0520	0.8520	0.6816	0.5292	0.3885	0.2553	0.1266
40	3.5510	2.7045	2.4233	2.2503	2.1229	2.0211	1.6839	1.3031	1.0500	0.8507	0.6807	0.5286	0.3881	0.2550	0.1265
45	3.5203	2.6896	2.4121	2.2411	2.1150	2.0141	1.6794	1.3006	1.0485	0.8497	0.6800	0.5281	0.3878	0.2549	0.1265
50	3.4960	2.6778	2.4033	2.2338	2.1087	2.0086	1.6759	1.2987	1.0473	0.8489	0.6794	0.5278	0.3875	0.2547	0.1263
55	3.4764	2.6682	2.3961	2.2278	2.1036	2.0040	1.6730	1.2971	1.0463	0.8482	0.6790	0.5275	0.3873	0.2546	0.1262
60	3.4602	2.6603	2.3901	2.2229	2.0994	2.0003	1.6706	1.2958	1.0455	0.8477	0.6786	0.5272	0.3872	0.2545	0.1262
65	3.4466	2.6536	2.3851	2.2188	2.0958	1.9971	1.6686	1.2947	1.0448	0.8472	0.6783	0.5270	0.3870	0.2544	0.1262
70	3.4350	2.6479	2.3808	2.2152	2.0927	1.9944	1.6669	1.2938	1.0442	0.8468	0.6780	0.5268	0.3869	0.2543	0.1261
75	3.4250	2.6430	2.3771	2.2122	2.0901	1.9921	1.6654	1.2929	1.0436	0.8464	0.6778	0.5266	0.3868	0.2542	0.1261
80	3.4163	2.6387	2.3739	2.2095	2.0878	1.9901	1.6641	1.2922	1.0432	0.8461	0.6776	0.5265	0.3867	0.2542	0.1261
85	3.4087	2.6349	2.3710	2.2071	2.0857	1.9883	1.6630	1.2916	1.0428	0.8459	0.6774	0.5264	0.3866	0.2541	0.1260
90	3.4019	2.6316	2.3685	2.2050	2.0839	1.9867	1.6620	1.2910	1.0424	0.8456	0.6772	0.5263	0.3866	0.2541	0.1260
95	3.3959	2.6286	2.3662	2.2032	2.0823	1.9853	1.6611	1.2905	1.0421	0.8454	0.6771	0.5262	0.3865	0.2541	0.1260
100	3.3905	2.6259	2.3642	2.2015	2.0809	1.9840	1.6602	1.2901	1.0418	0.8452	0.6770	0.5261	0.3864	0.2540	0.1260
125	3.3701	2.6157	2.3565	2.1951	2.0754	1.9791	1.6571	1.2884	1.0408	0.8445	0.6765	0.5257	0.3862	0.2539	0.1259
150	3.3566	2.6090	2.3515	2.1909	2.0718	1.9759	1.6551	1.2872	1.0400	0.8440	0.6761	0.5255	0.3861	0.2538	0.1259
200	3.3398	2.6006	2.3451	2.1857	2.0672	1.9719	1.6525	1.2858	1.0391	0.8434	0.6757	0.5252	0.3859	0.2537	0.1258
300	3.3233	2.5923	2.3388	2.1805	2.0627	1.9679	1.6499	1.2844	1.0382	0.8428	0.6753	0.5250	0.3857	0.2536	0.1258
400	3.3150	2.5882	2.3357	2.1779	2.0605	1.9659	1.6487	1.2837	1.0378	0.8425	0.6751	0.5248	0.3856	0.2535	0.1258
500	3.3101	2.5857	2.3338	2.1763	2.0591	1.9647	1.6479	1.2832	1.0375	0.8423	0.6750	0.5247	0.3855	0.2535	0.1257
∞	3.2925	2.5768	2.3271	2.1707	2.0543	1.9604	1.6452	1.2817	1.0365	0.8417	0.6745	0.5244	0.3853	0.2534	0.1257

*Generated by Stata, Version–9.1

Appendix 5 — Table of Values* of χ^2 Corresponding to Different Levels of Significance

df	\(P\)												
	0.9	0.8	0.7	0.6	0.5	0.4	0.3	0.2	0.1	0.05	0.02	0.01	0.001
1	0.0158	0.0642	0.1485	0.2750	0.4549	0.7083	1.0742	1.6424	2.7055	3.8415	5.4119	6.6349	10.8276
2	0.2107	0.4463	0.7133	1.0217	1.3863	1.8326	2.4079	3.2189	4.6052	5.9915	7.8240	9.2103	13.8155
3	0.5844	1.0052	1.4237	1.8692	2.3660	2.9462	3.6649	4.6416	6.2514	7.8147	9.8374	11.3449	16.2662
4	1.0636	1.6488	2.1947	2.7528	3.3567	4.0446	4.8784	5.9886	7.7794	9.4877	11.6678	13.2767	18.4668
5	1.6103	2.3425	2.9999	3.6555	4.3515	5.1319	6.0644	7.2893	9.2364	11.0705	13.3882	15.0863	20.5150
6	2.2041	3.0701	3.8276	4.5702	5.3481	6.2108	7.2311	8.5581	10.6446	12.5916	15.0332	16.8119	22.4577
7	2.8331	3.8223	4.6713	5.4932	6.3458	7.2832	8.3834	9.8033	12.0170	14.0671	16.6224	18.4753	24.3219
8	3.4895	4.5936	5.5274	6.4226	7.3441	8.3505	9.5245	11.0301	13.3616	15.5073	18.1682	20.0902	26.1245
9	4.1682	5.3801	6.3933	7.3570	8.3428	9.4136	10.6564	12.2422	14.6837	16.9190	19.6790	21.6660	27.8772
10	4.8652	6.1791	7.2672	8.2955	9.3418	10.4732	11.7807	13.4420	15.9872	18.3070	21.1608	23.2093	29.5883
11	5.5778	6.9887	8.1479	9.2373	10.3410	11.5298	12.8987	14.6314	17.2750	19.6751	22.6179	24.7250	31.2641
12	6.3038	7.8073	9.0343	10.1820	11.3403	12.5838	14.0111	15.8120	18.5494	21.0261	24.0540	26.2170	32.9095
13	7.0415	8.6339	9.9257	11.1291	12.3398	13.6356	15.1187	16.9848	19.8119	22.3620	25.4715	27.6883	34.5282
14	7.7895	9.4673	10.8215	12.0785	13.3393	14.6853	16.2221	18.1508	21.0641	23.6848	26.8728	29.1412	36.1233
15	8.5468	10.3070	11.7212	13.0298	14.3389	15.7332	17.3217	19.3107	22.3071	24.9958	28.2595	30.5779	37.6973
16	9.3122	11.1521	12.6244	13.9827	15.3385	16.7795	18.4179	20.4651	23.5418	26.2962	29.6332	31.9999	39.2524
17	10.0852	12.0023	13.5307	14.9373	16.3382	17.8244	19.5110	21.6146	24.7690	27.5871	30.9951	33.4087	40.7902
18	10.8649	12.8570	14.4399	15.8932	17.3379	18.8679	20.6014	22.7596	25.9894	28.8693	32.3462	34.8053	42.3124
19	11.6509	13.7158	15.3517	16.8504	18.3377	19.9102	21.6891	23.9004	27.2036	30.1435	33.6874	36.1909	43.8202
20	12.4426	14.5784	16.2659	17.8088	19.3374	20.9514	22.7746	25.0375	28.4120	31.4104	35.0196	37.5662	45.3148
21	13.2396	15.4446	17.1823	18.7683	20.3372	21.9915	23.8578	26.1711	29.6151	32.6706	36.3435	38.9322	46.7970
22	14.0415	16.3140	18.1007	19.7288	21.3371	23.0307	24.9390	27.3015	30.8133	33.9244	37.6595	40.2894	48.2679
23	14.8480	17.1865	19.0211	20.6902	22.3369	24.0689	26.0184	28.4288	32.0069	35.1725	38.9683	41.6384	49.7282
24	15.6587	18.0618	19.9432	21.6525	23.3367	25.1064	27.0960	29.5533	33.1962	36.4150	40.2704	42.9798	51.1786
25	16.4734	18.9398	20.8670	22.6156	24.3366	26.1430	28.1719	30.6752	34.3816	37.6525	41.5661	44.3141	52.6197
26	17.2919	19.8202	21.7924	23.5794	25.3365	27.1789	29.2463	31.7946	35.5632	38.8851	42.8558	45.6417	54.0520
27	18.1139	20.7030	22.7192	24.5440	26.3363	28.2141	30.3193	32.9117	36.7412	40.1133	44.1400	46.9629	55.4760
28	18.9392	21.5880	23.6475	25.5093	27.3362	29.2486	31.3909	34.0266	37.9159	41.3371	45.4189	48.2782	56.8923
29	19.7677	22.4751	24.5770	26.4751	28.3361	30.2825	32.4612	35.1394	39.0875	42.5570	46.6927	49.5879	58.3012
30	20.5992	23.3641	25.5078	27.4416	29.3360	31.3159	33.5302	36.2502	40.2560	43.7730	47.9618	50.8922	59.7031

P = Probability of getting a larger value of χ^2 by chance alone.

*Generated by Stata, Version—9.1

Appendix 6 — The Mann-Whitney Test (Wilcoxon Two-sample Test)*

Two-sided: ±α≤0.05   One-sided: ±α≤0.025

N/N_1	3	4	5	6	7	8	9	10	11	12	13	14
4	—	10-26	16-34	23-43	31-53	40-64	49-77	60-90	72-104	85-119	99-135	114-152
5	6-21	11-29	17-38	24-48	33-58	42-70	52-83	63-97	75-112	89-127	103-144	118-162
6	7-23	12-32	18-42	26-52	34-64	44-76	55-89	66-104	79-119	92-136	107-153	122-172
7	7-26	13-35	20-45	27-57	36-69	46-82	57-96	69-111	82-127	96-144	111-162	127-181
8	8-28	14-38	21-49	29-61	38-74	49-87	60-102	72-118	85-135	100-152	115-171	131-191
9	8-31	14-42	22-53	31-65	41-79	51-93	62-109	75-125	89-142	104-106	119-180	136-200
10	9-33	15-45	23-57	32-70	42-84	53-99	65-115	78-132	92-150	107-169	124-188	141-209
11	9-36	16-48	24-61	34-74	44-89	55-105	68-121	81-139	96-157	111-177	128-197	145-219
12	10-38	17-51	26-64	35-79	46-94	58-110	71-127	84-146	99-165	115-185	132-206	150-228
13	10-41	18-54	27-68	37-83	48-99	60-116	73-134	88-152	103-172	119-193	136-215	155-237
14	11-43	19-57	28-72	38-88	50-104	62-122	76-140	91-159	106-180	123-201	141-223	160-246
15	11-46	20-60	29-76	40-92	52-109	65-127	79-146	94-166	110-187	127-209	145-232	164-256
16	12-48	21-63	30-80	42-96	54-114	67-133	82-152	97-173	113-195	131-217	150-240	168-265
17	12-51	21-67	32-83	43-101	56-119	70-138	84-159	100-180	117-202	135-225	154-249	174-274
18	13-53	22-70	33-87	45-105	58-124	72-144	87-165	103-187	121-209	139-233	159-257	179-283

Appendix 6 — The Mann-Whitney Test (Wilcoxon Two-sample Test)*

N_2/N_1	3	4	5	6	7	8	9	10	11	12	13	14
						Two-sided: $\pm\,\alpha \leq 0.02$		*One-sided: $\pm\,\alpha \leq 0.01$*				
4	—	—	15-35	22-44	29-55	38-66	48-78	58-92	70-106	83-121	96-138	111-155
5	—	10-30	16-39	23-49	31-60	40-72	50-85	61-99	73-114	86-130	100-147	115-165
6	—	11-33	17-43	24-54	32-66	42-78	52-92	63-107	75-123	89-139	103-157	118-176
7	6-27	11-37	18-47	25-59	34-71	43-85	54-99	66-114	78-131	92-148	107-166	122-186
8	6-30	12-40	19-51	27-63	35-77	45-91	56-106	68-122	81-139	95-157	111-175	127-195
9	7-32	13-43	20-55	28-68	37-82	47-97	59-112	71-129	84-147	99-165	114-185	131-205
10	7-35	13-47	21-59	29-73	39-87	49-103	61-119	74-136	88-154	102-174	118-194	135-215
11	7-38	14-50	22-63	30-78	40-93	51-109	63-126	77-143	91-162	106-182	122-203	139-225
12	8-40	15-53	23-67	32-82	42-98	53-115	66-132	79-151	94-170	109-191	126-212	143-235
13	8-43	15-57	24-71	33-87	44-103	56-120	68-139	82-158	97-178	113-199	130-221	148-244
14	8-46	16-60	25-75	34-92	45-109	58-126	71-145	85-165	100-186	116-208	134-230	152-254
15	9-48	17-63	26-79	36-96	47-114	60-132	73-152	88-172	103-194	120-216	138-239	156-264
16	9-51	17-67	27-83	37-101	49-119	62-138	76-158	91-179	107-201	124-224	142-248	161-273
17	10-53	18-70	28-87	39-105	51-124	64-144	78-165	93-187	110-209	127-233	146-257	165-283
18	10-56	19-73	29-91	40-110	52-130	66-150	81-171	96-194	113-217	131-241	150-266	170-292

Appendix 6 — The Mann-Whitney Test (Wilcoxon Two sample Test)*

N_2/N_1	3	4	5	6	7	8	9	10	11	12	13	14
					Two-sided: $\pm\,\alpha \leq 0.01$		One-sided: $\pm\,\alpha \leq 0.005$					
4	—	—	—	21-45	28-56	37-67	46-80	57-93	68-108	81-123	94-140	109-157
5	—	—	15-40	22-50	29-62	38-74	48-87	59-101	71-116	84-132	98-149	112-168
6	—	10-34	16-44	23-55	31-67	40-80	50-94	61-109	73-125	87-141	101-159	116-178
7	—	10-38	16-49	24-60	32-73	42-86	52-101	64-116	76-133	90-150	104-169	120-188
8	—	11-41	17-53	25-65	34-78	43-93	54-108	66-124	79-141	93-159	108-178	123-199
9	6-33	11-45	18-57	26-70	35-84	45-99	56-115	68-132	82-149	96-168	111-188	127-209
10	6-36	12-48	19-61	27-75	37-89	47-105	58-122	71-139	84-158	99-177	115-197	131-219
11	6-39	12-52	20-65	28-80	38-95	49-111	61-128	73-147	87-166	102-186	118-207	135-229
12	7-41	13-55	21-69	30-84	40-100	51-117	63-135	76-154	90-174	105-195	122-216	139-239
13	7-44	13-59	22-73	31-89	41-106	53-123	65-142	79-161	93-182	109-203	125-226	143-249
14	7-47	14-62	22-78	32-94	43-111	54-130	67-149	81-169	96-190	112-212	129-235	147-259
15	8-49	15-65	23-82	33-99	44-117	56-136	69-156	84-176	99-198	115-221	133-244	151-269
16	8-52	15-69	24-86	34-104	46-122	58-142	72-162	86-184	102-206	119-229	136-254	155-279
17	8-55	16-72	25-90	36-108	47-128	60-148	74-169	89-191	105-214	122-238	140-263	159-289
18	8-58	16-76	26-94	37-113	49-133	62-154	76-176	92-198	108-222	125-247	144-272	163-299

* Extracted from "Critical Values and Probability Levels for the Wilcoxon Rank Sum Test and the Wilcoxon Singed Rank Test," by Frank Wilcoxon, S. K. Katti and Roberta A. Wilcoxon, *Selected Tables in Mathematical Statistics*, Vol- 1; 1973, Table I, pp. 177-235, by kind permission of Institute of Mathematical Statistics (IMS)

Appendix 7 — Critical Values for Wilcoxon Signed Rank Test

One tailed	$\pm\,\alpha \le 0.05$	$\pm\,\alpha \le 0.025$	$\pm\,\alpha \le 0.01$	$\pm\,\alpha \le 0.005$
Tailed two	$\pm\,\alpha \le 0.10$	$\pm\,\alpha \le 0.05$	$\pm\,\alpha \le 0.02$	$\pm\,\alpha \le 0.01$
5	0-15			
6	2-19	0-21		
7	3-25	2-26	0-28	
8	5-31	3-33	1-35	0-36
9	8-37	5-40	3-42	1-44
10	10-45	8-47	5-50	3-52
11	13-53	10-56	7-59	5-61
12	17-61	13-65	9-69	7-71
13	21-70	17-74	12-79	9-82
14	25-80	21-84	15-90	12-93
15	30-90	25-95	19-101	15-105
16	35-101	29-107	23-113	19-117
17	41-112	34-119	28-125	23-130
18	47-124	40-131	32-139	27-144
19	53-137	46-144	37-153	33-158
20	60-150	52-158	43-167	37-173
21	67-164	58-173	49-182	42-189
22	75-178	66-187	55-198	48-205
23	83-193	73-203	62-214	54-222
24	91-209	81-210	69-231	61-239
25	100-225	89-236	76-249	68-257
26	110-241	98-253	84-267	75-276
27	119-259	107-271	93-285	83-295
28	130-276	114-278	101-305	91-315
29	140-295	126-309	122-313	100-335
30	151-314	137-328	132-333	109-356

Extracted from "Critical Values and Probability Levels for the Wilcoxon Rank Sum Test and the Wilcoxon Singed Rank Test," by Frank Wilcoxon, S. K. Katti and Roberta A. Wilcoxon, *Selected Tables in Mathematical Statistics*, Vol. 1; 1973, Table II, pp 237-259, by kind permission of Institute of Mathematical Statistics (IMS)

Index

A

Abortion, 290
    induced, 291
    rate, 297
    ratio, 297
Accuracy, 12, 17, 62, 241, 315
    of a diagnostic test, 264
Adherence, 232
Adjacent bar diagram, 38, 39, 76
Ad hoc basis, 310
    approach, 233
    systems, 29
Age
    at first marriage, 289
    at last birthday, 290
    at marriage, 289
    average age at marriage, 297
    distribution, 286, 289
    heaping, 289
Agreement
    parameter, 333
    percentage, 333
Allocation, 221, 230, 241, 242, 243
Alternative inclusion, 222
Amenorrhea, 289
Analysis, 220, 230, 233, 236, 238, 239, 242, 243, 308
    ancillary, 241
    bivariate, 162, 163
    cluster, 164
    descriptive data, 234
    diagnostic, 2
    discriminant, 164
    epidemiological, 212
    exploratory, 233, 234, 240
    factor, 164
    intention to treat (ITT), 239, 243
    meta, 328
    method, 5, 6
    multiple variable, 308
    multivariable logistic regression, 173
    multivariate, 4, 163, 240, 324
    multivariate regression, 168, 169
    multi-way of variance, 234
    nonparametric, of variance, 157, 159, 234, 339
    of covariance, 132, 133
    of cross over design, 236
    of data, 233, 234, 239, 240, 243
    of phase III trials, 223
    of sample surveys, 320
    of variance (ANOVA), 122, 156, 157, 158, 234, 243
    of variance (independent samples), 334, 341
    one-way, of variance, 157, 159, 234, 235, 335, 336, 338, 339
    parametric, of variance, 234
    repeated-measures, variance, 235
Analytical methods, 110, 234, 235, 319
Ancillary analysis, 241
Association
    negative, 177, 178, 65
    non-linear, 65
    positive, 65
Average/mean, 35, 48, 66, 78, 222, 228, 230, 234, 235, 237, 238, 286, 292, 299, 306, 313, 327, 331, 335, 338, 340
    arithmetic, 35, 48, 49, 51, 52, 53, 54, 55, 56, 57, 59, 60, 61, 63, 66, 72, 76, 328, 329, 330, 340
    duration of hospital stay, 315, 317, 318
    geometric (G.M.), 53, 54, 76, 329, 330, 340
    harmonic, 54, 55, 330
    of binomial distribution, 87
    of the Poisson variate, 89

B

Balanced design, 243
Bar diagram, 37, 38, 39, 43, 76